T0291829

# Clinical case studies in physiotherapy

**Publisher:** Heidi Harrison
**Commissioning Editor:** Rita Demetriou-Swanwick
**Associate Editor:** Siobhan Campbell
**Development Editor:** Veronika Watkins
**Project Manager:** Andrew Palfreyman
**Designer:** Sarah Russell
**Illustrations Manager:** Kirsteen Wright

# Clinical case studies in physiotherapy

## *A guide for students and graduates*

Edited by

**Lauren Jean Guthrie** MCSP BSc (Hons)
Junior Physiotherapist,
Stobhill Hospital,
Glasgow, UK

CHURCHILL LIVINGSTONE
ELSEVIER

EDINBURGH LONDON NEW YORK OXFORD PHILADELPHIA
ST LOUIS SYDNEY TORONTO 2009

CHURCHILL
LIVINGSTONE
ELSEVIER

An imprint of Elsevier Limited

© 2009, Elsevier Limited. All rights reserved.

The right of Lauren Guthrie to be identified as an editor of this work has been asserted by her in accordance with the Copyright, Designs and Patents Act 1988.

No part of this publication may be reproduced, stored in a retrieval system, or transmitted in any form or by any means, electronic, mechanical, photocopying, recording or otherwise, without the prior permission of the Publishers. Permissions may be sought directly from Elsevier's Health Sciences Rights Department, 1600 John F. Kennedy Boulevard, Suite 1800, Philadelphia, PA 19103-2899, USA: phone: (+1) 215 239 3804; fax: (+1) 215 239 3805; or, e-mail: healthpermissions@elsevier.com.
You may also complete your request on-line via the Elsevier homepage (http://www.elsevier.com), by selecting 'Support and contact' and then 'Copyright and Permission'.

ISBN-13: 978-0-443-06916-1

**British Library Cataloguing in Publication Data**
A catalogue record for this book is available from the British Library

**Library of Congress Cataloging in Publication Data**
A catalog record for this book is available from the Library of Congress

**Notice**
Neither the Publisher nor the Editor assumes any responsibility for any loss or injury and/or damage to persons or property arising out of or related to any use of the material contained in this book. It is the responsibility of the treating practitioner, relying on independent expertise and knowledge of the patient, to determine the best treatment and method of application for the patient.

**The Publisher**

Working together to grow libraries in developing countries
www.elsevier.com | www.bookaid.org | www.sabre.org
ELSEVIER BOOK AID International Sabre Foundation

ELSEVIER your source for books, journals and multimedia in the health sciences
**www.elsevierhealth.com**

The publisher's policy is to use **paper manufactured from sustainable forests**

Printed in China

# CONTENTS

# PREFACE

When I was a student, which was not that long ago, starting placements was definitely the most terrifying thing that I did. Presentations and exams were pretty stressful and nerve racking. However, there is nothing like the realisation that you are going to be let loose on real people with real problems. Not just your mate pretending they have left-sided hemiplegia, and who coincidently can't talk or make eye contact (just to make your mock treatment even more difficult!). While at the same time you're trying to prove yourself as being all-knowing because your clinical educator is continually assessing you.

I've spent many a night frantically looking through textbook upon textbook, trying to memorise origins and insertions, normal values and special tests with thoughts like 'I'm never going to remember all of this stuff' and 'what am I supposed to do with all of this knowledge when I've got a patient sitting in front of me?'

So, during my fourth year at university a thought sprang to my mind while painstakingly trying to format my dissertation to the ridiculously detailed instructions in my module handbook. Your mind tends to wander – I'm sure you understand. I suddenly thought 'why isn't there a book out there for students that shows them how to apply the knowledge they desperately try to memorise to the clinical setting and that helps them to develop their clinical reasoning skills while helping them carry out a CPD activity? Shouldn't there be some resource that tells people in black and white what being on placement is like and how to prepare for said placement. This resource could also help graduates secure their first post!' Okay so maybe my thought wasn't as long-winded as that, but the initial idea was there!

The thing is, starting placement is never as bad or as scary as you think it will be. I was told this time and time again, and didn't believe it! Looking back now I realize it was the fear of the unknown that was the scariest thing. The not knowing what will be expected of you, not knowing what to know or what to revise, not knowing what it is really like to have your first patient. Most of all, not knowing how to use all of your knowledge in a clinical setting. With the information and case studies in this book I hope to remove some of the uncertainty for you.

The first chapter will outline how best to use this book to your advantage. The second chapter will take you through how to prepare for going on placement by starting with some general information. This chapter will then go through the most common placement areas and suggest topics to revise with corresponding recommended reading lists.

Chapter three will help you to understand what it is like to be on placement and what could be expected of you. I've tried to include as wide a range of settings as possible. However, as the NHS and thus clinical settings vary so much throughout the UK, use this as a rough guide. This chapter also provides tips on how to continue your learning throughout the placement.

Chapter four takes you through the whole job-hunting process starting with where to look for jobs. The chapter then gives tips and hints on writing your cover letter and CV, and on how to fill in application forms. How to survive the interview process is also covered, including ideas of interview questions you could get asked.

Chapters five to eleven take you through case studies related to various areas of physiotherapy. Each chapter is allocated to a certain area. These areas are: respiratory physiotherapy, orthopaedics, neurological physiotherapy, musculoskeletal out-patients, care of the elderly, mental health and women's health.

Each case study chapter includes a number of case studies, which will provide the subjective and objective assessment of the patient. This will be followed by a list of around eight questions that are designed to make you think about what the assessment means and clinically reason through what could be wrong with the patient, what their problems are and how you might deal with them. At the end of each chapter suggested answers to the questions posed will be given. This will allow you to test your knowledge and reasoning, hopefully without cheating!

So here is my creation. The vision I had in my cold student flat with a blanket wrapped round me and a dissertation deadline looming. I hope that it settles your butterflies and minimises the sweats you get on your first day of placement when you're sitting on a crammed bus thinking 'is this what 7.30am looks like? Who's decided it would be a good idea to start at 8.30am anyway?' Have confidence that it really won't be that bad. There is light at the end of the tunnel. Honest!

Good luck!

*Lauren Guthrie*

# ACKNOWLEDGEMENTS

Completing this project would not have been possible without the help and support of many people.

I would like to thank Amy Mellin, Kirsty Mosley, Ailidh Weddell, Jenni Calcraft, Nadia Kanoun, Sarah Murdin and Marty O'Docherty for filling out my long questionnaire and sharing their hints and tips and experiences of being on placement and finding a job. Thanks also to Gavin Hayden for his knowledgeable input and for reviewing chapters, Chris Seenan for reviewing chapters and listening to my ideas, and Ayaz Ghani for his helpful advice and listening to me in times of need.

I would also like to show appreciation to Heidi Harrison who had a good feeling about my book from the start, and Siobhan Campbell and Veronika Watkins for their much appreciated technical support. And also to Stuart Porter for kindly agreeing to help me out in the initial stages of editing this book.

Thanks also goes to all the people who have kindly contributed chapters and case studies to this book. You have all worked so hard in writing, amending and reviewing chapters and sections; without you the book wouldn't be what it is. Special thanks goes to Jeanette Haslam who gave up her own time to review and provide references for the women's health chapter.

And, finally, to all my amazing friends and family ... for being just that!

# LIST OF CONTRIBUTORS

**Josephine Bell BSc (Hons), MSc, MSCP**
Physiotherapy Team Leader,
Springfield University Hospital,
London, UK

**Mandy Dunbar BSc (Hons) Physiotherapy, MSc Rehabilitation Studies**
Senior Lecturer in Physiotherapy,
Department of Allied Health Professions,
University of Central Lancashire,
Preston, UK

**Maureen E. Gardiner DPT**
Senior Physiotherapist, Princess Royal Maternity Hospital,
Glasgow, UK

**Caroline Griffiths Grad Dip Phys**
Physiotherapy Team Leader,
Oxford and Buckinghamshire Mental Health Partnership NHS Trust, UK

**Sharon Greenshill MCSP, SRP, Dip RG & RT**
Clinical Specialist/Clinical Lead Physiotherapist Mental Health,
Rotherham Doncaster and South Humber Mental Health NHS Foundation Trust/Rotherham PCT,
Rotherham, UK

**Lauren Guthrie MCSP, BSc (Hons)**
Junior Physiotherapist, Stobhill Hospital, Glasgow, UK

**Janis Harvey BSc (Hons)**
Physiotherapy Clinical Specialist,
Western General Hospital,
Edinburgh, UK

**Anne-Marie Hassenkamp MSc (Health Psychology), MMACP**
Senior Lecturer,
School of Physiotherapy,
Kingston University/St. Georges University of London, UK

**Susan R. Hourigan BPhty (Hons), BSCApp, HMS-ExMan**
Physiotherapist,
PhD Candidate,
University of Queensland,
Australia

**Clare Leonard MCSP**
Head of Profession for Physiotherapy,
Avon and Wiltshire Mental Health Partnership Trust,
Victoria Hospital,
Swindon, UK

**Jamie Mackler BSc (Hons)**
Students' Advisor,
Chartered Society of Physiotherapy,
UK

**Sophia Mavraommatis MSc, AHP, MCSP**
Extended Scope Practitioner,
Clinical Specialist,
Physiotherapist

**Ken Niere BAppSc (Physio), Grad Dip Manip Ther, MManip/Ther**
Senior Lecturer,
School of Physiotherapy,
LaTrobe University,
Victoria, Australia

**Jennifer C. Nitz PhD MPhty BPhty**
Senior Lecturer,
Division of Physiotherapy,
The University of Queensland,
St. Lucia, Australia

**Jean Picton-Bentley MSCP**
Team Leader Physiotherapist, Maudsley Hospital, Denmark Hill, Camberwell, South London, UK

**Adrian M. M. Schoo PhysioD, MHlthSc, GradDip**
Senior Lecturer, Deputy Director, Greater Green Triangle University, Department of Rural Health, Flinders and Deakin Universities, Australia

**James Selfe PhD, MA, GD Phys, MCSP**
Professor of Physiotherapy, Department of Allied Health Professions,
University of Central Lancashire, UK; Visiting Academic, Physiotherapy Department, Satakunta Applied University, Pori, Finland

**Nicholas Taylor PhD, BAppSc (Physiotherapy), BSc**
Professor of Physiotherapy, La Trobe University, Victoria, Australia

**Diane Thomson PhD, MSc, MBACP (Accred)**
School of Biomedical and Health Sciences, Kings College, London, UK

**Kaye Walls MSc, MMACP, MCSP**
Superintendent Physiotherapist, Royal National Orthopaedic Hospital, London, UK

**Victoria Welsh Hamelin MCSP, BPhysio (Hons), BSc (Hons) Psych (Open)**
Physiotherapy and Exercise Service Team Leader, (North Somerset) Avon and Wiltshire Mental Health NHS Trust, UK

# LIST OF ABBREVIATIONS

| | |
|---|---|
| **_/12** | number of months, e.g. 3/12 = 3 months |
| **_/52** | number of weeks, e.g. 24/52 = 24 weeks |
| **_/7** | number of days, e.g. 1/7 = 1 day |
| **ABG** | arterial blood gas |
| **ACA** | anterior cerebral artery |
| **ACBT** | active cycle of breathing technique |
| **ACL** | anterior cruciate ligament |
| **ACLR** | anterior cruciate ligament repair |
| **ACPWH** | Association of Chartered Physiotherapists in Womens' Health |
| **ACT** | airway clearance technique |
| **AD** | autogenic drainage |
| **ADLs** | activities of daily living |
| **A & E** | Accident & Emergency |
| **AF** | arterial fibrillation |
| **AFO** | ankle foot orthosis |
| **ALS** | amyotrophic lateral sclerosis |
| **AP** | anterior posterior |
| **ARDS** | acute respiratory distress syndrome |
| **ASB** | assisted spontaneous breathing |
| **ASIA** | American Spinal Injuries Association |
| **ASIS** | anterior superior iliac spine |
| **AXR** | abdominal X-ray |
| **BE** | base excess |
| **BMI** | body mass index |
| **BNF** | *British National Formulary* |
| **BOS** | base of support |
| **BP** | blood pressure |
| **C_** | level at cervical spine, e.g. C3/4 |
| **CABG** | coronary artery bypass graft |
| **CAP** | community-acquired pneumonia |
| **CBT** | cognitive behavioural therapy |
| **CF** | cystic fibrosis |
| **CKC** | closed kinetic chain |
| **CMC** | current movement capacity |
| **CMHT** | community mental health team |
| **CNS** | central nervous system |
| **C/o** | complaining of |
| **COPD** | chronic obstructive pulmonary disease |
| **CP** | cerebral palsy |

| | |
|---|---|
| **CPA** | care programme approach |
| **CPAP** | continuous positive airway pressure |
| **cpd** | cigarettes per day |
| **CPN** | community psychiatric nurse |
| **CPR** | cardiopulmonary resuscitation |
| **CR** | controlled release |
| **CSF** | cerebrospinal fluid |
| **CSP** | Chartered Society of Physiotherapy |
| **CT Scan** | Computerized (axial) tomography scan |
| **CTS** | carpel tunnel syndrome |
| **CTSIB** | clinical test for sensory integration of balance |
| **CV** | closing volume |
| **CVA** | cerebrovascular accident |
| **CVP** | central venous pressure |
| **CVS** | cardiovascular system |
| **CXR** | chest X-ray |
| **DEXA Scan** | dual energy X-ray absorptiometry scan |
| **DH** | drug history |
| **DHS** | dynamic hip screw |
| **DoH** | Department of Health |
| **DRAM** | distress and risk assessment method |
| **DVLA** | Driver and Vehicle Licensing Agency |
| **DVT** | deep vein thrombosis |
| **E** | best eye response (component of GCS) |
| **ECG** | electrocardiogram |
| **ECRB** | extensor carpi radialis brevis |
| **ER** | end range |
| **ES** | electrical stimulation |
| **ETT** | endotracheal tube |
| **FABQ** | fear avoidance beliefs questionnaire |
| **FET** | forced expiratory technique |
| **$FiO_2$** | fraction of inspired oxygen |
| **FM** | fibromyalgia |
| **FRC** | functional residual capacity |
| **FROM** | full range of movement |
| **GCS** | Glasgow coma scale |
| **GMS** | gross motor function scale |
| **GP** | general practitioner |
| **GTN Spray** | glyceryl trinitrate spray (for angina) |
| **$H^+$** | hydrogen ion concentration |
| **$HCO_3^-$** | bicarbonate ion concentration |
| **HDU** | high-dependency unit |
| **HMEF** | heat moisture exchange filter |
| **HPC** | health professions council |
| **HR** | heart rate |
| **hr** | hour, e.g. mL/hour |
| **IABP** | intra-aortic balloon pump |
| **ICD** | intercostal drain |

| | |
|---|---|
| **ICF** | international classification of function and disability model |
| **ICU** | intensive care unit |
| **IPAP** | inspiratory positive pressure airway |
| **IPPB** | intermittent positive pressure breathing |
| **IV** | intravenous |
| **kg** | kilograms |
| **kPa** | kilopascals |
| **L** | litres |
| **L_** | lumbar vertebrae, e.g. L1 – first lumbar vertebra |
| **LBP** | lower-back pain |
| **LSA** | learning support assistant |
| **LSCS** | lower segment caesarean section |
| **M** | mucoid; *another meaning*: best motor response (component of GCS) |
| **MDT** | multidisciplinary team |
| **MFIQ** | modified functional index questionnaire |
| **MHI** | manual hyperinflation |
| **MI** | myocardial infarction |
| **mL** | millilitres |
| **MMSE** | mini mental state examination |
| **MND** | motor neurone disease |
| **MP** | mucopurulent |
| **MRI** | magnetic resonance imaging |
| **MRP** | motor relearning programme |
| **MRSA** | methicillin-resistant *Staphylococcus aureus* |
| **MS** | multiple sclerosis |
| **MSK** | musculoskletal system |
| **MSPQ** | modified somatic perception questionnaire |
| **MUA** | manipulation under anaesthetic |
| **NAD** | no abnormality detected |
| **NG** | nasogastric |
| **NHP** | Nottingham health profile |
| **NHS** | National Health Service |
| **NICE** | National Institute for Clinical Excellence |
| **NIV** | non-invasive ventilation |
| **NOF** | neck of femur |
| **NP** | nasopharyngeal |
| **NSAIDs** | non-steroidal anti-inflammatory drugs |
| **NSF** | national service framework |
| **NWB** | non-weight bearing |
| **OA** | osteoarthritis |
| **OKC** | open kinetic chain |
| **OP** | osteoporosis |
| **ORIF** | open reduction external fixation |
| **PA** | posterior anterior |
| **PC** | present complaint |
| **PCA** | patient-controlled analgesia |
| **PCL** | posterior cruciate ligament |

| | |
|---|---|
| **PCT** | Primary Care Trust |
| **PD** | Parkinson's disease |
| **PE** | pulmonary embolism |
| **PEEP** | positive end expiratory pressure |
| **PFM** | pelvic floor muscle |
| **PGP** | pelvic girdle pain |
| **pH** | inverse log of hydrogen ion concentration: a measure of hydrogen ions in solution |
| **PICU** | paediatric intensive care unit |
| **PIVD** | prolapsed intervertebral disc |
| **PMC** | preferred movement capacity |
| **PMH** | past medical history |
| **$pO_2$** | partial pressure of oxygen |
| **PRE** | progressive resisted exercise |
| **PRICE** | protection, rest, ice, compression, elevation |
| **Prn** | Pro renata |
| **PS** | pressure support |
| **PSIS** | posterior superior iliac spine |
| **PWB** | partial weight bearing |
| **RA** | rheumatoid arthritis |
| **RICE** | rest, ice, compression, elevation |
| **ROM** | range of movement |
| **RR** | respiratory rate |
| **RTA** | road traffic accident |
| **S_** | level at sacrum, e.g. S1/2 |
| **SAH** | subarachnoid haemorrhage |
| **Sats** | oxygen saturation by pulse oximetry |
| **SH** | social history |
| **SIJ** | sacroiliac joint |
| **SIMV** | synchronized intermittent mandatory breathing |
| **SLR** | straight leg raise |
| **SOB** | short of breath |
| **SP** | symphysis pubis |
| **SPADI** | shoulder pain and disability index |
| **SPD** | symphysis pubis dysfunction |
| **$SpO_2$** | oxygen saturation by pulse oximetry |
| **SV** | self ventilating |
| **T** | Intubated (component of GCS) |
| **T_** | Thoracic vertebrae, e.g. T2 – second thoracic vertebra |
| **TA** | achilles tendon |
| **TAQs** | toes, ankles, quads (circulation exercises) |
| **TCN** | subtalar-talocalcaneonavicular |
| **TEDs** | thrombo embolism deterrent stockings |
| **TENS** | transcutaneous electrical nerve stimulation |
| **THR** | total hip replacement |
| **TI** | technical instructor |
| **TKR** | total knee replacement |
| **TLSO** | thoracolumber spinal orthosis |

| | |
|---|---|
| **TMJ** | tempomandibular joint |
| **T*sk*** | skin temperature |
| **TUAG** | timed up and go |
| **Tv** | tidal volume |
| **UEFI** | upper extremity functional index |
| **UO** | urinary output |
| **UTI** | urinary tract infection |
| **V** | best vocal response (component of GCS) |
| **V/Q** | ventilation perfusion matching |
| **VAS** | visual analogue scale |
| **VEP** | visual evoked potentials |
| **VMO** | vastus medialis obligue |
| **WB** | weight bearing |
| **WH** | women's health |
| **WOB** | work of breathing |

CHAPTER ONE

# Introduction

*Lauren Guthrie*

Every person who trains as a physiotherapist has to go through it. You might be a first year physiotherapy student about to begin your first placement or you could be a final year student about to do your last placement. You might be a newly qualified junior physiotherapist looking for your first post or you might have been working for some time, in a rotational post. It's nerve racking but at the same time exciting and most defiantly full of unknowns. Don't know what I'm talking about yet? It's entering a clinical specialty of physiotherapy that you don't have much, or any experience in. Do not fear, help is at hand and this book aims to help and support you, and take away the unknowns in some of the many specialties within the physiotherapy profession.

Chapters two and three are aimed primarily at students preparing for a clinical placement as part of a training programme, but provide lots of references recommended by specialists in their field and may, therefore, be of use to any physiotherapist looking to find out more about other areas of physiotherapy. These chapters will tell you everything you need to know, from what your first day could be like to recommended texts and revision topics for the main physiotherapy specialties.

Chapter four is an excellent resource for students nearing the end of their study or recently qualified graduates who are trying to secure their first physiotherapy post. This chapter gives lots of hints and tips on where to look for jobs, how to fill an application form, how to compile your CV and how to survive that all-important interview when it comes along!

The remaining chapters of the book are case study chapters covering the main areas of physiotherapy along with two less common areas. Various clinical settings have been covered within each chapter, for example, community, acute hospital, rehabilitation hospital and out-patients. Each chapter also incorporates a range of patient age groups from paediatrics to the older adult. You may find that case studies from several chapters will be of benefit to you prior to and during placement, as, in reality, the various areas of physiotherapy can cross over. For example, on an orthopaedic ward you may have a patient with some respiratory complications post surgery. Or you may be working in the community dealing with a range of conditions from neurology to musculoskeletal.

The case studies are structured to help you develop problem solving and clinical reasoning skills as these are important once you are in the clinical setting. Each case will give details of a subjective and objective history of a patient. Take note of how the assessments have been structured in the case histories. They have been written out in more detail than would be expected when writing SOAP notes (the standard format of physiotherapy notes) in a clinical environment but include all the information that you should be looking out for, for example the patient's body language and behaviour. Getting used to the content of an assessment will be of great help once you start placement. Following the case history you will be presented with several questions relating to it, which will get you thinking about what the patient's diagnosis and main problems are as well as what types of treatment would benefit the patient. Questions relating to other health professionals are also included in some cases.

It is important to realise that the answers to the questions posed and suggested treatments are not a recipe for all patients with similar conditions. Every patient is individual and will cope with their condition differently and respond differently to treatments. What treatment is suitable for one patient may not be suitable for another patient with the same injury or condition. Therefore, use the case studies to give you a general idea and consider the patient's individual circumstances when assessing and treating them.

Working through the case studies can be useful prior to placement to get an idea of the clinical application of knowledge, in addition to during your placement as it may help you to see how everything fits together in the clinical setting. You may choose to revise your theory knowledge in a certain area then test that knowledge by working through a case study. Or, you could use case studies to identify your learning needs in a particular area, then form an action plan to address these needs and record it in your CPD (continuing professional development) portfolio.

When working through the case studies don't be alarmed or worried if you feel like you don't know or understand anything, it's normal. Use the suggested reading to help you or discuss it and think it through with some like-minded friends. Some of the techniques or approaches discussed within some of the case studies may be completely unfamiliar. Don't worry if after reading up on some of the techniques or approaches you are still unsure or are struggling with the questions, sometimes these things require practical experience to fully understand them but the case studies within this book will get your brain working in the right way and help you get started.

Unfortunately, it has been impossible to include everything that I would have liked to in this book. However, the recommended reading and sources of further information are really useful. Having a physiotherapy dictionary close to hand to look up any terms you are unfamiliar with will help, as it is outwith the scope of this book to provide definitions of physiotherapy terms.

# How to prepare for placement

*Lauren Guthrie*

Clinical placements are one of the most exciting and enjoyable parts of your training as a physiotherapist. Placements provide the opportunity to develop and enhance your patient handling, problem solving, communication and team working skills, and to apply all of your theoretical knowledge as well as gain lots of new knowledge.

The Chartered Society of Physiotherapy (CSP) states that to qualify as a physiotherapist you need a minimum of 1000 hours of practise-based learning to prepare you for professional practise (Chartered Society of Physiotherapy 2005). To some this may be adequate in order to build enough confidence in your own ability, get out there on your own and go for it. For the majority of others it just doesn't seem like enough time. Therefore, it is really important to make the most of every one of those 1000 hours and one way to achieve this is to do some placement preparation. Investing some time into getting ready for your placement will prevent you playing catch up on theoretical knowledge when you're working full time as a student physiotherapist, trying to process all the new clinical knowledge that you will be gathering daily.

## WHERE TO GET INFORMATION ON YOUR PLACEMENT

### Placement profiles

Some universities have a profile for each placement. This should give details of type of placement you are going on, the address of where the placement is and how to get there, the name and contact details of who your clinical educator(s) will be, hours of work, accommodation if applicable, educational facilities, local information (Chartered Society of Physiotherapy 2003), possibly some recommended reading, and the types of conditions you will be seeing.

### Ask your peers

Other students who have already been on placement there or have been on a placement in the same area will be able to give you first-hand advice.

### Your clinical educator

If he or she is happy to be contacted, call your clinical educator and make the most of the opportunity by writing down some specific questions before you phone. This is especially useful if the person you get on the other end of the phone is not volunteering much information. Examples of the things to ask about include: what types of patients or common injuries/conditions you will be dealing with; how many physiotherapists there are in the team; whether you will be seeing a patient on the first day or not; if there is anything they suggest you look over beforehand or any recommended textbooks or journal articles; what texts and other resources are available at the placement site; where and what time do you report on your first day; if there are any specific uniform requirements; what changing facilities are available and whether to bring a padlock. For infection control reasons you must change into uniform on site.

## WHAT DO YOU NEED TO KNOW BEFORE PLACEMENT?

- Housekeeping information, for example: address of hospital; how you are going to get there; if there is somewhere to get lunch or do you need to take it; what you are expected to wear as uniform.
- You are on placement to learn so remember you aren't expected to know everything for your first day. No matter what, you will learn things as you go along.
- Some departments will expect you to know more than others but know the basics and you can't go wrong – make notes in a notebook to keep in your pocket.
- Knowing too much will likely confuse you – know the basics to get a broad overview, then you will have a good knowledge base to build on when you start learning more on placement.
- How much time you allocate to revision prior to placement will depend on what placements you have already been on, what knowledge you already have, your development of transferable skills and how much confidence you have.
- Revision will help increase your self-confidence.
- Practising some practical skills, for example goniometry or carrying out other outcome measures, with a few friends will help you get used to handling patients when assessing them.

### Specific placement areas

Below is a general guide of topics to revise for some common placement areas. You may have to prioritize or concentrate on just some of the suggested revision when you find out more about your specific placement. Certain placements may even require you to look at a few of the sections. Ensure that you are aware of the basics of SOAP (Subjective, Objective, Assessment, Plan) notes and what you would write in each section. Revising some common abbreviations or making a list of them in a notebook will also be of great benefit while on placement.

***Recommended reading***

Kettenbach G 2004 Writing SOAP notes. F A Davis Company, Pennsylvania.

## Surgical respiratory

- Pre- and post-operative respiratory assessment, including chest X-ray interpretation and arterial blood gas normal values and interpretation.
- Find out common types of surgery you will encounter in your placement and be aware of what is involved and where the surgical incision is made as this can impact on physiotherapy input.
- Complications of surgery.
- Normal values for $SpO_2$ (blood oxygen levels), blood pressure, heart rate, respiratory rate, arterial blood gases.
- Basic understanding of types of mechanical ventilation and tracheostomy care.
- Thoracic anatomy, especially lung surface markings (helps with auscultation).
- Treatment options to clear secretions, decrease work of breathing and increase lung volume, e.g. mobilisation, positioning, ACBT (active cycle of breathing technique), manual techniques, incentive spirometry, suction (different types including via tracheostomy), IPPB (intermittent positive pressure breathing), oxygen therapy. Consider how you could assess for their effectiveness and how they may be modified and progressed.

***Recommended reading***

Harden B 2004 Emergency Physiotherapy. Churchill Livingstone, Edinburgh.
Hough A 2001 Physiotherapy in Respiratory Care – An Evidence Based Approach to Respiratory and Cardiac Management, 3rd edn. Nelson Thornes, Cheltenham.
Pryor J A, Prasad S A 2002 Physiotherapy for Respiratory and Cardiac Problems, 3rd edn. Churchill Livingstone, Edinburgh.
Kenyon J, Kenyon J 2004 The Physiotherapist's Pocket Book. Churchill Livingstone, Edinburgh.

## Medical respiratory

- Respiratory assessment, including chest X-ray interpretation.
- Knowledge of COPD (chronic obstructive pulmonary disease), asthma, brochiectasis, pneumonia, pneumothorax, acute bronchitis.
- Normal values for $SpO_2$, blood pressure, heart rate, respiratory rate, arterial blood gases.
- Thoracic anatomy, especially lung surface markings (helps with auscultation).
- Treatment options for potential respiratory problems, e.g. mobilisation, positioning, ACBT (active cycle of breathing technique), manual techniques, incentive spirometry, suction, IPPB (intermittent positive pressure breathing) oxygen therapy. Consider how you could assess for their effectiveness and how they may be modified and progressed.
- Pulmonary rehabilitation.

**Recommended reading**

Harden B 2004 Emergency Physiotherapy. Churchill Livingstone, Edinburgh.

Hough A 2001 Physiotherapy in Respiratory Care – An Evidence Based Approach to Respiratory and Cardiac Management, 3rd edn. Nelson Thornes, Cheltenham.

Pryor J A, Prasad S A 2002 Physiotherapy for Respiratory and Cardiac Problems, 3rd edn. Churchill Livingstone, Edinburgh.

Kenyon J, Kenyon J 2004 The Physiotherapist's Pocket Book. Churchill Livingstone, Edinburgh.

## Orthopaedics (trauma and elective)

- Pre- and post-operative assessment, and peripheral joint assessment (normal values for range of movement).
- Complications of fracture and surgical procedures.
- For any patients with chest complications – normal values for blood pressure, heart rate, respiratory rate, $SpO_2$, lung markings, auscultation, active cycle of breathing technique (ACBT).
- Types of gait patterns, gait re-ed and use of walking aids.
- Fracture classifications, mechanisms of injury.
- Basic knowledge of bone and soft tissue healing.
- Pathology of osteoarthritis.
- Common elective surgical procedures. Types of joint replacement (hip, knee, shoulder), internal and external fixation.
- Basic anatomy of hip, knee, wrist, shoulder and ankle.
- Principles of fracture management.



**Recommended reading**

Adams J C, Hamblen D L 1999 Outline of Fractures Including Joint Injuries, 11th edn. Churchill Livingstone, Edinburgh.

Atkinson K, Coutts F, Hassenkamp A M 2005 Physiotherapy in Orthopaedics: A Problem-Solving Approach, 2nd edn. Churchill Livingstone, Edinburgh.

www.shoulderdoc.co.uk Excellent website for pictures of knee and shoulder surgery.

Kenyon J, Kenyon J 2004 The Physiotherapist's Pocket Book. Churchill Livingstone, Edinburgh.

## Neurological

- Neurological assessment, i.e. assessing tone, joint range of movement, sensation, muscle power, posture, functional abilities (sit-to-stand, gait, etc.), balance.
- Awareness of outcome measures: Tinetti, Berg balance scale, motor assessment scale, elderly mobility scale.

- Depending on the type of neurological placement, know about the most likely neurological conditions you will encounter including pathology, signs and symptoms, overview of medical management. For example, Parkinson's disease, multiple sclerosis, stroke, motor neurone disease, Guillain–Barré syndrome.
- The types of treatment physiotherapists may use with the types of conditions you will come across in your placement. For example, balance re-education, gait re-education, exercise prescription.
- Find out the approach adopted by the physiotherapists at that particular site. For example, Bobath, motor re-learning, etc.

***Recommended reading***

Carr J H, Shepherd R B 1998 Neurological Rehabilitation. Optimizing Motor Performance. Butterworth-Heinemann, Oxford.
Carr J H, Shepherd R B 2003 Stroke Rehabilitation Guidelines for Exercise Training to Optimize Motor Skill. Butterworth-Heinemann, Edinburgh.
Davis P M 2000 Steps to Follow, 2nd edn. Springer, Berlin, London.
Stokes M 2004 Physical Management in Neurological Rehabilitation. Mosby, London.
Kenyon J, Kenyon J 2004 The Physiotherapist's Pocket Book. Churchill Livingstone, Edinburgh.



## Musculoskeletal out patients

- Anatomical knowledge primarily of the peripheral joints including major muscle groups and ligaments. Depending on the placement, you may also be required to know about the spinal column.
- Subjective assessment is usually more important to know prior to placement. Having an awareness of the objective assessment of peripheral joints (and spinal column) including pain assessment, neurological assessment (myotomes, dermatomes, reflexes, nerve tension tests) and appropriate special tests will give you a good head start, but a lot of this knowledge will be picked up on placement.
- Normal range of movement for peripheral joints and capsular patterns.
- Outcome measures for peripheral joints and pain, for example goniometry, Oxford muscle scale.
- Red and yellow flags of back pain.
- Electrotherapy (including ultrasound, TENS, heat and cold application – PRICE regime).
- Timescales for healing of muscle, tendon, ligaments, bone.

***Recommended reading***

Adams J C, Hamblen D L 1999 Outline of Fractures Including Joint Injuries, 11th edn. Churchill Livingstone, Edinburgh.

Brunker P, Khan K 2006 Clinical Sports Medicine, 3rd edn. McGraw Hill, Australia.
Kendall F P, McCreary E K, Provance P G 1993 Muscles Testing and Function, 4th edn. Lippincott Williams & Wilkins, Philadelphia.
Kenyon J, Kenyon J 2004 The Physiotherapist's Pocket Book. Churchill Livingstone, Edinburgh.
Kesson M, Atkins E 1998 Orthopaedic Medicine: A Practical Approach. Butterworth Heinemann, Somerset.
Magee D J 2006 Orthopaedic Physical Assessment, 4th edn. Saunders, Edinburgh.
Petty N J 2005 Neuromusculoskeletal Examination and Assessment: A Hand Book for Therapists, 3nd edn. Churchill Livingstone, Edinburgh.
Petty N J 2004 Principles of Neuromusculoskeletal Treatment and Management: A Guide for Therapists. Churchill Livingstone, Edinburgh.
www.shoulderdoc.co.uk Excellent website for pictures of knee and shoulder surgery.
Vlaeyen J, Crombez G 1999 Fear of movement, re-injury, avoidance and pain disability in chronic low back pain patients. Manual Therapy 4:187–195.



## Care of the elderly

- Common conditions/pathology: Parkinson's disease, increased falls risk/balance problems, osteoarthritis, rheumatoid arthritis, stroke, dementia, confusion, fractures, joint replacements.
- Principles of palliative care (if applicable to your specific placement).
- Effects of ageing on the body including muscle strength, and strength training and cardiovascular system.
- Holistic assessment of the older person that considers individual physical, social and behavioural aspects, which may include neurological assessment, functional gait analysis.
- Balance re-education, prescription of mobility aids and gait re-education, exercise prescription and pre-cautions of exercise with the elderly.
- Awareness of outcome measures – Tinetti, Berg balance scale, elderly mobility scale, 10-m walk, 6-minute walk, motor assessment scale.

### *Recommended reading*

Davis P M 2000 Steps to Follow, 2nd edn. Springer, Berlin, London.
Pickles B, Compton A, Cott C, Simpson J M 1995 Physiotherapy with Older People. Bailliere Tindall, London.
Stokes M 2004 Physical Management in Neurological Rehabilitation. Mosby, London.
Wagstaff P, Coakley D 1988 Physiotherapy and the Elderly Patient. Croom Helm, London.

## Mental health

- Read up on causes, signs and symptoms and treatment (including medication) of: dementia (including Alzheimer's, Lewy-body and vascular) bi-polar disorder; depression; anxiety disorders; schizophrenia; addictive behaviours including alcohol, prescribed and non-prescribed medication (how substances affect the body, neuropathy, vestibular problems); eating disorders (anorexia, bulimia).
- Relaxation techniques.
- How exercise affects mood.
- Communication theory – motivational techniques (goal setting).
- Outcome measures. For example, HAD scale (hospital anxiety and depression scale), Becks depression/anxiety assessment.

***Recommended reading***

Donaghy M, Everett T, Feaver S (eds) 2005 Interventions for Mental Health: An Evidence Based Approach for Physiotherapists and Occupational Therapists. Butterworth Heinemann, London.
Bernstein D A 2005 Psychology, 7th edn. Houghton Mifflin Co, Boston.
The Chartered Society of Physiotherapy. Outcome Measures for People with Depression (a working document) February 2002 Available from www.csp.org.uk.

***Useful websites***

www.mentalhealthcare.org.uk.
www.mind.org.uk This site is great for giving a user/carer view.



## Women's health/obstetrics

- Anatomy of the lumbar spine and pelvis including the sacro-iliac joints, symphsis pubis, pelvic floor muscles and ligaments.
- Knowledge of the physiological changes to the body associated with pregnancy, and problems that can arise as a result.
- The three stages of labour.
- Types of delivery including: spontaneous vertex delivery, forceps, ventouse, caesarean section.
- Complications of delivery including perineal tears and episiotomy.
- Gynaecological conditions and surgery.
- Assessments and treatment of common MSK problems; SPD, diastasis recti, LBP.
- General physiotherapy management of pelvic floor disorders.

***Recommended reading***

Mantle J, Haslam J, Barton S, Polden M 2004 Physiotherapy in Obstetrics and Gynaecology, 2nd edn. Butterworth-Heinemann, China.
Sapsford R, Bullock-Saxton J, Markwell S 1997 Womens Health: A Textbook for Physiotherapists. Bailliere Tindall, London.

Visit The Association of Chartered Physiotherapists in Women's Health Website for general information about working in this area. www.acpwh.org.uk.

## Paediatrics

A placement in paediatrics could involve respiratory, musculoskeletal or neurological conditions; therefore, preparation for a placement in this specialty should reflect the type of conditions you will encounter and referring to the appropriate section above should get you started on revision topics. Many of the above textbook references will cover paediatric conditions. See below for a specific paediatric title.

***Recommended reading***

Eckersley P M 1993 Elements of Paediatric Physiotherapy. Churchill Livingstone, Edinburgh.

***References***

Chartered Society of Physiotherapy 2003 Clinical Education Placement Guidelines. CSP, London.

Chartered Society of Physiotherapy 2005 Learning in the Practise Environment in Qualifying Programmes of Physiotherapy, Guidance on its Organisation, Delivery and Recognition. CSP, London.

***Other useful websites***

www.csp.org.uk
http://www.interactivecsp.org.uk/
www.physioroom.com
http://www.mckenziemdt.org/
www.physiostuff.com

# What to expect when on placement

*Lauren Guthrie*

## FIRST DAYS AND FIRST IMPRESSIONS

So you have done some preparation for your placement, you have found out what time you start and all the other small details and you turn up on your first day, then what happens?

The first day is often quite laid back and will let you suss out the environment you will be working in. You should be shown round the department and introduced to the physiotherapy team and any other people you will be working with. You should get information, where appropriate, regarding: bleep system, emergency telephone numbers, fire procedures/exits, departmental policies and procedures, profile and staffing structure (Chartered Society of Physiotherapy 2003). You might discuss your learning objectives, observe patient treatments or possibly assess a patient on your own.

It's very normal to be nervous when starting a new placement, especially if it's your first placement or even a placement in an area that's new to you. The likelihood is that it won't be as bad or as scary as you think once you get there and get started. Try to relax as much as possible and don't panic. You usually get lots of support especially if it's your first placement. Be safe in the knowledge that you aren't expected to know everything, even as a junior. It is expected that you will be asking questions and seeking help from your seniors. If you weren't asking questions they would probably be wondering why. Even seniors don't know everything. As mentioned in chapter two, knowing the basics will give you a good knowledge base to build on.

### Getting along with your clinical educator

Most people will get on really well with their Clinical Educators (CE). CEs usually choose to take on students and are therefore very willing to teach you and share their knowledge and experience.

Showing that you are enthusiastic about learning and interacting with the team and the patients will always go down well. Don't be afraid to ask questions and admit it if you don't know something, even when you're a junior. They are there to help you and make you a better physiotherapist so take advantage of it. Bear in mind that it's not unusual for your CE to ask you a question back to help you work out the answer yourself. Therefore, put a little bit of thought into your question first. If you really don't know the answer, then mention that you will look it up that night, and then if you get asked again you'll know the answer.

Also be aware of the variation between CEs when it comes to marking. There are variations between universities on the marking scheme as well. Try to gauge at the start what your CE expects of you. If you have any problems or don't agree with their appraisal then try to resolve this with them as soon as possible, for example at a mid-way review. If the issue still isn't resolved then your university should be able to provide the appropriate support.

## WHAT EACH ENVIRONMENT IS LIKE

Every placement you complete will be very different and individual. The environment that you will be working in will vary across individual hospitals within the same Trust/Health Board and will vary between Trusts/ Health Boards. The people that you work with and your CE will also have a significant impact on your working environment. Even the time of year can affect the number of patients needing care. It is, therefore, impossible to explain what every placement is going to involve but the sections below should help you get some sort of idea.



It is likely that you will be working alongside other health professionals as part of a multidisciplinary team (MDT) including nursing staff, health care assistants, specialist nurses, ward clerk, occupational therapist, speech therapist, podiatrist, dietician, social worker, ward doctors and consultants. The MDT may work closely with each other and have regular planned meetings or you may be expected to liaise with them as appropriate. Whatever the set up on your particular placement it is useful to know what role other members of the team have. You may also be involved with referring patients to other teams or services, for example, community rehabilitation or pain team, falls or osteoporosis service. Each hospital will vary in the services it offers; however, your CE should be able to inform you of what is available in your area.

To read more about the daily working experiences of physiotherapists log onto the Physio buddies blogs at www.physiobuddies.co.uk

### Acute hospital environment

This might include placements in surgical or medical respiratory, orthopaedics, combined assessment or acute receiving unit and other regional specialties. The physiotherapy team that you will be part of may cover a number of wards depending on the set up of the hospital. This environment tends to be very fast paced and busy due to bed demand. Depending upon what year you are in and how many placements you have done you may be given a list of a few patients to see by yourself. The number of patients will be at the discretion of your CE and depend upon how they feel you are getting on in the placement.

## Rehabilitation ward

This could be an elderly rehabilitation ward, stroke rehabilitation ward or spinal injuries ward for example. Within this environment the pace may be a bit slower depending on staffing levels and patient numbers. It's likely that you will have a bit more time to spend with patients and will therefore see fewer patients during the course of a day than you would in a busy acute ward.

## Community/domiciliary setting

Placements in the community are generally varied. It may involve seeing patients with neurological conditions, orthopaedic problems and elderly people with mobility problems. As a student you will always be with your CE, visiting people in their homes. The placement may also involve attending an orthopaedic clinic in the hospital for example. You can see anything from 4 to 12 patients a day, spending between 15 minutes and 1 hour with a patient.

It can be a very different experience from seeing patients in hospital as it is important to consider all aspects of the patient and address any psychosocial issues. This may involve liaising with GPs, nurses, occupational therapists and social workers. You also have to adapt your assessment and treatment to suit the patient in their home. Household tasks can be utilized as treatment to make rehabilitation more functional.



## Out-patients setting

Out-patient departments in hospitals tend to be quite big and very busy with lots of physiotherapists in the team. Departments in community health centres may have just two or three physiotherapists with a fairly limited space.

In this environment your day will be more rigidly structured as patients will be booked in at set times. Again, depending on what year you are in, you may be left on your own to assess and treat a patient with a helping hand close by if required. Or else you may be seeing a patient together with your CE. How much time allocated to each patient will depend on department policy and what your CE decides on. It can vary from 1 hour for new patients and 45 minutes for return patients to 45 minutes for new patients and 30 minutes for return patients.

Your caseload will be very varied. The number of patients you see in a day will depend on your level at university and how well your CE thinks you are doing. You will generally be given extra time each day to write your notes and reflect on the patients you have seen. This can be variable depending on the department.

## Intensive care unit (ICU)

Working within this environment would usually be part of a placement in surgical respiratory or cardiothoracic for example.

The number of ICU beds will vary depending on the size of hospital. The ICU can be very scary the first time you go in as patients are usually very ill. They will have lots of lines and drips in situ and are closely monitored so expect to hear alarms go off regularly when patient observations go over their respective limits.

This can be daunting initially but remember that the ICU is a safe place with highly skilled nursing staff very close by who are used to dealing with the unexpected. They will always be near by if you have any questions. Your CE is unlikely to ever leave you on your own in the ICU, but see this as an advantage to learn from them at every opportunity.

## WHAT IS EXPECTED OF YOU WHILE ON PLACEMENT?

While on placement be expected to do a bit more than just turn up everyday and float along without paying much attention to anything.

You will be expected to:

- write physiotherapy SOAP notes for all your patients as per the CSP standards (Chartered Society of Physiotherapy 2005a) and have them countersigned by a qualified physiotherapist. Writing your notes will probably be quite difficult to begin with until you get used to the terminology. Different places use different abbreviations as well so just try to pick it up as you go along, but know the basic layout and content
- abide by the CSP Rules of Professional Conduct (Chartered Society of Physiotherapy 2005b) and Core Standards of Physiotherapy Practise (Chartered Society of Physiotherapy 2005a)
- have good communication skills and acceptable bedside manner
- work as part of a physiotherapy team and MDT when appropriate and communicate with other professionals regarding your patients
- clinically reason everything you do. Always be aware of the reasons why you are doing what you are doing for safety and ethical reasons, but also in case your clinical educator asks you questions about it
- observe and comply with Health and Safety and infection control policies
- use the evidence base where possible to inform your practise
- carry out CPD activity
- form prioritized problem lists for your patients and set appropriate goals for them
- plan treatment programmes and progress and modify them as appropriate
- use outcome measures to ensure your practise is clinically effective.

You could be expected to:

- see a patient by yourself on the first day, with help close at hand if required

- set yourself learning objectives and goals
- read up on conditions/injuries/surgeries that you come across during your day. Doing this anyway will help you get more out of the placement
- prepare a presentation for your physiotherapy colleagues as part of in-service training or lead a journal club meeting (i.e. find and critique a research article and present it)
- undertake a small project, for example revamp a patient information leaflet
- take an exercise class. You should get help with this so don't panic too much
- observe surgical or investigative procedures (for example, bronchoscopy or abdominal surgery) if you choose to. This can be a fantastic opportunity to learn more about anatomy and help you understand what the patient has to go through
- take part in a home visit
- represent your patients at a case conference or a MDT meeting.



## LEARNING THROUGHOUT PLACEMENT

The CSP Rules of Professional Conduct state that 'Every physiotherapist must keep up to date and must engage actively in a constant process of learning and development.'

It is also CSP policy that physiotherapy students must 'begin to collect evidence of learning for your CPD' (http://www.csp.org.uk). When you qualify it is required by law to register with the Health Professions Council (HPC). To stay registered you may be asked to provide evidence of your learning and professional development. Therefore, being on placement is an excellent place to start building up your CPD portfolio. It will also help you get more out of your placement and bring together the theory that you have covered in university.

Quite often you will get reading time throughout the day so make sure you use this time wisely to read up on the things you are seeing clinically or carry out other CPD activity such as a SWOT (Strengths, Weaknesses, Opportunities, Threats) analysis or reflection. Including a copy of your assessment form or placement appraisal completed by your CE in your CPD portfolio is also useful for future reference, especially when it comes to applying for jobs as it will help you to identify your strengths. Refer to the Careers and Learning section on the CSP website for more details.

Other tips:

- Carrying a notebook in your pocket is a good way to remember things to look up in your free time.
- Carryout a weekly SWOT analysis and set your self SMART (Specific, Measurable, Appropriate, Realistic, Time specific) goals.

- Use the CSP CPD proformas to help structure your learning and help you reflect on your experience and enhance your practise (visit www.csp.org.uk). The department you are working in may have some of these as well so ask around.
- Remember CPD isn't just about reflection. Other activities include critical appraisals, attending in-services or lectures and working though a case study. This list is not exhaustive!
- Use feedback from your CE constructively and don't take any negative feedback to heart, just see it as a way to improve your skills.
- Be confident as patients will tend to trust a therapist who demonstrates their knowledge, by explaining procedures and treatments for example.
- Don't be hard on yourself and try not to compare yourself with your co-workers or feel you have to work at their level. They will all have a lot more experience than you and it is impossible for you to have the knowledge base that they do by the end of your placement.
- There will be times when you feel a bit lost or overwhelmed by everything, but don't worry about it, even experienced physiotherapists feel the same from time to time.



## WHO TO ASK FOR HELP

- Your university should provide you with someone who you can get in contact with if you have any problems while on placement.
- Don't be afraid to ask clinical educator for help. Ask questions at every opportunity even when you're a junior!
- Ask for a tutorial on things you are struggling with or not sure about. For example, how to use specialised equipment/machines or how to carry out treatment techniques.
- Other staff in the team, for example junior members of staff are usually happy to help and it is sometimes easier to approach them.

### *References*

Chartered Society of Physiotherapy 2003 Clinical Education Placement Guidelines. CSP, London.

Chartered Society of Physiotherapy 2005a Core Standards of Physiotherapy Practise. CSP, London.

Chartered Society of Physiotherapy 2005b Rules of Professional Conduct. CSP, London.

Harden B 2004 Emergency Physiotherapy. Churchill Livingstone, Edinburgh.

### *Useful websites*

www.eventphysio.com
www.physiobuddies.co.uk
www.practisebasedlearning.org
www.csp.org.uk

CHAPTER FOUR

# Obtaining your first physiotherapy post

*Jamie Mackler*

After graduation, there may be opportunities for work within the National Health Service in hospitals and also within the community, in the private sector, professional sport, industry or overseas. There are also ever-increasing opportunities for postgraduate study and research. Most graduates start their careers in the NHS, although more and more are beginning to look outside this area of employment. Physiotherapy is at a very exciting point in its development and the profession is well placed to take advantage of increasing opportunities that are being presented. The role of Consultant Therapist has been established and rehabilitation teams are being developed in intermediate care and in the community, with therapists taking the lead role in many instances.

While studying you will most likely have benefited from an interprofessional approach to learning in which some modules were shared with other students from nursing, social work, midwifery and occupational therapy. This type of learning will help to prepare you for work in the current dynamic nature of the health care environment.

Your job hunt begins in earnest when you have your examination results. You may need to be flexible when looking for your first physiotherapy post but no matter what the job situation, the hints and tips contained within this chapter should help you to get to the front of the job queue.

## REGISTRATION WITH THE HEALTH PROFESSIONS COUNCIL (HPC)

In order to practise as a physiotherapist in any capacity in the UK, you need to be registered with the HPC. Registration must be renewed every 2 years and you must meet CPD standards.

For further information visit www.hpc-uk.org

## CHARTERED SOCIETY OF PHYSIOTHERAPY (CSP) MEMBERSHIP

In order to call yourself a Chartered Physiotherapist rather than simply a physiotherapist, you must join the CSP. They are the UK's only trade union, professional body and educational organisation for people working in, or studying physiotherapy.

Some of the benefits of CSP membership include:

- Supporting members through: a comprehensive professional liability insurance; workplace representation; professional and practice advice; negotiating the best possible pay and conditions; representing your interests to the government, NHS and private sector employers; free legal advice and representation
- Developing learning through clinical advice, CPD and qualifying education
- Helping you stay in touch through Interactive CSP, specialist interest groups, events such as Congress and newsletters
- Keeping you informed through the Physiotherapy Journal, Frontline magazine, fact sheets and resource materials
- Promoting the profession and influencing for change by talking regularly to ministers and key decision makers as well as boosting the professions profile in national, regional and international media.

Visit the societies website www.csp.org.uk for further information.

## Where to look for your first post

- The Chartered Society of Physiotherapy (CSP) jobs website: http://www.jobescalator.com/
- www.healthjobsuk.com/jobs is a useful site, as it tends to have the jobs that are advertised on individual trust websites and not the NHS site.
- http://www.physiobob.com
- Job ads in *Frontline*, the CSP's fortnightly publication.
- There are web-based NHS job sites in all four countries where vacant posts are advertised:
  - England: www.jobs.nhs.uk/for/juniorphysiotherapists
  - Scotland: www.jobs.scot.nhs.uk
  - Wales: www.wales.nhs.uk/jobs/index.cfm
  - Northern Ireland: www.n-i.nhs.uk which has a link on the home page to the job vacancies section
- At times of job shortages the CSP often offers managers a free service whereby they can send in details of vacant posts suitable for new graduates. All graduates will then automatically be sent details of these posts until they inform the CSP they have secured a post.
- NHS Trusts' circulars, which are sometimes sent to schools and colleges Trust websites (many Trusts have a 'job shop' on their website).
- Write speculative letters to every hospital within the area you wish to work, requesting any information on Open Days.
- It's important to also look away from the large acute trusts as many primary care trusts are organising new physio posts in community settings.
- Private hospitals (including BUPA) have also started recruiting newly qualified physiotherapists.

- Contact past placements? Maybe you could visit/volunteer or shadow perhaps (if you can afford to). Also see CSP's guidelines on volunteering.

## Choosing where to apply to

You should consider the issues raised in the CSP's information paper 'CPD2 The New Chartered Physiotherapist: Guidelines of good practice for new entrants to physiotherapy' when selecting a Trust in which you wish to work:

- It is not necessarily an advantage to look for a job in a large acute Trust - smaller Trusts, and primary care Trusts, can offer a good range of experience and, increasingly, therapy managers are being encouraged to combine junior rotational posts across both sectors.
- Check there are enough senior people to ensure there will be adequate support and teaching in the different clinical areas. Remember even static, temporary or part-time positions still provide valuable experience if a rotation is not available.
- Make an informal visit to the Trust. Talk to as many staff as possible. The CSP steward is a good source of information, or talk to students who have been to the Trust on placement. What about the attitude of the people you would be working with? Are they forward thinking and progressive? What's the atmosphere like? Do people appear friendly and supportive?
  Find out about:
- the type of rotations available
- terms and conditions of employment, e.g. are they implementing the Agenda for Change band 5 to 6 run through (not necessarily the same in each Trust)
- the staffing and resource levels
- any specialties in the Trust
- attitudes and opportunities for continuing professional development (CPD)
- policies of the Trust, for example, equal opportunities
- medical library facilities
- whether pre-qualifying students attend clinical placements
- Open Days—if they are being organised make sure you attend
- what the managers recommend you do in order to make your application as attractive as possible
- the DH Allied Health Professions Bulletins on the Department of Health website, where you can look for up to date initiatives as well as on the CSP website.

## JUNIOR ROTATIONS

The Chartered Society of Physiotherapy firmly believes that physiotherapists from the beginning of their career can be employed across the whole of the health, social, educational, voluntary and independent sectors given the appropriate support. The CSP identifies the kind of supervision and considerations that are necessary in developing new graduate posts and rotations within a range of health care settings (CSP PA52 2006). You should also look at the CSP guidance on developing and supporting new graduates in the community and other non-traditional settings.

## PRIVATE PRACTICE

In the past, private practice is generally not something that the CSP have encouraged for newly qualified physiotherapists due to, amongst other things, their lack of clinical experience, the potential lack of senior support or access to a structured CPD programme and a potentially limited career development pathway.

However, as a result of the expanding scope of physiotherapy and since some graduates have struggled to find jobs within the NHS, it is clear that some people were starting to look at beginning their careers outside traditional employment, which includes private practice.

Given appropriate mentorship; access to immediate help and advice when required; a structured training programme, including business and clinical training days; peer support and a clear understanding about working within their scope of practice, it is something that cannot be dismissed out of hand.

With the backing of senior colleagues willing to mentor and share their knowledge, regular meetings with peers and structured CPD training, there is a possibility of newly qualified physios developing in the same way that they would in a junior role within the NHS.

If you feel you are ready to take on the challenge and responsibility of private practice, it may be helpful to contact Physio First on: Telephone: 01327 354 441 Email: towcester@physiofirst.org.uk



## JOB APPLICATIONS

The easy bit is locating where to apply; the hard bit is actually managing to secure a post.

### Phoning for a job

Some advertisements invite you to telephone for more details or for an informal chat about the post. This may be so the employer can ask a few general questions and, on the basis of your responses, tell whether it will be worth your while making a formal application.

### Hints and tips on application forms

Departments that receive many applications will usually use the application form as the first stage of their selection process and draw up a short-list of people to invite for interview. It is therefore essential to take time and care when completing an application form and complete it electronically if possible.

- Always read the job description and person specification carefully, and address in your application how you meet all aspects of the person specification.
- Photocopy your completed application form so you don't forget what you said on the form at interview.
- Be precise about your work/placement experience.
- It is particularly important to make sure you can demonstrate learning experiences from a wide variety of conditions/areas of practice. For example, if you were unable to have a neurology placement during your degree, you are strongly advised to record evidence of learning from treating patients with neurological problems in other placements, e.g. community paediatric.
- When discussing your outside interests, be specific and don't make them up. It's possible that you could get asked about them in an interview. Think about how they are related to physiotherapy, how they will make you a better physiotherapist and what you have learned from them.
- Mention some specific reasons why you want to work for the place you are applying to.
- Demonstrate how you have acquired the necessary skills for the job. For example, communication, team working, problem solving, clinical reasoning, analytical, etc., and remember to give examples.



## Cover letters

- The cover letter is just as important as the CV as its purpose is to give an overview of your skills and qualities that make you perfect for the position.
- One side of A4 with 3–4 paragraphs is suitable and should be tailored to every job.
- Begin by introducing yourself and explain what you are currently doing.
- Explain why you are interested in working for this employer by researching them and providing specific reasons.
- Pull out the key points from your CV and give relevant examples to show how you are ideal for the job.
- Explain how everything mentioned in your CV is relevant in physiotherapy and also to the job description for the post you are applying to.
- End with a short positive sentence that may include thanking them for their time and saying that you look forward to hearing from them in the near future for example.

## Compiling a CV

There are many examples on the Internet and in books on how to produce covering letters as well as putting together great CVs, such as those used by Shellenbarger & Chunta (2007) and Littlewood (2005). There is deliberately no example of a 'good' CV in this book as everyone's CV must be individual to them and reflect their personality, otherwise it wouldn't stand out from all the others:

- The way in which information is organised in a CV could mean the difference between rejection and being offered an interview.
- It's important to have your CV up to date and accessible, so that you can apply for posts with minimal notice, e.g. ½ hour. The reason being is many jobs disappear within a few hours of them appearing due to high numbers of applicants.
- Refer to the AHP Employability guide, especially for transferable skills. http://www.cihe-uk.com/docs/SEP/AlliedHealth.pdf
- Your CV should give an overview of what you can offer an employer and leave them wanting to learn more at an interview. Therefore, use just two sides of A4 and don't cram too much in.
- Headings you might want to consider including are: personal and contact details, education and training (including a list of placements), relevant experience; recent achievements, skills profile, other interests.
- Write in the first person and use short sentences and bullet points to make the CV easier to read.
- Don't just rely on the computer to check spelling and grammar. Check through it yourself and ask someone else for a second opinion.
- If you send your CV in to a place and don't hear back from them for a while, follow it up with a phone call. Do some research so you know the correct person to speak to. Always make sure you send them an updated version if your circumstances or experiences change.
- Also, don't lie! It will eventually catch up with you.

It is worth reading the article by Shellenbarger & Chunta (2007) who write that when reviewing CVs, it becomes clear that some CV information provides a better reflection of work completed than others do. They provide a description of common CV errors, propose strategies to avoid such problems, and suggest methods for developing an accurate and clear CV that highlights accomplishments and clearly represents the work. Tips for updating CV and suggestions for electronic formats are also provided.

## Surviving an interview

It is worth preparing yourself as much as possible. It's been tried and tested, so thinking about possible interview questions before you actually have an interview will help you feel more confident, which will come across in the interview.

When you do get that interview for your first job the chances are you will probably feel really nervous about it, so read on to learn how to get yourself ready for the big day.

Interviews may be individual or group, or in some cases both. Your interview may also require you to deliver a presentation on a chosen or given topic, or complete a written test; it may involve a practical test. Preparation for each type of interview should be very similar, but some extra tips for group interviews are also given below as well as what to expect from doing a practical test.

If you have any particular needs for the interview (e.g. if you are visually impaired, hard of hearing, use a wheelchair, etc.), let them know. Interview panels should provide support/access for candidates where required.

**Before interview:**

- Always call to confirm your attendance and show you are still interested in the job.
- Look clean, smart and presentable. Plan your journey and be on time!
- Remember to take along any important documents such as your degree certificate and HPC registration certificate.
- Research the employer and the physiotherapy department via the Internet, personal contact, the organisation's annual report, etc.
- If applying to the NHS, get yourself up to date with key government policies for the NHS and the contribution that physiotherapists can make, now and in the future.
- Make sure you are clear about your understanding of clinical governance and its implications for the physiotherapy service, have a good understanding of the legal responsibilities of the profession and ensure you can demonstrate use of reflective practice.
- Know the job description for the post you are being interviewed for inside out, as you may get asked a question about issues surrounding the job. For example, what do you think your role as a junior would be within this trust/health board? Also, notice any current topical issues in the specific job setting you are applying for.
- Find out as much as possible about your potential employer. This will impress the employer and show initiative and enthusiasm.
- Read through your application form and CV, and think of things they may ask you about them. Be prepared to expand on and give further examples of anything you have included.
- Practise saying your answers with a friend or stage a mock interview.
- Take your CPD portfolio with you. In advance it's a good idea to identify possible items as evidence from your portfolio. This is useful to show to interviewers to back up any examples you give, although make sure you can find them easily. Remember your portfolio is private and personal and you can always remove the reflections you do not want others to see.

**During interview:**

- Establish rapport: show a positive attitude, smile, relax, be enthusiastic, polite and friendly, and address interviewers by name. A panel of at least two people normally conducts interviews.
- Make eye contact with the interview panel, especially the person asking the question, but don't hold it long so that the person is forced to look away to break the contact.
- Try not to fiddle with pens, your hands, etc., or shift around in your chair too much as this is distracting to interviewers.
- Interviewers will normally write notes during the interview – don't be put off by this, it is so that they have a record of the interview to refer to at the end – it is not a sign that you have said anything particularly good or bad!
- Good interviewers will ask open questions, i.e. questions that don't elicit a one-word answer. They tend to begin with 'How..', 'Tell me about...', 'What...', 'Why....', etc.
- Take time to think about the question you have been asked – it's better to do this than to rush in and realise afterwards that you could have given a better response.
- If your mind goes blank in response to a particular question, be honest about this and ask if you can return to the subject later in the interview.
- Show humour during the interview, but don't overdo it.
- Speak clearly, and try not to rush. Be alert to verbal/non-verbal prompts from the panel, which may indicate that you need to either give more information, or have already given enough. Don't talk too much! If the panel do want you to expand further they will use prompts, asking open, probing questions.
- Concentrate on your achievements, experience and strengths. Give examples in your answers wherever you can. If you are asked about your weaknesses, try to turn this into a strength, e.g. 'I can sometimes be overly critical of myself if I make a mistake – but I'm conscious of this, and on the positive side it means I always work to as high a standard as possible.'
- Use every opportunity to show you are interested in this particular job/Trust.
- Remember, a good panel will do their best to put you at your ease to ensure you present yourself as well as possible. They want to find the best candidate for the job, so there should be no trick questions or attempts to make things difficult for you. Try to relax!

CHAPTER FOUR

**At the end**

- The panel may ask you if you have any questions for them. Have one or two prepared – about the job or place of work – as this demonstrates your interest in the post. But there is unlikely to be time for a long list of questions. This could also be an opportunity for you to tell the panel anything important that you think you have missed or didn't have an opportunity to say during their questions.

- The panel will normally tell you when you are likely to be given the result. If they don't, it is perfectly acceptable to ask.

## After

- Analyse what you did well.
- Note down anything you were not prepared for, and think about how you might answer differently in the future.
- If you aren't successful, ask for feedback.
- Every interview could go better, and there will always be something you could improve upon. Just remember that everyone who has been interviewed will probably be feeling the same way.

## Group interviews

- Preparation should be the same or similar to that required for an individual interview.
- The aim of group interviews is to see how each individual participates in a group setting. Interviewers will be looking at your communication skills, how you voice your opinion, your manners and your interaction with the group.
- The set up of group interviews will vary greatly across the NHS. You may be in a group with five to ten other candidates with two or three people interviewing or observing.
- Usually you will be given a topic to discuss, for example, how to plan a MDT meeting relating to a patients discharge, an on-call scenario, a list of patients that need prioritized or the issue of continuing professional development.
- A few people may then be picked for individual interview or everyone may get the chance.
- Alternatively, you may be asked individual questions that you must then answer in front of the group, or there may be members of the physiotherapy team that you can have a chat with and ask questions to.
- Whatever the set up of the interview, just remember to be yourself and don't just focus on simply getting your voice heard.
- Have opinions on different topics and make sure you can explain yourself in a concise way. Don't be afraid to disagree with someone, just explain why you disagree.
- Avoid repeating what others have said. If you agree with them say so, but elaborate on their answer to show further thinking.
- Encourage quieter members of the group to talk. If someone was interrupted, go back and ask them what they were going to say. Listening is just as important as talking!

- Aim to make the group summarize main points at the end to show initiative and organisation or offer to be scribe.

## Practical tests

- Normally you will be told prior to the interview if you will be asked to carry out a practical task.
- They aren't as scary as they sound. Its just like answering a clinical question.
- Examples of tasks people have been asked to carry out include: teaching the active cycle of breathing technique; mobilizing a patient for the first time post operatively; teaching the use of a walking aid; analysing arterial bold gases and interpreting a chest X-ray; carrying out an outcome measure on a patient, for example the elderly mobility scale.
- Just take your time and picture it as a real-life situation.
- Consider if there is anything you would do prior to carrying out the physical task, i.e. reading medical notes, consulting nursing staff, checking observations.
- During the task always be aware of your own safety as well as the patients.
- At the end consider whether you would reinforce what you have done with the patient by providing literature, for example.



## Interview question topics

It's great preparation to think about all the possible questions they might ask you or speak to people who have been on interviews before. Littlewood (2005) explains that the key to interview success is thorough preparation and gives advise on how to excel at job interviews. The sections below break down the types of question topics you could be asked.

Refer to the Interview Questions section on www.redgoldfish.co.uk for further hints and tips.

### *University related questions*

These questions could include what placements you have been on, what ones you have and haven't liked and why. You could get asked about your research project or dissertation, what were its aims, limitations or why you chose that topic.

### *Clinical questions*

Clinical questions tend to scare people a lot. In reality though you probably know the stuff, you just don't realise it. So try to think up clinical scenarios that you may get asked about. How to prioritise patients in various settings is popular. For example, how to prioritise a number of respiratory patients when you only have time to see one of them. Questions beginning with 'what would you do if...' are also common. Generally speaking there is no right and wrong answer to this type of question.

As long as you explain your reasoning behind what you are saying you will show consideration of all the possibilities and a good insight and awareness into clinical situations.

You may also be asked a direct question regarding your clinical knowledge, such as 'what complications would you give for someone who has had a fracture?' or 'can you give me some examples of red and yellow flags for back pain?' or 'what are the contraindications for suctioning?' So, remember to revise general clinical knowledge as well especially in the areas of respiratory, musculoskeletal and neurology.

When you first start employment you will never be expected to begin being on-call until you are fully trained and have demonstrated competency in the appropriate areas. However, it is not unheard of to be asked an on-call-related question. *Emergency Physiotherapy* by Harden (Churchill Livingstone 2004) is a good resource to revise topics related to being on-call.

### Topical questions

Topical questions could relate to any current issues happening within the profession and the NHS. Have a good read of recent *Frontline* issues and look up the CSP website. Discuss things with friends and form opinions of what is happening in the profession.

### Personal questions

Know what your strengths and weaknesses are, how you identified them, how to improve your weaknesses and how to make the most of your strengths. Be prepared to explain why you chose physiotherapy as a career and what your ambitions are within the profession. Know how to answer questions relating to how you work as part of a team, how you would cope with stressful situations, an aggressive patient, disagreement with another health professional, confrontation, etc.

### Professional questions

Questions relating to the profession might include questions about:

- the Chartered Society of Physiotherapy (CSP)
- Continuing professional development (CPD)
- reflective practise, including a request for examples of how you have used this during your training and how it has improved your practise
- role differences between levels of physiotherapists and clinically effective practice
- clinical governance and what you understand by the term
- clinical audit and what you understand by the term
- the impact, if any of 'Agenda for Change' on physiotherapists
- the term CPD and how it may be acquired?

For more detailed questions log onto http://www.interactivecsp.org.uk and choose the newly qualified network. Then go to the discussion form on interview questions. There are lots of examples, which will be invaluable in your interview preparation.

## WHO CAN HELP YOU MAINTAIN YOUR CONTINUING PROFESSIONAL DEVELOPMENT (CDP) WHILE SEEKING THAT FIRST POST?

### Clinical interest and occupational groups

They often include reduced or free membership for out of work newly qualified physiotherapists as well as reduced or free entry to courses, CI/OG workshops and conferences. Some may even arrange mentoring or even some kind of shadowing so that you can keep your CPD up to date.

There is a complete list of groups and their areas of interest, with contact details, on the CSP website: http://www.csp.org.uk/director/groupandnetworks/ciogs.cfm

### Graduate workshops

When graduates are without their first physiotherapist post, it is suggested that final year students from each university group together, meet their universities and ask them if they will help arrange workshops for after they graduate. In this way there is more chance of skills being kept up to date.

Some of these, such as Cardiff University, have been on a 1-day a week basis over a period of weeks, while others are one-off days. In general, these focus on the core skills of musculoskeletal, cardio respiratory and neurology. They are designed to maintain clinical reasoning as well as practical skills. Others are offering graduates assistance with CVs and interview techniques while some have developed 6–12 month teaching and research assistant posts for graduate applicants.



### CSP boards

You could get in touch with your local CSP Board. Previously one graduate volunteered to help out the Board Secretary write up the notes of the meeting, etc. This got her known and she was subsequently offered work shadowing and then an actual job.

### Trusts

A number of Trusts have supported graduates in a variety of ways, in particular through involvement in in-service training sessions and work shadowing. Some have put on practical skills refresher days.

Please note there aren't any Trusts in Scotland. These were dissolved some years ago and have been replaced by Divisions and Community Health Partnerships.

If Trusts are unable to help, you could try contacting the Strategic Health Authorities and see if they can assist; after all, they are supposed to be proactive in supporting newly qualified physios.

### Private practitioners

You should look at physio first (formerly known as the Organisation of Chartered Physiotherapists in Private Practice website) (http://www.physiofirst.org.uk/) for contact details of thousands of private practitioners. You could then contact them to see if they will offer you any shadowing opportunities.

For details on HPC return to practice requirements and its impact on physiotherapy graduates not currently employed/working as physiotherapists, contact the Chartered Society of Physiotherapy.

## SUMMARY

This chapter has outlined the different areas you can look at to first find your physiotherapy post, what you can do to maintain your CPD until you secure your first job and, ultimately, how to put yourself in the best possible position to secure it.

Your time at university will most probably have been one of the most memorable experiences of your life. You've expanded your skills in a host of different ways, for example, learning how to care for others' health and wellbeing, to relieve or resolve their symptoms and disabilities. You are now an independent learner and an autonomous practitioner.

It's recommended to remain a member of the Chartered Society of Physiotherapy when you graduate. They offer lots of help and assistance, not only when you get your first job, but also when you are trying to secure it. They also offer Professional Liability Insurance as standard with their membership, which will be essential if you are working or volunteering. Not only that but also many trusts put CSP membership down as 'desirable' on their person specification.

Don't forget though to check with the CSP to see if they have any discounted rates of membership available until you secure your first post.

It's important to remember that due to inadequate planning within the NHS, new graduates are sometimes unable to find a job in the NHS. Sometimes it really can be down to being in the right place at the right time. However, with the massive expansion in physiotherapy, there are many other areas of work that can be explored. By following the tips in this chapter and being as proactive in your search as possible, you will be putting yourself in the best possible position to enable you to fulfil your dream of being a Chartered Physiotherapist.



### *References*

CSP PA52, 2006, A CSP briefing paper PA 52 Guidance for Developing New Graduate Posts and Rotations Within a Range of Health Care Settings.

Littlewood S 2005 Careers. How to excel at a job interview. Nursing Times 101(6): 66–67.

Shellenbarger T, Chunta K S 2007 The curriculum vitae: sending the right message. Nurse Educator 32(1): 30–33.

## FURTHER INFORMATION

### NHS policy and health reform websites

NHS Policy: websites to look at: http://www.dh.gov.uk/en/Policyandguidance/index.htm
Policy on health and social care, includes things like NSFs and clinical governance http://www.dh.gov.uk/en/Policyandguidance/Healthandsocialcaretopics/index.htm

Commissioning:

http://www.dh.gov.uk/en/Policyandguidance/Organisationpolicy/Commissioning/index.htm
Commissioning a patient-led NHS:
http://www.dh.gov.uk/en/Policyandguidance/Organisationpolicy/Commissioning/CommissioningapatientledNHS/index.htm

Health Reform – reorganization of ambulance trusts, SHAs and PCTs

http://www.dh.gov.uk/en/Policyandguidance/Organisationpolicy/Healthreform/DH_4135663.

Payment by results:

http://www.dh.gov.uk/en/Policyandguidance/Organisationpolicy/Financeandplanning/NHSFinancialReforms/index.htm.

### *CSP resources*

Website: http://www.csp.org.uk Find out latest developments in the profession.
Interactive CSP: http://www.interactivecsp.org.uk/ The newly qualified network has lots of information from the latest job situation to typical questions asked at interview.

CSP Survival Guide in obtaining your first physiotherapy post can be found on iCSP newly qualified network/

Job Escalator: http://www.csp.org.uk/director/careersandlearning/physiotherapyjobs.cfm
Frontline: http://www.csp.org.uk/director/newsandevents/frontline.cfm

Library and Information Services: http://www.csp.org.uk/director/librar-yandpublications/libraryandinformationservices.cfm

### Library resources

National Library for Health: http://www.library.nhs.uk/Default.aspx Includes specialist libraries information, including Health Management: http://www.library.nhs.uk/specialistlibraries/

### Assistance interview

M Messmer 1999 Job Hunting For Dummies, 2nd edn. Hungry Minds Inc, U.S.A. This book guides you through CV writing, cover letters and interview technique.
www.redgoldfish.co.uk Has a really good detailed document regarding interview questions and the interview process.
www.physiobuddies.co.uk Visit this site for information on interviews that have taken place as different hospitals across the country.
www.flyingstart.scot.nhs.uk/CVsandInterviews.htm Has activities that can help you get started writing your CV.
www.careers-scotland.org.uk Has tips on interviews and CV writing.

# Case studies in respiratory physiotherapy

*Lead author Janis Harvey, with contributions from Sarah Ridley, Jo Oag, Elaine Dhouieb, Billie Hurst*



## INTRODUCTION

The area of respiratory physiotherapy reaches a number of patient groups, both in the in-patient and out-patient settings. The case studies that follow are based predominantly in the in-patient environment; however, the components of a respiratory assessment and the subsequent identification of physiotherapy problems and treatment plan could be applied to any patient with respiratory compromise in any clinical setting.

Like all other areas of physiotherapy practice, respiratory physiotherapy involves accurate patient assessment in order to identify patient problems. Respiratory assessment should include certain key elements: general observations of the patient; consideration of trends in physiological observations (e.g. HR, BP, oxygen saturations); patient position; auscultation, palpation and, where available, analysis of arterial blood gases and chest X-ray (CXR).

Patient problems identified from the assessment generally fall into three main categories: loss of lung volume, secretion retention and increased work of breathing. The extent of any resulting respiratory compromise can vary greatly between patients and may not always be reflected by the ward area in which the patient is being treated. On occasion the most acutely unwell patients are in the general ward areas and not within critical care as expected.

A problem-orientated treatment plan may include a combination of a number of interventions such as mobilisation, positioning, breathing techniques (e.g. ACBT, AD), manual techniques (percussion, vibrations), mechanical aids (e.g. IPPB, CPAP) or more invasive measures (e.g. airway suctioning).

A respiratory assessment is mainly indicated for patients who have undergone surgery, those with medical respiratory conditions, e.g. exacerbation of COPD, and those requiring critical care. Cardiothoracic surgery and paediatrics are other specialist clinical areas that physiotherapists are involved in providing respiratory care. However, it must be remembered that patients requiring such care may not be in these ward areas exclusively. Physiotherapists working in any clinical area may be required to undertake a respiratory assessment and provide respiratory care. For example, assessment of a stroke patient who has aspirated or an oncology patient who develops respiratory failure following chemotherapy. It is important, therefore, that all physiotherapists are familiar with respiratory assessment and intervention.



Another key area of work where physiotherapists are required to undertake respiratory care is in the provision of emergency duty/on-call services. Such services are available to patients who have a condition amenable to physiotherapy, which has either deteriorated or is likely to deteriorate without intervention before daytime service resumes (Scottish Intercollegiate Guideline Network 2004). This can be a very challenging area of work for the physiotherapist on-call, who needs to think clearly while being faced with an acutely unwell patient who is in need of their attention, whatever the time of day. Guidance is available to support the clinician involved in providing such care and to aid ongoing assessment of competence (Chartered Society of Physiotherapy 2002).

## CASE STUDY 1 RESPIRATORY MEDICINE – BRONCHIECTASIS OUT-PATIENT

### Subjective assessment

| | |
|---|---|
| PC | 35-year-old female<br>Attending routine multidisciplinary bronchiectasis clinic appointment |

| | |
|---|---|
| HPC | Diagnosed 6/12 ago with bronchiectasis following an in-patient admission with community-acquired pneumonia (CAP) in her right lower lobe. This resulted in the development of bronchiectatic changes. Since diagnosis the patient reports daily production of mucopurulent secretions with excessive coughing and feelings of fatigue |
| PMH | CAP<br>Gastric oesophageal reflux |
| SH | Married with two children<br>Lifelong non-smoker<br>Full-time employment as drug company representative, involving frequent travel around the United Kingdom<br>Normally leads an active lifestyle with two to three visits a week to the gym, although this has decreased over the past 3/12 |
| DH | Omeprazole |
| **Consultant handover** | Patient is currently stable but is concerned about the impact of her cough and increased sputum on everyday life, especially in relation to her work, where she frequently does formal presentations |

## Objective assessment

| | |
|---|---|
| Respiratory | *Ventilation*<br>SV room air $SpO_2$ 99% RR 12<br>*CXR*<br>Bronchiectatic changes present in right lower lobe<br>*ABG*<br>Not appropriate to be taken as stable |
| CVS | Temp 37°C HR 70 BP 120/70 |
| CNS | Nil of note |
| Renal | Nil of note |
| MSK | Nil of note |
| Microbiology | *Staphylococcus aureus* in sputum sample 6/12 ago |
| Patient position | Sitting in chair |

CHAPTER FIVE

| | |
|---|---|
| **Observation** | Looks well, good colour, breathing pattern normal<br>Patient actively trying to suppress cough and noise of secretions |
| **Auscultation** | Breath sounds throughout both lung fields with mid inspiratory crackles right lower lobe |

## Questions

1. You feel this lady seems a little vague regarding her diagnosis, how will you deal with this issue?
2. Following discussion it is now evident that the patient's knowledge about her condition is sparse. How will you resolve this issue?
3. What is the range of airway clearance techniques commonly taught to this group of patients?
4. Considering this patient's condition and lifestyle what would be the advantages and disadvantages to each of the treatments mentioned in the previous question?
5. Your patient seems reluctant to undertake airway clearance management, how will you motivate your patient to undertake regular treatment?
6. What frequency and duration may you suggest to this patient for performing airway clearance techniques?
7. What signs and symptoms would you highlight to your patient to recognize at the start of an exacerbation?
8. Your patient asks what she should do if she has an exacerbation, what advice do you give her?
9. Why would you consider asking this patient if she has any urinary stress incontinence problems?



## CASE STUDY 2 RESPIRATORY MEDICINE – LUNG CANCER PATIENT

### Subjective assessment

| | |
|---|---|
| PC | 70-year-old male<br>Non-small-cell lung cancer (NSCLC) in the right main bronchus<br>Admitted with an acute deterioration in condition and the family are no longer able to cope with the patient at home |
| HPC | Diagnosed 9/12 ago following a 3/12 history of increasing shortness of breath and cough. Two episodes of frank haemoptysis also reported. Following diagnosis, patient was deemed appropriate for a course of chemotherapy, but had limited response to intervention. As an out-patient he had |

| | |
|---|---|
| | a CT scan, which showed brain and spinal metastases, and he has been suffering uncontrollable pain. As a result he has been bed bound for the past month and has required increasing support from Macmillan oncology nurse specialists |
| **PMH** | Nil of note |
| **SH** | Lives with wife in a bungalow<br>Smokes 40 cpd<br>Retired teacher<br>Close family network<br>Until 2/12 ago independent with walking stick, able to walk to local shops approximately 100 m |
| **DH** | Paracetamol<br>Co-codamol<br>Oramorph<br>Lactulose<br>Build up drinks |
| **Handover** | Patient admitted with a decreased GCS, frail, emaciated<br>Family very concerned, emotional and distressed by patient's breathing pattern and audible secretions<br>Pain management sub-optimal |

## Objective assessment

| | |
|---|---|
| **Respiratory** | ***Ventilation***<br>SV 4L $O_2$ via non-venturi system mask, unhumidified $SpO_2$ 95% RR 10–22<br>***CXR***<br>No CXR taken on admission<br>Previous CXR (1/12 ago): white out of right lung field, secondary to bronchus obstruction<br>***ABG***<br>None available |
| **CVS** | Temp 39°C HR 120 BP 105/65 |
| **CNS** | GCS fluctuating between 5 and 8 |
| **Renal** | Catheterised on admission |
| **MSK** | Pain at lower back region in keeping with spinal metastases |
| **Microbiology** | None |

| | |
|---|---|
| **Patient position** | Supine |
| **Observation** | Flushed, drowsy, intelligible speech with audible secretions. Agitated at times, with arms flailing and pulling at oxygen mask<br>Normal chest shape with altered breathing pattern illustrated by Cheyne–Stoking |
| **Auscultation** | Breath sounds diminished throughout right lung field with widespread coarse inspiratory/expiratory crackles transmitting throughout left lung field |
| **Palpation** | Decreased chest excursion on right with palpable secretions over trachea and left apex |

## Questions

1. How would you describe Cheyne–Stoking?
2. If a patient is performing a Cheyne–Stoke breathing pattern, what does this indicate?
3. Prior to assessing and treating this patient, what further information do you require?
4. What are the main physiotherapy problems?
5. What are the associated problems for this patient that may affect your physiotherapy intervention?
6. How will you treat the problems that you have highlighted?
7. What outcome measures will you use to evaluate the effectiveness of your intervention?
8. In this scenario, which medical and physiotherapy interventions are inappropriate and why?
9. What do you see as the role of the palliative care team in this scenario?

# CASE STUDY 3 RESPIRATORY MEDICINE – CYSTIC FIBROSIS PATIENT

## Subjective assessment

| | |
|---|---|
| PC | 19-year-old female<br>Admitted with acute exacerbation of cystic fibrosis (CF) |
| HPC | Diagnosed at birth. Multiple hospital admissions over last 3 years due to exacerbation of CF. On admission patient reporting 1/52 history of increased breathlessness, sputum volume and cough. These symptoms have not responded to a 2/52 course of intravenous antibiotics. In respiratory distress. Dehydrated. Recent weight loss and current BMI 17. |

| | |
|---|---|
| | Under review for lung transplantation assessment. Patient previously agreed to perform twice daily ACBT in alternate side lying/supine for 20 minutes, but generally non-compliant with suggested airway clearance programme and prescribed medications |
| **PMH** | Asthma<br>Osteoporosis |
| **SH** | Lives at home with parents and sister (non-CF)<br>Unemployed and sedentary lifestyle due to health status |
| **DH** | Ventolin via nebuliser<br>Becotide via inhaler<br>Dnase via nebuliser<br>Colomycin via nebuliser<br>Azithromycin<br>Creon<br>Alendronate<br>Vitamins A, D, E, K<br>Long-term oxygen therapy |
| **Handover** | Patient exhausted and only able to clear small amounts of very thick, purulent bronchial secretions with difficulty. Pyrexial and requiring intravenous fluids. C/O nausea following overnight feed via PEG tube |

## Objective assessment

| | |
|---|---|
| *Respiratory* | ***Ventilation***<br>SV 28% $O_2$ via venturi system mask $SpO_2$ 85% RR 34<br>***CXR* (Figure 5.1)**<br>Hyperinflated, chronic bronchiectatic/fibrotic changes throughout upper and mid zones bilaterally<br>Intravenous access device in situ<br>***ABG***<br>$H^+$ 50 nmol/L $pCO_2$ 13 kPa $pO_2$ 7 kPa<br>$HCO_3^-$ 30 mmol/L BE −9.0 |
| **CVS** | Temp 38.5°C HR 129 BP 100/85 |
| **CNS** | Nil of note |
| **Renal** | Nil of note |
| **MSK** | Kyphotic with history of osteoporosis |
| **Microbiology** | *Pseudomonas* in sputum |

| | |
|---|---|
| **Patient position** | Sitting upright in bed holding onto cot sides |
| **Observation** | Pale with signs of central cyanosis. Unable to speak due to SOB and excessive cough. Looks distressed. Breathing pattern shallow, apical with active expiration |
| **Auscultation** | Coarse inspiratory crackles transmitting throughout chest on background of high-pitched expiratory wheeze |
| **Palpation** | Limited chest excursion on inspiration (right = left) Secretions palpable upper, anterior chest wall |

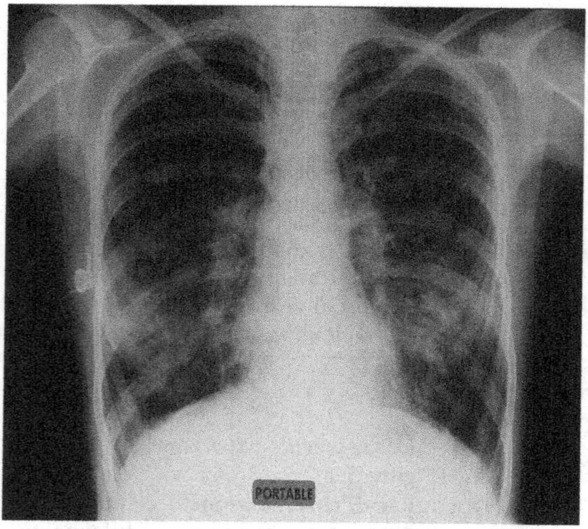


**FIGURE 5.1** X-ray for Case Study 3 showing hyperinflated, chronic bronchiectatic/fibrotic changes throughout upper and mid zones bilaterally. Intravenous access device *in situ*.



## Questions

1. Considering the above information, list this patient's physiotherapy problems.
2. What information from the objective assessment led you to this problem list?
3. What does the ABG result tell you?
4. What are the specific signs of hyperinflation on this patient's X-ray (Figure 5.1)?

5. During this admission, how might you initially modify this patient's normal daily routine of alternate side lying and ACBT for 20 minutes twice a day?
6. Having decided on an acceptable airway clearance technique, what else would you include in your initial treatment plan?
7. Following two physiotherapy sessions with modified ACBT that morning, you feel that the patient is becoming more exhausted and unable to clear her secretions effectively. How might you change your physiotherapy management and with whom would you want to discuss these potential changes?
8. How might your treatment/management change if your patient was commenced on NIV?
9. Why would it be inappropriate to introduce activity/exercise at this stage?

## CASE STUDY 4 RESPIRATORY MEDICINE – COPD PATIENT

### Subjective assessment

| | |
|---|---|
| PC | 65-year-old male<br>Admitted to respiratory ward with acute exacerbation of COPD |
| HPC | Diagnosed 5 years ago with severe emphysema. Recent viral illness that has resulted in a dry cough, wheeze and breathlessness for 1/52. Has been house bound last few days. Normally 1–2 exacerbations per year that are managed by GP. No previous hospital admissions for COPD |
| PMH | Hypertension |
| SH | Retired engineer. Lives alone in third-floor flat. No lift. Normally manages all ADL independently. Exercise tolerance 50 m on flat – no aid required. Drives a car. No family living locally. No social services required. Smokes 30 cpd |
| DH | Salbutamol inhaler<br>Becotide inhaler<br>Atenolol<br>GP letter states that patient has not picked up repeat prescription for inhalers from 1/12 ago |
| Handover | Admitted overnight. Patient noted to be drowsy but able to be roused for short periods. When awake, able to talk in short sentences but appears slightly disorientated. Breathing pattern laboured and has a dry, spontaneous cough. Dehydrated but receiving IV fluids |

CHAPTER FIVE

## Objective assessment

| | |
|---|---|
| Respiratory | *Ventilation*<br>SV 6 L $O_2$ via a simple face mask $SpO_2$ 97% RR 9<br>*CXR*<br>Hyperinflated lung fields with flattened diaphragms<br>Emphysematous bullae upper zones<br>No focal signs of collapse/consolidation<br>*ABG*<br>$H^+$58 mmol/L $pCO_2$ 12 kPa $pO_2$ 12 kPa<br>$HCO_3^-$ 30 mmol/L<br>BE +9 |
| CVS | Temp 37.5°C HR 115 BP 130/90 |
| CNS | Drowsy but able to be roused for short periods Disorientated and confused. Moving all four limbs |
| Renal | Nil of note |
| MSK | Nil of note |
| Microbiology | None available |
| Patient position | Slumped lying in bed |
| Observation | Obese man with barrel shaped chest and large abdomen. Colour – flushed. Breathing through an open mouth. Predominately a shallow, apical breathing pattern with increased use of accessory muscles. Also demonstrating in-drawing of his lower chest wall on inspiration. Active expiration |
| Auscultation | Quiet BS generally with end expiratory polyphonic wheeze throughout |
| Palpation | Decreased expansion bi-basally (right = left). No palpable secretions |

## Questions

1. The patient is drowsy with a RR of 9. What may be the contributing factors?
2. What is the difference between fixed and variable oxygen therapy?
3. Which type of oxygen therapy would be more suitable for the patient at this point?
4. What is this patient's main physiotherapy problem?
5. What led you to this conclusion?
6. What factors may be contributing to this increased WOB?
7. How might your initial treatment plan address this problem of increased WOB?

8. Consider this patient's CXR report, chest shape and breathing pattern. Would he benefit from lower lateral costal breathing exercises to improve basal chest excursion once he was less drowsy?
9. What goals would you hope to have achieved before this patient was discharged home?

## CASE STUDY 5 SURGICAL RESPIRATORY – ANTERIOR RESECTION

### Subjective assessment

| | |
|---|---|
| PC | 63-year-old male<br>Day 2 post-laparotomy for anterior resection (end to end anastomosis) |
| HPC | Emergency admission yesterday with increasing abdominal pain<br>2/12 altered bowel habit |
| PMH | Nil of note- previously fit and well |
| SH | Lives with wife, recently retired, independent with ADL, plays golf three times a week, smoker 5 cpd |
| DH | Nil of note |
| Handover | Acute desaturation this morning. Patient has been coughing – effective and occasionally moist, nil expectorated. Otherwise stable<br>Not been out of bed as yet |

### Objective assessment

| | |
|---|---|
| Respiratory | *Ventilation*<br>SV 4 L $O_2$ via nasal cannulae $SpO_2$ 90% RR 12<br>*CXR*<br>Right basal collapse<br>*ABG*<br>None available |
| CVS | Temp 37.4°C HR 80 BP 130/60 |
| CNS | GCS E4 V5 M6<br>Pain score VAS 2/10 at rest 4/10 on movement/coughing<br>Morphine PCA |
| Renal | UO 20–30 mL/hr +1.5 L cumulative balance to date |
| MSK | Nil of note |

| | |
|---|---|
| **Microbiology** | Nil of note |
| **Patient position** | Slumped in bed |
| **Observation** | Talking freely |
| **Auscultation** | Breath sounds throughout, fine end inspiratory crackles right base |
| **Palpation** | Reduced expansion right base, no secretions palpable |

## Questions

1. Is this patient adequately oxygenated? What suggestions might you make?
2. List this patient's physiotherapy problem(s).
3. What information from the objective assessment led you to this problem list?
4. Why are patients who have undergone surgery/anaesthetic at risk of developing respiratory compromise?
5. What are the treatment options for this patient?
6. What would your initial treatment plan include?
7. How would you progress this patient?
8. HDU patients can have many attachments including monitoring (ECG, sats probe), oxygen therapy, catheter and wound drains. What considerations would you have to give before mobilising such a patient?



# CASE STUDY 6 SURGICAL RESPIRATORY – DIVISION OF ADHESIONS

## Subjective assessment

| | |
|---|---|
| PC | 74-year-old female<br>Day 3 post-laparotomy and division of adhesions |
| HPC | Existing ileostomy – no output for 48 hours, vomiting and no significant fluid intake |
| PMH | Small bowel resection and formation of ileostomy 2 years previous for incarcerated hernia<br>COPD<br>Right axillary node clearance<br>Previous pulmonary TB |
| SH | Lives alone, housebound, home help three times/day, smokes 10 cpd |
| DH | Ventolin inhaler<br>Seretide inhaler |

| | |
|---|---|
| Handover | Initially in intensive care, intubated and ventilated. Extubated yesterday and transferred to HDU. Stable overnight, difficulty clearing secretions |

## Objective assessment

| | |
|---|---|
| Respiratory | *Ventilation*<br>SV $FiO_2$ 0.28 via face mask cold humidification RR16 $SpO_2$ 89%<br>***CXR – taken prior to extubation* (Figure 5.2)**<br>Scoliosis, rotated, hyperinflated, nil focal<br>*ABG*<br>$H^+$ 36.35 nmol/L $pCO_2$ 5.91 kPa $pO_2$ 7.42 kPa $HCO_3^-$ 28.2 mmol/L $BE^+$ 4.7 |
| CVS | Temp 36.5°C HR 85 BP 110/50 Noradrenaline 8 mL/hr |
| CNS | GCS E4 V5 M6<br>Pain score VAS 3/10 at rest 8/10 on movement/coughing<br>Morphine PCA |
| Renal | UO 50 mL/hr +3.2 L cumulative balance to date |
| MSK | Nil of note |
| Microbiology | Nil of note |
| Patient position | Sitting upright in bed, frail |
| Observation | Hyperinflated chest, looks well, chatting freely, dry mouth |
| Auscultation | Breath sounds throughout, coarse expiratory crackles throughout |
| Palpation | Expansion equal, palpable secretions bilateral upper zones |

## Questions

1. Describe the advantages and disadvantages of patient-controlled analgesia (PCA).
2. Considering this patient's CXR (Figure 5.2), what additional hardware/monitoring is visible?
3. List this patient's physiotherapy problem(s).
4. What information from the assessment led you to this problem list?
5. From the assessment information, what suggestions should the physiotherapist make before physiotherapy care commences?

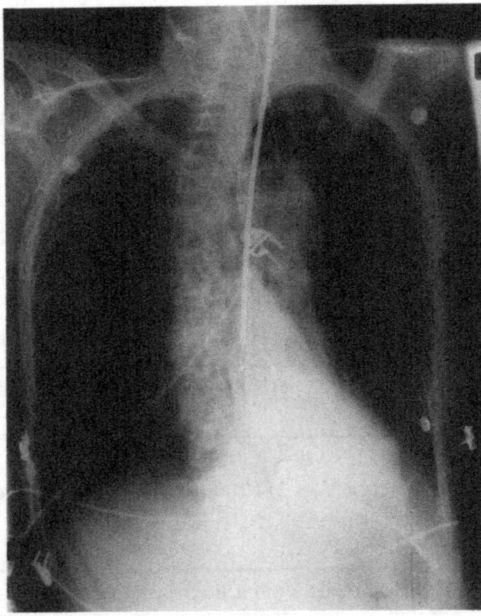

**FIGURE 5.2** X-ray for Case Study 6 taken prior to extubation showing the patient has a scolosis with hyperinflated lungs and nil focal in lung fields.



6. What would be your initial treatment plan?
7. Given this patient's present condition and past history, how might you need to modify the treatments delivered?
8. How would you know if your treatment had been effective (outcome measures)?
9. If the initial treatment plan were to be unsuccessful in clearing secretions, how would you modify your treatment?

## CASE STUDY 7 SURGICAL RESPIRATORY – HEMICOLECTOMY

### Subjective assessment

| | |
|---|---|
| PC | 55-year-old male<br>Day 2 post laparotomy for right hemicolectomy (end to end anastomosis) |
| HPC | Elective admission for bowel resection – investigated 6/12 ago due to altered bowel habit and weight loss. Tumour identified and biopsy taken during colonoscopy |
| PMH | Nil of note |

| | |
|---|---|
| SH | Lives alone, independent with ADL, non-smoker |
| DH | Nil of note |
| Handover | Acute desaturation this morning requiring increased $FiO_2$, not been out of bed as yet due to reduced blood pressure, otherwise stable |

**Objective assessment**

| | |
|---|---|
| Respiratory | *Ventilation*<br>SV $FiO_2$ 0.6 via face mask cold humidification<br>RR 12 $SpO_2$ 96%<br>*CXR*<br>Left lower lobe collapse<br>*ABG*<br>None available |
| CVS | Temp 37.4°C HR 80 BP 80/45 |
| CNS | GCS E4 V5 M6<br>Pain score VAS 2/10 at rest 3/10 on movement/ coughing<br>Epidural analgesia (Bupivacaine and Morphine mix) |
| Renal | UO 30 mL/hr +1.5 L cumulative balance to date |
| MSK | Nil of note |
| Microbiology | Nil of note |
| Patient position | Slumped in bed |
| Observation | Looks well, talking freely |
| Auscultation | Breath sounds throughout, reduced at left base |
| Palpation | Reduced expansion left base, no secretions palpable |

**Questions**

1. What does the procedure of a right hemicolectomy involve?
2. Why can the presence of an epidural lead to hypotension?
3. List this patient's physiotherapy problem(s).
4. What information from the objective assessment led you to this problem list?
5. What would be your initial treatment plan?
6. After identifying an appropriate treatment plan, what information/ instructions would you handover to the nursing staff caring for the patient?

7. How would you determine if your treatment plan had been effective (outcome measures)?
8. What goals would you hope to have achieved before this patient was discharged home?

## CASE STUDY 8 SURGICAL RESPIRATORY – BOWEL RESECTION

### Subjective assessment

| | |
|---|---|
| PC | 80-year-old male<br>Day 3 post-laparotomy for bowel resection |
| HPC | Presented to A&E with painful distended abdomen. Bowels not opened for 2/7 previous. Distended loops of bowel and sigmoid volvulus on AXR. Attempted decompression by colonoscopy unsuccessful therefore proceeded to theatre for open procedure |
| PMH | Hypertension |
| SH | Lives with wife, independently mobile |
| DH | Atenolol |
| Handover | Patient confused and drowsy since return from theatre. Has a moist, ineffective cough that is not productive |

### Objective assessment

| | |
|---|---|
| Respiratory | ***Ventilation***<br>SV 2L $O_2$ via nasal cannulae RR 17 $SpO_2$ 94%<br>***CXR* (Figure 5.3)**<br>Reduced lung volume bibasally<br>***ABG***<br>$H^+$ 49.8 nmol/L $pCO_2$ 4.87 kPa $pO_2$ 10.16 kPa $HCO_3^-$ 18.0 mmol/L BE –8 |
| CVS | Temp 37°C HR 100 BP 160/70 CVP +9 |
| CNS | GCS E3 V4 M5<br>Pain score – unable to score reliably |
| Renal | UO 35 mL/hr +6 L cumulative fluid balance to date |
| MSK | Nil of note |
| Microbiology | Nil of note |
| Patient position | Slumped in bed |

| | |
|---|---|
| **Observation** | Drowsy, audible added sounds at mouth |
| **Auscultation** | Breath sounds throughout reduced bibasally, expiratory crackles upper zones |
| **Palpation** | Expansion equally reduced bilaterally, no secretions palpable |

## Questions

1. Explain the patient's drug history in relation to the past medical history.
2. Why do post-operative patients tend to have a significant positive fluid balance?
3. Why is metabolic acidosis a common finding when analysing the ABG of a post-operative patient?
4. List this patient's physiotherapy problem(s).
5. What information from the objective assessment led you to this problem list?
6. Systematically analysing this patient's CXR (Figure 5.3), what signs do you find that would confirm bibasal loss of lung volume?
7. What would be your initial treatment plan?
8. What could be suggested as a management strategy if the patient required regular suctioning and why?



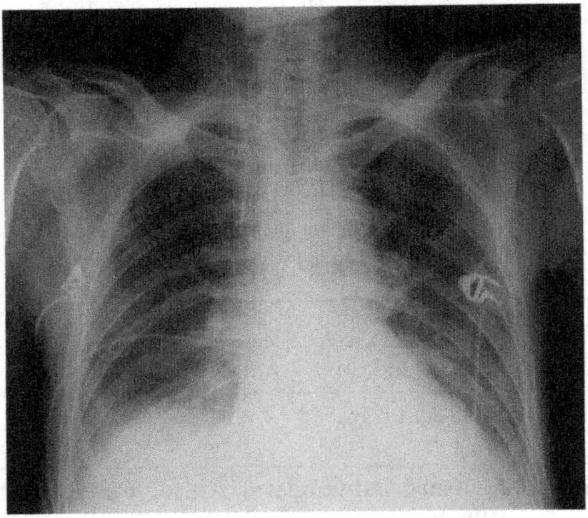

**FIGURE 5.3** X-ray for Case Study 8 showing reduced lung volume bi-basally.

## CASE STUDY 9 INTENSIVE CARE – PATIENT FOR EXTUBATION

### Subjective assessment

| | |
|---|---|
| PC | 55-year-old female<br>Day 7 post-laparotomy for subtotoal colectomy and extensive bowel resection, formation of ileostomy |
| HPC | Emergency admission from A&E in shock with reduced BP, abdominal pain<br>Unwell for 3–4 days, intermittent diarrhoea and vomiting<br>Theatre findings – patchy infarction of small and large bowel |
| PMH | Hypertension |
| SH | Lives with son, 10 cpd smoker |
| DH | Bisoprolol |
| Handover | Stable overnight<br>Possibly for extubation. Just weaned to ASB from SIMV |



### Objective assessment

| | |
|---|---|
| Respiratory | *Ventilation*<br>ASB (PEEP 5 PS 5) ETT size 7.0 $FiO_2$ 0.35 RR 19 Tv 0.46 L $SpO_2$ 97% M1 secretions<br>*CXR*<br>Nil focal<br>*ABG*<br>$H^+$ 39.7 nmol/L $pCO_2$ 5.06 kPa $pO_2$ 14.15 kPa $HCO_3^-$ 23.1 mmol/L BE –1.5 |
| CVS | Temp 38.6°C HR 135 BP 169/88 CVP +11 |
| CNS | GCS E3 VT M4 Propofol 10 mL/hr Alfentanil 2 mL/hr |
| Renal | UO 50 mL/hr overall +500 mL |
| MSK | Nil of note |
| Microbiology | Sputum and urine – no growth |
| Patient position | Head-up tilt in bed |
| Observation | Intubated and ventilated, settled, relaxed breathing pattern |

| | |
|---|---|
| **Auscultation** | Breath sounds throughout, no added sounds |
| **Palpation** | Expansion equal, no secretions palpable |

## Questions

1. Define and explain the difference between SIMV and ASB modes of ventilation.
2. What would you look for in a patient assessment that might indicate to you a patient is ready for extubation?
3. The Glasgow Coma Scale (GCS) is used to assess level of consciousness. What are the components of the scoring system?
4. On assessment this patient GCS is E3 VT M5. What is the patient 'doing' and what are the implications of this for the patient with regard to readiness to extubate?
5. List this patient's physiotherapy problem(s).
6. What information from the objective assessment led you to this problem list?
7. What would be your initial treatment plan?
8. How would you assess as to whether the deep breaths the patient was attempting to take were effective?



## CASE STUDY 10 INTENSIVE CARE – SURGICAL PATIENT

### Subjective assessment

| | |
|---|---|
| PC | 51-year-old female<br>Day 1 post laparotomy – drainage of pelvic abscess and over sew of serosal tears |
| HPC | Admitted previous day with abdominal pain and distension. CT revealed free gas, fluid and faeces in the abdomen and a pelvic collection |
| PMH | Ischaemic colitis<br>Hartmans procedure 1 year ago |
| SH | Lives with husband<br>Independent with all ADL |
| DH | Nil |
| Handover | Problems with cuff leak on repositioning. Aiming to place NG tube then reduce sedation |

### Objective assessment

| | |
|---|---|
| Respiratory | *Ventilation*<br>SIMV ETT size 7.0 $FiO_2$ 0.35 PEEP 5 PS 10 Tv 0.419 L RR 14 $SpO_2$ 92% HMEF brown secretions |

| | |
|---|---|
| | *CXR*<br>Nil focal<br>*ABG*<br>$H^+$ 52.19 nmol/L $pCO_2$ 4.6 kPa $pO_2$ 10.96 kPa $HCO_3^-$ 16.6 mmol/L BE –9.8 |
| CVS | Temp 36.5°C HR 100 BP 140/90 CVP +10 |
| CNS | GCS E3 VT M5 Propofol 7 mL/hr Alfentanil 2 mL/hr |
| Renal | UO 35 mL/hr +2.5 L cumulative balance |
| MSK | Nil of note |
| Microbiology | Nil of note |
| Patient position | Head-up tilt in bed |
| Observation | Intubated, ventilated, settled |
| Auscultation | Breath sounds throughout, coarse expiratory crackles right upper/middle zones |
| Palpation | Expansion equal, palpable secretions right upper zone |



## Questions

1. Analyse the ABG presented.
2. On handover the presence of a cuff leak has been highlighted. What is the significance of this information?
3. List this patient's physiotherapy problem(s).
4. What information from the objective assessment led you to this problem list?
5. Positioning is integral to all respiratory physiotherapeutic input. Which position would you choose for this patient and why?
6. What would be your initial treatment plan?
7. If your initial treatment was unsuccessful in clearing the secretions, how might you modify your treatment?
8. What are the potential hazards associated with endotracheal suctioning?

## CASE STUDY 11 INTENSIVE CARE – MEDICAL PATIENT

### Subjective assessment

| | |
|---|---|
| PC | 72-year-old male<br>Bilateral pneumonia and sepsis, 4 hours post ICU admission |

| | |
|---|---|
| HPC | Presented to Acute Receiving Unit today. Poor oral intake for 1/52 – dehydrated and weak |
| PMH | Mild learning difficulties, irritable bowel syndrome |
| SH | Lives with partner, home help twice a week, otherwise independent |
| DH | Nil of note |
| Handover | Stable since admission; plan to keep sedated for at least 24 hours |

## Objective assessment

| | |
|---|---|
| Respiratory | *Ventilation*<br>Uncut ETT size 8.0 SIMV $FiO_2$ 0.65 PEEP 10<br>$SpO_2$ 96% RR 25/0 mandatory/spontaneous<br>Tv 0.55 L nil-M1 secretions<br>*CXR*<br>Collapse consolidation left lower zone, patchy changes right middle zone<br>*ABG*<br>$H^+$ 53.8 nmol/L $pCO_2$ 6.9 kPa $pO_2$ 10.7 kPa<br>$HCO_3^-$ 24 mmol/L BE –1.2 |
| CVS | Temp 38°C HR 90 BP 95/55 CVP +12<br>Noradrenaline 26 mL/hr |
| CNS | Pupils 2+ 2+ GCS E2 VT M4<br>Sedation – Propofol 10 mL/hr, Alfentanil 2 mL/hr |
| Renal | UO 30+ mL/hr +1 L balance |
| MSK | Nil of note |
| Microbiology | No result as yet, commenced on broad-spectrum antibiotics |
| Patient position | Head-up tilt in bed |
| Observation | Intubated, ventilated, sedated |
| Auscultation | Breath sounds throughout, bronchial breathing left lower zone |
| Palpation | Reduced expansion left base, no secretions palpable |

## Questions

1. The patient is septic. What information from the objective assessment indicates this?
2. Analyse the ABG presented.
3. Describe bronchial breathing.
4. List this patient's physiotherapy problems(s).
5. What information from the objective assessment led you to this problem list?
6. What could be your initial treatment plan for each of these problems?
7. Clinically reason through whether MHI would be appropriate for this patient.
8. What would be your short-term goals for this patient?

## CASE STUDY 12 INTENSIVE CARE – PATIENT MOBILISATION

### Subjective assessment

| | |
|---|---|
| PC | 50-year-old male<br>Community-acquired pneumonia<br>Day 41 in ICU |
| HPC | Admitted via A&E drowsy, sweaty and 'unwell'. Quickly deteriorated with respiratory failure, requiring intubation and ventilation<br>Complicated ICU stay with ARDS and two failed extubations |
| PMH | Alcohol excess (½ bottle vodka a day)<br>Previous IV drug abuser<br>Previous ICU admission with pneumonia |
| SH | Lives alone, first floor flat |
| DH | Nil of note |
| Handover | Been on CPAP overnight via tracheostomy, now on speaking valve<br>Patient is keen to mobilise |



### Objective assessment

| | |
|---|---|
| Respiratory | *Ventilation*<br>Trache size 8.0 (with inner tube, non-fenestrated)<br>Speaking valve in situ. 2 L $O_2$ $SpO_2$ 96% RR 20<br>MP2 secretions on suction<br>*CXR*<br>No recent |

| | |
|---|---|
| | *ABG*<br>$H^+$ 39.42 nmol/L $pCO_2$ 5.34 kPa $pO_2$ 11.5 kPa<br>$HCO_3^-$ 24.1 mmol/L BE −0.2 |
| **CVS** | Temp 36.5°C HR 80 BP 140/80 |
| **CNS** | GCS E4 V5 M6 |
| **Renal** | UO 100 mL/hr overall negative balance |
| **MSK** | Nil of note |
| **Microbiology** | MRSA +ve in sputum |
| **Patient position** | High sitting in bed |
| **Observation** | Looks well, strong clear voice |
| **Auscultation** | Breath sounds throughout, no added sounds |
| **Palpation** | Expansion equal, no secretions palpable |

### Questions

1. This patient developed ARDS due to severe pneumonia. What is ARDS?
2. This patient failed two attempts at extubation and so had a tracheostomy inserted to facilitate weaning. What other indications are there for tracheostomy tube insertion?
3. Tracheostomy tubes vary depending on purpose and manufacturer. What is the benefit of a tracheostomy tube that has an inner cannulae?
4. This patient is receiving CPAP overnight via his tracheostomy. Define and describe this form of respiratory support.
5. Speaking valves allow a patient with a tracheostomy to vocalise and communicate. How do such valves enable this to occur?
6. The patient has expressed that he would like to mobilise out of bed. What preliminary checks would you undertake?
7. What would be your initial treatment plan?
8. What would be your short-term goals for this patient?

## CASE STUDY 13 CARDIOTHORACIC SURGERY – SELF VENTILATING PATIENT

### Subjective assessment

| | |
|---|---|
| PC | 65-year-old male elective admission for coronary artery bypass grafting (CABG). Underwent CABG X 3 via median sternotomy 1/7 ago. Left internal mammary artery graft to left anterior descending coronary artery, |

| | |
|---|---|
| | radial artery graft to right coronary artery, savenous vein graft to circumflex coronary artery. Currently in cardiothoracic intensive care. You are routinely assessing and treating |
| **HPC** | 2-year history of increasing angina. Coronary angiogram identifies three-vessel disease with preserved left ventricular function. Patient reports a decreasing exercise tolerance with angina on climbing two storeys or walking briskly on flat |
| **PMH** | Hypertension<br>Hyperlipidaemia |
| **SH** | Married, lives with wife in a two-storey house<br>Retired civil servant<br>Stopped smoking 2 years ago |
| **DH** | (On admission)<br>Atenolol<br>Simvastatin |
| **Handover** | Nursing staff report patient stable post-operatively is for transfer to cardiothoracic ward later today |

## Objective assessment

| | |
|---|---|
| **Respiratory** | ***Ventilation***<br>SV $FiO_2$ 0.35 via venturi mask $SpO_2$ 95%<br>***CXR***<br>Raised diaphragms bilaterally, sternal wires visible, mediastinal and left pleural drains *in situ*<br>***ABG***<br>$H^+$ 44 nmol/L $pCO_2$ 5.8 kPa $pO_2$ 12 kPa $HCO_3^-$ 23 mmol/L |
| **CVS** | Temp 37.4°C HR 90 BPM sinus rhythm BP 110/76 CVP 5<br>Observations stable |
| **CNS** | Patient alert, cooperative and gives consent for treatment<br>Pain score VAS 3/10 at rest and 5/10 on moving<br>PCA connected (morphine) |
| **Renal** | Good diuresis post-operatively<br>UO 30 mL/hr |

| | |
|---|---|
| **MSK** | Slight swelling of left hand<br>Moving all limbs well |
| **Microbiology** | Nil of note |
| **Patient position** | Slumped in bed with head up 30° |
| **Observation** | Breathing pattern shallow<br>Not using accessory muscles<br>Inter costal drains swinging, drained 100 mL in past 6 hours |
| **Auscultation** | Reduced breath sounds bi-basally with few fine crackles left base |
| **Palpation** | Reduced expansion bi-basally |
| **Cough/ secretions** | Cough effort fair, dry<br>No secretions expectorated |

### Questions

1. What are the common physiotherapy post-operative problems following coronary artery bypass grafting?
2. What conduits are frequently used for coronary artery bypass grafting and what are the implications for physiotherapists?
3. What is an intercostal chest drain and its implications for physiotherapists?
4. What are this patient's clinically reasoned physiotherapy problems?
5. What are the physiotherapy initial treatment goals?
6. What would be the physiotherapy initial treatment plan for this patient?
7. If the patient failed to respond to the initial treatment plan what are other physiotherapy treatment options for this patient?
8. What physiotherapy discharge advice would be important for this patient?

## CASE STUDY 14 CARDIOTHORACIC SURGERY – INTENSIVE CARE PATIENT

### Subjective assessment

| | |
|---|---|
| PC | 70-year-old lady transferred from the cardiology unit for urgent cardiac surgery. Pre-operative unstable angina on maximum treatment. Underwent CABG × 3 via median sternotomy 1/7 ago. Left internal mammary artery graft to left anterior descending coronary artery, radial artery graft to right coronary artery, savenous |

| | |
|---|---|
| | vein graft to circumflex coronary artery. Currently in cardiothoracic intensive care. You are assessing the patient on the first post-operative day |
| HPC | 3-year history of angina<br>Significant myocardial infarction 1 year ago – coronary angiogram identified triple vessel disease with moderately impaired left ventricular function |
| PMH | Hypertension<br>Bilateral cataracts (removed 2 years ago)<br>Left total hip replacement 8 years ago<br>Total abdominal hysterectomy 20 years ago |
| SH | Lives alone in ground floor flat, retired teacher, smoker until 2/12 ago |
| DH | (On admission)<br>Labetalol<br>Furosemide<br>Captopril<br>Paracetamol |
| Handover | The patient required large amounts of support to come off the cardiopulmonary bypass machine. An intra-aortic balloon bump was inserted in theatre. Initially unstable on return to the cardiac intensive care unit but for past 10 hours more stable with no change in cardiac support |

**Objective assessment**

| | |
|---|---|
| Respiratory | *Ventilation*<br>Intubated with endotracheal tube SIMV $FiO_2$ 0.6<br>Preset tidal volume 0.45 L measured at 0.51 L respiration rate set 20 measured at 22 PEEP 5<br>*CXR*<br>Slight increased opacity in left basal zone, sternal wires visible, mediastinal, pericardial and left pleural drains in situ<br>*ABG*<br>$H^+$ 48 nmol/L $pCO_2$ 6.0 kPa $pO_2$ 10 kPa $HCO_3^-$ 24 mmol/L |
| CVS | Temp 37.8°C HR 95 fixed pacing BP 90/50<br>CVP +8<br>Adrenaline 15 mL/hr Nor-adrenaline 20 mL/hr<br>Intra-aortic balloon pump augmenting every heart beat |

CHAPTER FIVE

| | |
|---|---|
| **CNS** | Sedated on Propofol 10 mL/hr<br>Patient settled, responding to pain |
| **Renal** | Moderate diuresis post-operatively with the help of diuretics<br>UO 25 mL/hr |
| **MSK** | Nil of note |
| **Microbiology** | Nil of note |
| **Patient position** | Supine |
| **Observation** | Sedated, intubated and ventilated, synchronizing well with ventilator<br>Intercostal chest drains swinging, drained 150 mL in last 6 hours |
| **Auscultation** | Some bilateral central crackles with reduced breath sounds in basal zones |
| **Palpation** | Reduced expansion bases |
| **Secretions** | Small amount of purulent thick secretions on endotracheal suction |

## Questions

1. What is cardiac output and blood pressure dependent on?
2. How is the cardiovascular system monitored?
3. What is an intra-aortic balloon pump (IABP)?
4. How do adrenaline and nor-adrenaline support the cardiovascular system?
5. How can cardiorespiratory physiotherapy potentially affect patients with compromised cardiovascular systems?
6. What are this patient's clinically reasoned physiotherapy problems?
7. What are the physiotherapy initial treatment goals?
8. What is the physiotherapy initial treatment plan?

# CASE STUDY 15 PAEDIATRIC RESPIRATORY CARE – MEDICAL PATIENT

## Subjective assessment

| | |
|---|---|
| PC | 3/12-old baby admitted overnight with chest infection |
| HPC | 3/7 history of irritability, poor feeding, cough, runny nose (coryzal symptoms), pyrexia |

| | |
|---|---|
| PMH | Previously well, normal vaginal delivery at term (39/40 weeks), no neonatal problems, discharged at 6 hours |
| SH | Third baby, lives at home with family, siblings and parents have upper respiratory tract symptoms |
| DH | Intravenous flucloxacillin, paracetamol via nasogastric tube |
| Handover | Increased work of breathing, several apnoeas overnight, thick mucopurulent secretions on nasopharyngeal suction |

## Objective assessment

| | |
|---|---|
| Respiratory | *Ventilation*<br>SV 4 L $O_2$ via nasal cannulae $SpO_2$ 95% (87% in air) RR 60–80 bpm Occasional apnoeas resolve with stimulation<br>*CXR*<br>Right lower lobe collapse/consolidation<br>*ABG*<br>pH 7.2 $pCO_2$ 7.2 kPa $pO_2$ 9.4 kPa BE +2 |
| CVS | Temp 38.9°C HR 160 BP 90/60 |
| CNS | Lethargic but awake and rousable |
| Renal | Several wet nappies, urine dark |
| MSK | Normal tone |
| Microbiology | *Staphylococcus aureus* |
| Patient position | Lying supine on flat cot |
| Observation | Pale but well perfused, working hard, nasal flaring, tracheal tug, and intercostal indrawing. Fed via nasogastric tube hourly |
| Auscultation | Widespread inspiratory and expiratory crackles |
| Palpation | Secretions palpable |

## Questions

1. Why is birth history important?
2. What could you change in oxygen delivery?
3. What else may be contributing to increased work of breathing and what could you do to reduce this?

4. The infant's parents are very stressed and anxious and wish to stay during treatment sessions. How would you deal with this?
5. What other factors would you take into consideration about the stability of the baby with regards to the objective assessment and the baby's observations?
6. What would your treatment plan be?
7. What would be your handover to nursing staff?
8. How frequently would you see this patient in the day?

## CASE STUDY 16 PAEDIATRIC RESPIRATORY CARE – INTENSIVE CARE PATIENT

### Subjective assessment

| | |
|---|---|
| PC | 8-year-old boy with non-progressive dystrophy admitted with possible aspiration pneumonia today |
| HPC | 5/7 history of being generally unwell, lethargic and off food/ liquids. Vomited and sudden increase of work of breathing at home. Presented to A&E in severe respiratory distress. Transferred to PICU intubated and ventilated |
| PMH | Frequent respiratory infections, parents do daily chest clearance, non-ambulatory, uses electric wheelchair, no independent sitting, decreased tone, swallowing, cough and speech deteriorating, although still taking fluid and diet orally. Levels of intervention discussed with parents, not ready to decide whether for resuscitation or not |
| SH | Lives at home with parents and older brother. Attends mainstream school, seen by physiotherapist, occupational therapist and liaison nurse. Input from community child health consultant |
| DH | Morphine<br>Midazolam<br>Broad-spectrum antibiotics<br>IV fluids<br>Hyoscine patches |
| Handover | Cardiovascularly stable post intubation. Well sedated. CXR changes and thick MP secretions |

## Objective assessment

| | |
|---|---|
| Respiratory | *Ventilation*<br>SIMV Pressure control/pressure support 25/6 bpm 25<br>RR 25 $FiO_2$ 0.60<br>*CXR*<br>White out right lung field, mediastinal shift to right, hyperinflated left lung<br>*ABG*<br>pH 7.4 $pCO_2$ 7.2 kPa $pO_2$ 10 kPa BE −3 |
| CVS | Temp 37.5°C core; 34°C peripherally HR 110<br>BP 95/50 CVP 6 |
| CNS | Sedated but not paralysed |
| Renal | Just catheterised, passing small volumes dark urine |
| MSK | Low tone, sedated, scoliosis |
| Microbiology | Sent but no results |
| Patient position | Patient in supine |
| Observation | Intubated, ventilated, sedated. Radial and femoral arterial lines. Peripheral cannulae left wrist |
| Auscultation | Bronchial breathing right side, scattered crackles on left |
| Palpation | Decreased movement right side of chest visible from bedside |

## Questions

1. The patient may be dehydrated as CVP is low and urine is small in volume and dark. This may be making secretions thicker and more difficult to move. Why could this be and what would help?
2. The patient has probably vomited and aspirated. He also has weak muscles and low tone. What risks does this present?
3. What do we mean by SIMV pressure control support/pressure control ventilation?
4. This patient has a non-progressive dystrophy. Why might he be getting more frequent chest infections?
5. What might your treatment be?
6. What are the risks after extubation and how might they be addressed?
7. What are the other considerations in total long-term care?

# ANSWERS TO CHAPTER 5: CASE STUDIES IN RESPIRATORY PHYSIOTHERAPY

## Case Study 1

1.
- Establish the source and the reliability of patient's knowledge, i.e. written information, respiratory consultant or the Internet.
- Establish the patient's actual knowledge and understanding regarding bronchiectasis and its effects.
- Read her medical notes for conformation and evidence of other diagnostic factors.

2.
- Offer patient information leaflets and discuss the following topics with the patient: definition, diagnosis, causes, disease development.
- Offer website links or other sources of information that the patient could utilise.
- Explain the role of physiotherapy and the importance of airway clearance techniques in the management of bronchiectasis.
- Further information on this disease can be found at the British Lung Foundation website www.lunguk.org

3.
- Active cycle of breathing technique (ACBT)
- Autogenic drainage (AD)
- Postural drainage (PD)
- Manual techniques – percussion, vibrations, shakings.
- Flutter/Acapella/Cornet – positive expiratory pressure (PEP) oscillatory device
- PEP device.

4.
- ACBT–easy to perform, no equipment, performed in sitting or side lying, independent and quick to learn.
- AD–easy to perform once technique learnt, although it can take longer to learn correct technique, no equipment, can be performed in lying or sitting and done independently.
- PD–need bed or plinth to lie on, appropriate pillows or device to tip bed, tipping frame and there is a risk of reflux with this technique. With this intervention you must check if the patient suffers from any gastric oesophageal reflux as this would be a possible contraindication.
- Manual techniques–percussion can be done independently but can become tiring for the patient, assistance required for vibrations and shaking. Performing percussion can be noisy.
- Cornet/Flutter/Acapella–easy to use but maintenance and cleaning/drying of equipment is required. When using the flutter you must be upright for the device to work.
- PEP–easy to use but maintenance and cleaning/drying of equipment required. Can only be done in a seated position.

5. 
- Further emphasise to the patient the benefits of performing regular airway clearance techniques.
- Explain that by performing effective and efficient self-treatment there will be a reduction in the pooling of peripheral secretions.
- Less potential risk of infection and therefore a reduction in the number of exacerbations.
- With fewer exacerbations there will be less demand for antibiotics and hospital contact of an in-patient and out-patient nature.
- Improved management of secretions will reduce the frequency of her cough.
- Airway clearance techniques can be done flexibly when required. For this patient's lifestyle she could perform chest clearance techniques prior to delivering a presentation. This would ensure that her chest is clear and therefore reduce the anxiety and stress levels she experiences about needing to clear her secretions during the delivery of her presentation.
- Regular exercise is encouraged for cardiovascular benefits, but specific airway clearance techniques might be required to access and clear peripheral secretions.

6. 
- Ideally for this patient you would want her to perform airway clearance techniques twice a day for a minimum of 20 minutes per session or until her secretions have been cleared.
- However, to improve compliance as mentioned above you may say that she only needs to do one session on the days that she attends the gym.
- It should also be highlighted again that as well as her formal sessions for airway clearance, she can utilise the techniques at any time she feels secretions are present.

7. 
- Increased temperature
- Chest discomfort
- Flu-like symptoms
- Change in sputum colour
- Change in sputum volume expectorated/swallowed
- Change in tenacity of sputum
- Increased levels of fatigue
- Increased shortness of breath
- Decreased exercise tolerance.

8. 
- Increase the duration and frequency of performing her airway clearance techniques.
- Ensure adequate hydration.
- Acquire a sputum sample in a universal container and hand it into her GP for microbiology testing.

- Attend GP as soon as she becomes aware that she has an infection, to ensure she receives prompt treatment with a prescription for antibiotics if required.

9. • This lady has had two children and therefore has the potential for already weakened pelvic floor muscles secondary to childbirth.
   - The patient has a newly diagnosed chest condition and is performing airway clearance techniques including a forced expiratory technique and cough to clear secretions on a daily basis. This in turn can result in increased pressure on the pelvic floor and further weaken the muscles resulting in urinary stress incontinence.
   - It is important to establish if this is a problem to allow appropriate advice to be given and a referral to an obstetric and gynaecological physiotherapist if necessary.

## Case Study 2

1. Cheyne–Stoking refers to an irregular breathing pattern of rate and depth. Generally the patient's breathing cycle consists of a few relatively deep breaths, which progressively become shallower. This can continue until the patient has a period of apnoea. Following this episode their depth of breath gradually starts to increase again.

2. Cheyne–Stoking is usually associated with end-stage heart failure due to the impaired blood supply to the respiratory centre. Therefore, it is a sign that the patient is at the end stage of their disease and often nearing end of life.

3. • Resuscitation status of a patient should always be known prior to treatment so as to ensure in the event of an arrest or acute deterioration that the correct procedure can be followed. If a patient is not suitable for resuscitation, unnecessary calling of the CPR team can be very distressing for patients and their relatives.
   - Is the patient for active treatment? Liaise with the medical staff for the answer to this question. When patients reach end stage in such diseases as lung cancer, the decision is often made to keep the patient comfortable and not to actively treat any infections.
   - If a patient is for active intervention the appropriate degree of escalation should be established.
   - As the patient's pain control is sub-optimal, what additional analgesia can be introduced should be established.

4. • Secretion retention – the patient has audible secretions and is unable to clear them independently. This is compounded by inappropriate positioning, supine in bed.

- Risk of hypoxaemia – due to poor compliance at keeping oxygen mask *in situ*.

5.
- Pain
- Drowsiness
- Agitation
- Metastases.

6. Position:
- Re-position the patient to either semi-supine or side-lying supported by pillows.

Hypoxaemia:
- Change the oxygen mask to nasal cannulae to recruit better compliance with keeping the oxygen therapy in situ.

Secretion retention:
- Liaise with senior physiotherapy colleagues
- Oral hygiene as required
- Initially try yankeur suction to establish if secretions were pooling in the patient's mouth
- If yankeur suction was unsuccessful you may then progress to attempting oral suction, with the appropriate equipment and sterile technique
- If the patient was gagging on this approach or you were confident to try this first you would perform nasopharyngeal (NP) suction, again with all the appropriate equipment and sterile technique
- Only perform as many suctions as required to clear the secretions, or as many as the patient will tolerate
- If secretions have been cleared successfully and the patient is not for any active treatment then you may wish to discuss with your senior colleague the use of hyoscine and then take this forward as an option to medical staff
- If hyoscine was to be unsuccessful in drying up the secretions, consider the possibility of using an NP airway to allow easy access for the nursing staff to suction the patient on an as-required basis

7.
- Decreased audible secretions
- Decreased added sounds on auscultation
- Decreased agitation as patient is no longer distressed by the secretions
- Oxygen therapy has remained *in situ*
- Maintenance of appropriate position.

8.
- Manual techniques – as the patient has known spinal and bony metastases, by performing manual techniques you could cause the patient further pain and distress or even a fracture.

- Intermittent positive pressure breathing (IPPB) – due to the location of the tumour, you would not want to give positive pressure as this could lead to air trapping. Also, if the patient is having difficulty tolerating an oxygen mask they are unlikely to tolerate an IPPB mask.
- Non-invasive ventilation (NIV) – this is a form of escalation of treatment and commonly not appropriate in this situation.
- Postural drainage would not be utilised as the patient is unlikely to tolerate such a position due to retention of secretions and it may also worsen their breathing pattern and increased work of breathing.
- Intubation – this patient is end stage and is now a palliative patient and as such should be made comfortable. The patient is not suitable for intervention like intubation.
- NP airway would generally be inappropriate as you have requested an agent to dry up the secretions and if this works effectively there should be no requirement to perform the invasive technique of suction.

9.
- The palliative care team play a vital role in the cancer patient journey. They are instrumental in the palliation of symptoms and ensuring that the patient is in as comfortable a state as can be achieved.
- This is achieved by the use of a syringe pump, which will include medications to assist in reducing patient agitation, pain and breathlessness. This is done by ensuring the correct combination of medications, are included in the syringe pump.
- They also play a vital role in liaising with family and ensuring that they have their needs met.
- Support to the MDT.



## Case Study 3

1.
- Increased WOB
- Secretion retention
- Associated problems – osteoporosis and nausea.

2.
- Increased WOB – respiratory rate of 34, inability to speak, high oxygen requirement but low oxygen saturation levels, ABGs (acidotic with low $pO_2$), auscultation findings indicating airway obstruction.
- Retention of secretions – audible, palpable secretions, auscultation findings indicating possible presence of secretions and airway obstruction, ABGs (high $pCO_2$), handover report indicating patient's difficulty in expectorating.
- Associated problems – osteoporosis listed in PMH and nausea mentioned in handover.

3. The patient is in type II respiratory failure: acute respiratory acidosis with high $pCO_2$, low $pO_2$ with partial metabolic compensation showing a high bicarbonate and base excess.

4. 
   - 7th rather than 6th rib crosses the right mid hemi-diaphragm
   - Angle of posterior ribs are more horizontal
   - Long thin heart
   - Increased rib spacing.

5. 
   - As the patient is breathless, positions such as alternate high side lying or upright long sitting with head, arms and knees supported may be more acceptable.
   - Modifying the ACBT by emphasising and increasing the breathing control phase. Only one slightly deeper breath at a time, if the patient is able, may also be indicated. Breath hold at the end of inspiration would be inappropriate with this level of breathlessness. Effective forced expiration technique (FET) may be enhanced by use of a peak flow tube facilitating an open glottis. The patient could also be shown how to suppress her excess coughing to conserve energy.
   - Shorter, more frequent treatment sessions may be less exhausting for the patient and appropriate timing of inhaled therapies must be considered.
   - The addition of manual techniques or head-down postural drainage positions may not be appropriate in a patient in respiratory distress and a history of osteoporosis.
   - Considering the introduction of autogenic drainage, with or without the addition of manual holds, may be beneficial but would depend on patient's ability to respond to a new technique at this stage.

6. 
   - Humidify oxygen
   - Time input appropriately with feeds and medications including anti-emetics
   - Liaise with emergency duty physiotherapist to highlight the patient's problems and arrange a visit with the patient to observe current management if necessary.

7. 
   - The patient is in type II respiratory failure and is not responding favourably to your initial input therefore possibly requires assistance with ventilation and expectoration in the form of IPPB or NIV.
   - This would require discussion with the CF team as the introduction of NIV in this patient group is sometimes not in the best interest of the patient. If the patient is nearing end of life with no prospect of a transplant then prolonging of life via assisted ventilation may not be appropriate. However, in this case, the patient is being considered for lung transplantation and may

benefit in this acute phase and as an ongoing bridge to surgery if necessary.

- If NIV had been deemed inappropriate, then IPPB may have facilitated secretion removal in the short term, but may not have addressed patient fatigue as effectively due to its intermittent application.
- Naso or oro-pharyngeal suction is rarely indicated in this patient group. The chronic problem of daily sputum overproduction would not be resolved through a potentially distressing technique, such as suctioning, in the short term.

8. 
   - Hopefully once the patient's WOB has reduced, due to the introduction of NIV, they may be able to tolerate lying in flatter positions.
   - The patient may also be able to take deeper breaths at a slower rate during ACBT on the machine and possibly achieve a comfortable end inspiratory breath hold.
   - The patient's expired tidal volume and RR may now be continuously determined from the NIV display panel and used as outcome measures.
   - It may be indicated, following discussion with medical staff, to agree an increase in IPAP during airway clearance.
   - It may be preferable to manually hold the soft seal mask to the patient's face, rather than repeatedly removing the straps during therapy, to facilitate ease of expectoration.

9. 
   - The patient is in acute respiratory acidosis requiring assisted ventilation
   - The patient has a high temperature
   - The patient is requiring high flow oxygen
   - The patient is exhausted.



## Case Study 4

1. 
   - The patient is receiving variable oxygen therapy via a simple facemask at 6 L/minute which will be raising his $pO_2$.
   - If the patient normally has a raised $pCO_2$ and is dependent on a hypoxic drive to breathe, then his $pO_2$ of 12 may be too high.
   - If his $pCO_2$ continues to rise, this may further increase the drowsiness and lower his RR.

2. 
   - Fixed oxygen therapy is delivered through fixed performance devices, such as a venturi system mask, that delivers a known fraction of inspired oxygen. A sufficiently high flow of premixed gas, aiming to be in excess of the patient's peak inspiratory flow rate, will ensure a set percentage of oxygen that does not vary according to the patient's respiratory rate or tidal volume.

- Variable oxygen therapy may be delivered via variable performance devices such as a simple mask or nasal cannulae (1–4 L/minute) or non-venturi system masks (1–15 L/minute) but the percentage of oxygen inspired will vary dependent on the patient's breathing pattern. A higher flow rate can be delivered via nasal cannulae but it is generally accepted that a flow greater than 4 L/minute would compromise patient comfort.

3. This patient would benefit from fixed oxygen therapy via a venturi system mask with an oxygen percentage as prescribed by the medical staff. By simply delivering the appropriate amount of oxygen via a fixed oxygen system, the patient's respiratory drive may be increased, thus reducing the $CO_2$ retention, acidosis and subsequent drowsiness. Venturi system masks delivering 24% or 28% oxygen are commonly appropriate for patients in acute type II respiratory failure within the acute clinical setting.

4. Increased work of breathing (WOB).

5. 
   - Breathing pattern – mouth breathing/active expiration/increased use of accessory muscles
   - Auscultation findings – indicate airway obstruction/bronchospasm.

6. 
   - Slumped lying position
   - Large abdomen pushing up against his diaphragm
   - Inefficient lung mechanics secondary to his emphysematous bullae and hyperinflated lungs.

7. 
   - Changing the patient's position from slumped lying to one of the following options:
     High side lying or side lying, with abdomen well forward to facilitate diaphragmatic excursion. Appropriate support/position for head, uppermost arm and leg.
     Half lying with head and forearms supported by pillows and knees in supported flexed position – patient may not tolerate being too upright due to size of abdomen.
     Forward lean sitting in bed or chair would probably not be appropriate at this stage as the patient is drowsy.
   - Encourage breathing control with relaxation of shoulder girdle/upper limbs if patient able to participate/follow requests.
   - Consider appropriate timing of bronchodilator therapy in relation to physiotherapy input.
   - Discuss potential benefits of fixed oxygen therapy delivery system with medical staff due to reasons highlighted in question 2.
   - Discuss with medical staff whether non-invasive ventilation is being considered.

8. No – this patient has in-drawing of his lower chest wall on inspiration because he has flattened diaphragms secondary to hyperinflation. The altered mechanics of his diaphragm will be the cause of this paradoxical movement and the patient will be unable to alter this aspect of his breathing pattern.

9.
   - Patient able to manage his breathlessness independently on room air at rest, walking on the flat over 50 m and on three flights of stairs.
   - Patient aware of importance of pacing and energy conservation.
   - Patient aware of importance of correct inhaler technique and administration as prescribed.
   - Patient aware of effects of smoking and the support available if willing to stop.
   - Patient aware of local pulmonary rehabilitation programme/ support groups/patient information sources.

## Case Study 5

1.
   - Normal oxygen saturation levels are above 95%. Given that the patient is saturating poorly on oxygen therapy the patient is probably not as well oxygenated as he could be.
   - As the patient is talking, suggestion of oxygen delivery via facemask may improve delivery. When oxygen is delivered via nasal cannulae $FiO_2$ will be higher if the mouth is closed (Hough 2001). If the patient is talking/mouth breathing an amount of the oxygen delivered is lost therefore a facemask may be more appropriate.



2.
   - Reduced lung volume (right lung)
   - Reduced mobility post operation
   - Potential for secretion retention.

3.
   - Lung volume – changes on CXR, fine end inspiratory crackles on auscultation and reduced expansion at the right base on palpation. Fact that the patient is post operative is also a contributing factor.
   - Mobility – post operative and not yet been out of bed/mobilised.
   - Secretions – post operative smoker, possible ineffective cough (from handover).

4. There are many contributing factors:
   - Anaesthetic. Under normal circumstances the functional residual capacity (FRC) of the lungs exceeds the lung volume below which small airways in dependent regions close (closing volume, CV). FRC reduces by approximately 20% for the duration of anaesthesia. During anaesthetic, mucociliary clearance mechanisms are depressed or abolished. The inflated cuff of the endotracheal tube further interrupts cilial beating. Subsequently, there is pooling

peripherally of uncleared secretions. Blockages in small airways result and trapped air is absorbed contributing to the development of atelectasis.

- Recumbency. Typically for general surgical procedures patients are positioned supine with the legs separated, flexed and supported in raised stirrups. The cardiopulmonary consequences of such a position include reduced FRC due to cephalad movement of the diaphragm secondary to abdominal content movement (Barnas et al 1993, West 2000 as cited in Blanchard 2006).
- Immobility. Loss of gravitational stimulus to the cardiovascular system while immobile leads to fluid shift from the legs into the thoracic compartment, displacing a proportion of air in the lung reducing lung volume.
- Pain. Typically post-operative pain results in a monotonous shallow breathing pattern and reduced respiratory movement and tidal volumes. The patient does not inspire or expire adequate air volumes, reducing lung expansion and FRC, leading to airway closure and low V/Q. Due to fear of inducing pain, occurrence and effectiveness of coughing is reduced and may allow secretions to accumulate.
- Other factors include dehydration (affecting consistency of secretions and therefore ease of expectoration), abdominal distension (further compressing lower lobes of the lungs), nausea and anxiety (which will both affect compliance with physiotherapy input).



5.
- Mobilisation would be an appropriate treatment option for all the stated problems – it will contribute to increasing lung volume (if done in conjunction with deep breathing exercises as demonstrated by Orfanos et al (1999), will aid in redistribution of pulmonary secretions if there are any to clear, optimise V/Q and ultimately will aid in regaining pre-operative level of mobility.
- Reduced lung volume – thoracic expansion exercises, incentive spirometry.
- Reduced mobility – graded exercise.
- Potential secretion retention – ACBT, supported cough, ensure adequate hydration, humidification of inspired gases and adequate pain relief.

6.
- Mobilise into chair
- Instruct through thoracic expansion exercises with inspiratory holds
- Instruct through supported coughing, ensure adequate pain relief.

7. - Aim for mobilising increasing distances with decreasing assistance, until pre-operative mobility achieved.
   - Monitor for signs of secretion retention/clearance issues.

8. - Cardiovascular stability – it will be easier to mobilise with as few attachments as possible but they should only be removed if safe to do so. Liaise directly with the bedside nurse to establish patient stability and agree what can and shouldn't be removed.
   - Attachments – make sure everything that can't be removed is accounted for and comes with you when you leave the bed space!
   - Oxygen requirements – mobilisation is only beneficial to cardiopulmonary function if the oxygen supply meets the increased demand with exercise. Monitor sats and consider the need for mobilising with portable oxygen.
   - Equipment – the level of assistance required to achieve mobilisation will need to be assessed. Be prepared to use hoists, frames and sticks/drip stands to support your patient while mobile. Check that equipment that is unplugged but needs to stay with the patient has battery back up.
   - Other resources – with all this to consider it can take time to mobilise such a patient so be prepared. You will also more than likely need assistance from another team member (physio or nursing staff) to achieve your goal.



## Case Study 6

1. Advantages:
   - Patient administers analgesia as they perceive they need it, rather than having to request and wait for nursing staff to administer.
   - 'Lock out' function on the syringe driver ensures that there is a minimum period between bolus deliveries. Each time the patient presses the button a bolus of medication is given, unless it is within the 'lock out' period.
   - Drowsiness due to overuse of, or sensitivity to PCA should be limited as patient will become sleepy and therefore not press the handset.

   Disadvantages:
   - If patients do not understand the principle of self-administration, pain relief may be inadequate.
   - The handsets can be difficult to use, limiting its suitability for patients with hand/upper limb weakness, e.g. arthritis (easy trigger handsets are available).
   - Respiratory depression can occur with opiate-based analgesia, particularly if administration is assisted, e.g. by relatives.
   - Hallucinations can occur with opiate-based analgesia which may lead to the patient restricting their use of the PCA leading to

ineffective pain relief (alternative PCA based analgesia should be considered, e.g. Tramadol).
- Patients can also experience nausea and vomiting with opiate-based analgesia. Anti-emetic medication can be administered.

2.
- Endotracheal tube and spring of cuff inflation valve/pilot balloon
- ECG leads
- Central line (right internal jugular approach)
- Oesophageal Doppler probe
- Nasogastric tube
- Clips from axillary node clearance.

3.
- Secretion retention
- Reduced mobility post operation
- Associated problem – pain.

4.
- Secretion retention – moist, ineffective cough (from handover), coarse expiratory crackles on auscultation, palpable secretions, dry mouth. Also is post operation, has PMH of COPD and increased VAS for pain which are all contributing factors.
- Reduced mobility – not been out of bed or mobile since operation.
- Pain – significant VAS at rest and on movement despite PCA.

5.
- Pain control – this is likely to be the issue that overarches the actual physiotherapy-specific problems. The level of pain the patient is experiencing is limiting their ability to cough/deep breathe effectively, increasing the risk of atelectasis and secretion retention. Progression of mobilisation will also be hindered increasing risk of DVT or PE. Discussion with the multidisciplinary/pain team to address establishing effective pain relief should be instigated.
- Hypoxaemia – as the patient has normal $pCO_2$, could potentially increase $FiO_2$. Bearing in mind the patient has COPD, if oxygen therapy is increased, must monitor for signs of $CO_2$ retention, e.g. drowsy, flapping tremor.
- Humidification – the patient is currently receiving cold humidified oxygen therapy. The capacity of a gas to carry humidity is affected by its temperature. The warmer the gas the more moisture it can carry. Changing this patient from a cold humidification system to a heated system may help secretion clearance, as more humidity will be carried into the airways by the warmed gas.
- Hydration – the patient has a dry mouth that will hinder expectoration of secretions. Fluid intake may be restricted due to surgery but would be balanced by IV fluids. Good mouth care (wet mouth sponges, sips of water for comfort) and possibly saline nebulisers will be appropriate to keep the mouth moist.

6. • Ensure adequate pain relief.
   • Ensure adequately hydrated.
   • Assist out of bed to sit in chair.
   • Instruct through ACBT.

7. • Pain – ensure timing of intervention such that pain relief has been administered, and given time to be effective pre-treatment. Patient has a PCA so should be encouraged to utilise this as required.
   • Hydration – fluid intake should be encouraged but be aware that fluid restrictions may be in place as part of the post-operative regime.
   • Mobilisation – care with attachments (drips, drains, catheters, monitoring), ensure appropriate patient monitoring is in place so significant changes can be quickly identified, e.g. postural hypotension. Must also take into account the fact that the patient is receiving noradrenaline to support blood pressure which may also limit the extent of mobilisation that can be undertaken.
   • ACBT – FET component will need to be taught in conjunction with support over the abdominal wound.

8. • Expectoration of secretions
   • Reduced/eliminated added sounds on auscultation
   • Reduced/eliminated palpable secretions
   • Improvement in $SpO_2$.

9. • Progress mobility – actual mobilisation, rather than just into the chair, may be beneficial in aiding secretion clearance due to the redistribution of bronchial secretions, improvements in tidal volume and often spontaneous coughing that occur (assuming cardiovascular stability).
   • Incorporate manual techniques – expiratory vibrations during the thoracic expansion component of ACBT may be useful to aid expiratory flow and secretion clearance assuming pain relief is adequate. But, must consider that patient is at risk of osteoporosis given steroid use for COPD and also metastatic rib and lung disease given previous axillary node clearance.
   • Introduce IPPB – intermittent positive pressure breathing delivers a positive pressure on inspiration, augmenting tidal volume. It may therefore be indicated for the patient who is unable to do thoracic expansion component of ACBT effectively. Positive pressure may, however, compromise blood pressure due to potential reduction in venous return so cardiovascular monitoring must be continued at all times.
   • Suction – if the patient's cough/FET is ineffective and secretion retention is compromising gas exchange, airway suctioning may

CHAPTER FIVE

be indicated. Either nasopharyngeal or oropharyngeal routes can be used, with or without insertion of an airway.

## Case Study 7

1. The large intestine consists of the cecum proximally, ascending, transverse and descending colon then sigmoid colon. A right hemicolectomy refers to the resection of a portion of the large intestine. It can involve removal of the cecum, ascending colon and the right side of the transverse colon (with a few centimetres of the terminal ileum/small intestine). Continuity of the tract is restored by end to end anastomosis of the cut ends at the ileum and transverse colon. Alternatively a colostomy is formed.

2. Epidural analgesia provides a sensory block to provide the patient with a 'band' of pain relief at the operation site. The local anaesthetic introduced via the epidural route can also block sympathetic vasoconstrictor fibres in the cardiovascular system. This will reduce peripheral resistance leading to venous pooling and a fall in blood pressure, particularly when the legs are positioned over the bed edge, e.g. when attempting to mobilise (postural hypotension).

3. 
   - Reduced lung volume (left lung)
   - Reduced mobility post operation.

4. 
   - Reduced lung volume (left lung) – day 2 post laparotomy, signs on CXR, reduced breath sounds on auscultation and reduced expansion on palpation.
   - Reduced mobility post operation – not been out of bed or mobilised since operation.

5. 
   - Mobilisation – this would address both of the identified physiotherapy problems. However, given that this patient is hypotensive it is not an appropriate inclusion for the initial treatment plan. This should be reconsidered on a daily basis at least.
   - Enhanced recovery programmes for surgical patients focus on an integrated multimodal approach to peri and post-operative care. Early mobilisation is part of this care programme, as is epidural analgesia. If hypotension associated with the epidural is limiting early mobilisation, oral ephedrine can be administered 30 minutes prior to movement (to augment blood pressure).
   - Reposition high sitting or right side lying – the patient is currently slumped in bed, which is not beneficial for improving lung volume. Moving the patient into high sitting would relieve pressure on the diaphragm from the abdominal contents and improve the distribution of ventilation through the lungs. Right side lying would improve V/Q matching in the lower most lung

and encourage re-expansion of the uppermost lung due to the weight of tissue being pulled down under the effect of gravity. Left side lying could be considered. This would place the affected lung lowermost, into a position where the compressed, lower lung has better potential to ventilate and so aid in increasing lung volume. However, in this position, the affected lung area is also in the area of better perfusion. As a result V/Q match may actually be compromised further in this position, compounding the established problems with oxygenation. If attempted, and desaturation occurs, prompt repositioning of the patient would be necessary.

- Instruct through thoracic expansion exercises – inclusion of an inspiratory hold to encourage collateral ventilation, would be appropriate given the extent of compromise in gas exchange.
- Introduce incentive spirometry – the visual feedback given from the device can encourage a more effective, slow and controlled deep breath. For this patient, as their oxygen therapy will have to be removed to enable use, supplementary oxygen may need to be given via nasal cannulae to maintain oxygen saturations.

6.
- Feedback on treatment session – what the intervention involved and how well the patient tolerated it.
- To regularly reposition, preferably into either high sitting or right side lying.
- To encourage hourly deep breathing or use of incentive spirometer (if introduced) – once inflated, alveoli stay open for about 1 hour therefore breathing exercises should be repeated hourly to maintain volume (Hough 2001).
- If using the incentive spirometer ensure the nurse involved in patient care is familiar with the technique so they can supervise the patient's use if necessary.
- Depending on the ward setting that the patient is in, ask if the nurse can document on the patient's chart when deep breathing/incentive spirometer is carried out.

7.
- Improved breath sounds on auscultation
- Improvement in expansion on palpation
- Improvement in $SpO_2$
- Reduced $FiO_2$ requirements.

8.
- Equal breath sounds throughout on auscultation
- Equal expansion on palpation
- Maintenance of normal oxygen saturations (>95%) in room air
- Independently mobile in ward area
- Safe and independent on climbing an appropriate number of stairs.

## Case Study 8

1. Atenolol is a cardioselective beta-adrenoreceptor blocking drug indicated for management of hypertension. The mode of action of such drugs in hypertension is not understood but they reduce cardiac output, alter baroreceptor reflex sensitivity and block adrenoreceptors (*British National Formulary* 2006).

2. 
   - The amount of fluid a surgical patient is given is related to an estimation of pre- and post-operative fluid losses. The baseline requirements for young adults is 30mL/kg/day of water which is probably an overestimation for the obese, elderly and women. Fluid management of surgical patients needs to take into account this basal requirement, any pre-existing deficits (e.g. from fasting, bowel preparation or diarrhoea and vomiting pre-operatively), replace fluid losses intra-operatively (e.g. blood loss) and then account for losses in the post-operative stages, e.g. from surgical drains, possible restricted oral fluid intake, NG aspirates and also account for insensible losses. With this in mind, the fluid balance of an early post-operative patient can appear significantly positive while these losses are trying to be managed.
   - Accurate assessment of a patient's needs in relation to fluid can be difficult and so must be individualised and reviewed frequently to avoid volume depletion or overload.
     (Scottish Intercollegiate Guidelines Network 2004).
   - The metabolic and hormonal changes associated with the stress response to surgery influence metabolism of salt and water. These changes support preservation of adequate body fluid volumes, which could contribute to overall fluid-management difficulties (Desborough 2000).

3. 
   - Metabolic acidosis in the post-operative patient is usually due to hypovolaemia, poor tissue perfusion, and the subsequent development of lactic acidosis (due to inadequate oxygen delivery to the tissues).
   - Hypovolaemia can occur due to a number of factors such as unrecognized or uncorrected pre-operative hypovoleamia, inadequate intra or post-operative fluid replacement
     (Scottish Intercollegiate Guidelines Network 2004).

4. 
   - Secretion retention
   - Reduced lung volume (bibasally)
   - Reduced mobility post operation.

5. 
   - Secretion retention – ineffective moist cough, audible added sounds at mouth and expiratory crackles on auscultation.

- Reduced lung volume (bibasally) – CXR findings and reduced expansion on palpation.
- Reduced mobility post operation – not been out of bed or mobile since operation.

6. Shift of structures is the key change which occurs:
   - The hemidiaphragms are elevated
   - As a result, the rib level at the diaphragm will be less
   - There is rib crowding i.e. narrowing of rib spaces, at the lower lobes.

7. - Reposition – the patient is currently slumped in bed, which is not of any physiological benefit. As the problems are bilateral in nature, repositioning to a more upright position will improve lung expansion by displacing the abdominal contents and will encourage better V/Q matching. It may also stimulate the patient to be more alert. Time in high side lying may also be considered. Given the patient's confusion (GCS V4) and inability to follow commands (GCS M5), mobilisation is possibly not appropriate at this time.
   - IPPB – as the patient is not obeying commands attempting ACBT (to aid secretion clearance) or thoracic expansion exercises/incentive spirometry (to improve lung volume) is not appropriate. If available, IPPB would be a suitable alternative, as the positive pressure delivered on inspiration would increase lung volume, and also affect secretion clearance by opening collateral channels allowing air behind secretions to mobilise them. IPPB may also potentially trigger a spontaneous cough.
   - Suction – gas exchange has been compromised by the patient's secretion retention and as the patient has an ineffective spontaneous cough and is unable to follow commands, effective clearance of secretions may involve suction. This can be achieved either by nasopharyngeal or oropharyngeal routes.
   - Review oxygen therapy – the patient is currently receiving dry oxygen therapy via nasal cannulae. The ABG demonstrate the patient is hypoxic on the current therapy. As the $pCO_2$ is within normal range, oxygen therapy should be increased. Consideration should also be given to the method of delivery – the patient is drowsy and could be mouth breathing. If this is the case, a facemask may be a more appropriate means of delivery. Humidification of the oxygen should also be considered given the problems with secretion retention.

8. - Short term – insertion of nasopharyngeal or oropharyngeal airway to allow access for suctioning while reducing the trauma of repeated suctioning.

- Long term – minitracheostomy could be indicated. Regular repeated suctioning via nasopharyngeal or oropharyngeal routes can be unpleasant and uncomfortable for the patient but can also cause damage to the upper airway. A minitracheostomy involves the passing of a short narrow catheter surgically into the trachea offering direct access to clear secretions. It does not provide a means to ventilate, protect the airway or directly enable delivery of oxygen therapy to a patient.

## Case Study 9

1. 
   - Synchronized Intermittent Mandatory Ventilation is a mandatory mode – the ventilator delivers a set number of breaths per minute at a set tidal volume. The ventilator will accommodate any spontaneous effort made by the patient, either by bringing the next mandatory breath forward or by augmenting the spontaneous effort with pressure support (confirm locally as ventilator manufacturers vary).
   - Assisted spontaneous breathing (also known as CPAP and Pressure Support or Pressure Support Ventilation) differs in that the patient is breathing spontaneously, setting their own respiratory rate and to a certain extent their tidal volume. The patient's breathing efforts are supported by a positive end expiratory pressure (PEEP) splinting open the airways/alveoli and facilitating oxygenation. Inspiratory effort and so tidal volume is augmented by pressure support.

2. 
   - The indication for intubation has resolved.
   - Patient is alert, cooperative and able to follow simple commands.
   - The patient is able to control own airway – cough reflex present (preferably on command, if not then on suction) and able to swallow.
   - Manageable bronchial secretions.
   - Respiratory function has improved enough that spontaneous ventilation could be sustained indefinitely. There is now a significant body of evidence to support the use of weaning protocols. Such protocols will be locally agreed and guide the MDT to make an objective assessment as to whether extubation will be successful. It should include simple objective measures such as rapid shallow breathing index as indicators of potential extubation success/failure.
   - The presence of an air leak around endotracheal tube cuff should be demonstrated to be confident that the airway is patent and not potentially going to be an issue post extubation. (Hinds & Watson 1996, Hough 2001)

3. Eyes
    1. No eye opening to painful stimuli
    2. Eyes open only to painful stimuli
    3. Eyes open to speech
    4. Spontaneous eye opening
    C. Closed, e.g. due to swelling

    Vocal
    1. No verbal response
    2. Incomprehensible sounds
    3. Inappropriate speech
    4. Converses, but confused
    5. Orientated in time, person and place
    T. Intubated/tube

    Motor
    1. No motor response to painful stimuli
    2. Extension to painful stimuli
    3. Abnormal flexion to painful stimuli
    4. Flexion to painful stimuli
    5. Localizes to painful stimuli
    6. Obeys simple commands

    (Hickey 1992)



4.
    - This patient is opening her eyes when spoken to (E3), is localising to a painful stimulus, e.g. the presence of the endotracheal tube (M5) and due to that tube is unable to vocalize (V T).
    - The patient is rousable by speech but not necessarily awake enough that she is able to follow commands. The concern is that once the painful stimulus she is localising to is removed, her GCS would deteriorate. If so, she will be less able to protect her own airway, increasing the risk of requiring re-intubation. She is also not obeying commands and we would want to be sure she was able to deep breathe and cough to command – essential for airway clearance once extubated.

5.
    - This patient has no physiotherapy-specific, respiratory-related problems.
    - Reduced mobility post operation and potential for soft tissue shortening.
    - Associated problems include reduced GCS, most likely related to sedation.

6.
    - There are no signs of secretion retention – there are no added sounds on auscultation, nil focal on CXR, minimal secretions on suction, no secretions are palpable and there is adequate gas exchange on minimal oxygen therapy.

- There are no signs of loss of volume – there are breath sounds throughout on auscultation, expansion is equal on palpation, nil focal on CXR and there is adequate gas exchange.
- There are no signs of increased work of breathing – the respiratory rate is acceptable and there is no mention of accessory muscle use.
- The patient has been 7 days in bed post operation and as a result is likely to have potential for soft tissue shortening and muscle weakness (compounded by presence of a laparotomy wound).

7. - If extubation is imminent, sit patient as upright as possible in the bed.
   - Assess ability to follow simple commands, e.g. deep breathe.
   - Assess ability to cough against endotracheal tube or, whether a cough is stimulated on endotracheal suction.
   - Should a patient show signs of secretion retention or loss of lung volume on assessment, other techniques such as positioning, manual hyperinflation and suction may be indicated to optimise respiratory function prior to extubation.
   - Assessment of joint range of movement should have been made by this stage and any joint stretches indicated should have been performed. Could assess muscle strength with a view to potentially assisting the patient out of bed at a later stage.

8. - Monitoring ventilator display for demonstration of increase in tidal volume.
   - Palpation of lateral expansion as an indicator of increase in tidal volume.



## Case Study 10

1. Metabolic acidosis with hypoxaemia.

2. - The presence of the cuff on an endotracheal tube (ETT) is to take up the space between the ETT and the tracheal wall. It is inflated with air by way of an external port on the ETT itself. As the patient is receiving positive pressure ventilation, the inflated cuff ensures ventilation of the lungs by preventing the gas taking the path of least resistance, i.e. back up the trachea and leaking out of the mouth. The inflated cuff also minimises aspiration of gastric contents.
   - If the cuff is not sufficiently inflated there will be an audible 'leak' at the patient's mouth. Tidal volumes from the ventilator may be more difficult to achieve and the risk of aspiration is increased.

- For this particular patient, potential aspiration of gastric contents could have occurred given that there is no NG tube in place (to enable aspiration of gastric contents) and ETT secretions on suction are brown.

3. - Secretion retention (right lung)
   - Potential for soft tissue shortening.

4. - Secretion retention – probable aspiration of gastric contents, coarse expiratory crackles right upper/middle zones on auscultation, palpable secretions right upper zone.
   - Soft tissue shortening – patient is sedated, limited independent mobility and has been immobile since surgery.

5. - Left side lying. This position will use gravity to encourage drainage of secretions from the right lung, i.e. postural drainage. Given that this patient has possibly aspirated, a head down variation is not appropriate.
   - As this patient is desaturating the use of repositioning can also be used to influence gas exchange. In a ventilated patient, ventilation and perfusion gradients are altered – the ventilation gradient reversed and the perfusion gradient exaggerated. In a ventilated patient with unilateral lung changes/disease, positioning the patient with the affected lung uppermost (in this case left side lying) will allow the clearer lung to participate more effectively in gas exchange despite the V/Q mismatch due to mechanical ventilation.

6. - Repositioning – left side lying
   - Suction – without saline in first instance
   - Assessment of joint range of movement/passive movements.

7. - Instillation of saline. There is controversy as to whether the introduction of saline into an artificial airway is of benefit or detriment to the patient. Jackson (2006) lists the suggested beneficial effects to include dilution and mobilisation of secretions, ETT lubrication and cough stimulation, and adverse effects include nosocomial pneumonia and decreased oxygen saturations. Conclusive evidence is lacking but, if used when indicated rather than routinely, saline instillation may have its place in aiding secretion clearance. Local policy may be in place with regard to saline instillation and should be followed.
   - Introduce MHI. During MHI technique, the increased tidal volume and inclusion of an inspiratory hold will aid secretion clearance by enhancing collateral ventilation. A quick release of the bag on expiration may also aid secretion clearance by mimicking forced expiration.

- Introduce manual techniques. Expiratory vibrations may enhance expiratory flow and aid clearance of secretions.
- Consider humidification. This patient has an HMEF in situ for humidification of inspired gas from the ventilator. Moisture lost during expiration is trapped in the filter, conditioning gases on the following inspiratory phase. Although there is evidence to suggest that HMEF is just as effective as heated humidification for conditioning inspired gas, there are patients who do benefit from heated water bath systems to aid delivery of adequate humidification. Saline nebulisers may also be an option to decrease secretion viscosity. Systemic hydration may also need addressed.

8.
- Hypoxaemia. By suctioning an intubated patient the ventilation being delivered will be interrupted which may precipitate desaturation/hypoxaemia episode. Patients requiring significant amounts of PEEP and/or oxygen may also be susceptible. The use of closed suction systems enable suctioning to be done without significant disruption to ventilation, which may reduce the incidence of hypoxaemia. It can also be minimised by hyper-oxygenation of the patient prior to suctioning or by incorporating manual hyperinflation. Selecting the correct catheter size should prevent against excessive negative pressures and potential atelectasis (ETT size –2 × 2) (Odell et al 1993).
- Cardiovascular instability. Changes in heart rate and blood pressure as a result of suctioning can be caused by vagal nerve stimulation. This response can also be due to hypoxaemia. Such side effects could be minimised by hyper-oxygenation prior to suctioning. Arrhythmias that cause cardiovascular compromise will require prompt medical attention.
- Mucosal damage. Damage to the mucosa can be minimised by a good technique (pass catheter to end point/resistance/cough stimulated, withdraw catheter 1 cm then apply continuous suction on withdrawal), use of appropriate suction pressures (13–20 kPa (Young 1984 as cited in Donald et al 2000) and by using a catheter of suitable design (rounded tip, multiple side eyes). Damage is, however, more likely due to repetition of suction and negative pressures rather than type of catheter (Jung & Gottlieb 1976 as cited in Fiorentini 1992).
- Patient anxiety. Minimised by explanation to the patient about what is about to happen and why. The patient may require a bolus of sedation in order to tolerate the technique. Another factor, which may need to be considered in this particular case, is pain on coughing and the need for adequate pain relief.

## Case Study 11

1. Sepsis is a systemic response to infection. The patient is pyrexial at 38°C. The way in which the body tries to control this temperature is by vasodilation of blood vessels which subsequently causes a reduction in blood pressure. This patient requires noradrenaline, a vasoconstrictor to augment blood pressure and so maintain perfusion to the vital organs.

2. Respiratory acidosis and hypoxaemia.

3. Normal breath sounds are generated by turbulent airflow in the proximal airways. Airflow becomes less turbulent in the narrower airways creating less noise at the periphery due to large cross sectional area of the peripheral zones. Where the periphery is not air filled, such as in consolidation, the airflow cannot pass into the narrower airways and become less noisy. A sound more turbulent and hollow in tone, is transmitted from the more proximal patent airways, down through the solid lung tissue. This is what is heard at the periphery on auscultation as bronchial breathing.

4. 
   - Reduced lung volume (left)
   - Potential for secretion retention
   - Potential for soft tissue shortening
   - Associated problem – cardiovascular instability.

5. 
   - Reduced lung volume – changes on CXR, bronchial breathing on auscultation and reduced expansion on palpation at the left base.
   - Potential for secretion retention – minimal secretions currently but patient has an uncut ETT. This may mean that a cough reflex is not stimulated on suction, as the suction catheter may not pass down far enough in the airway to do so. The patient is currently in an unproductive phase of pneumonia, but as antibiotic therapy continues, this may change to a more productive phase.
   - Potential for soft tissue shortening – as the patient is sedated and not moving spontaneously, he is at risk of developing soft tissue shortening.

6. 
   - Reduced lung volume – reposition right side lying (to optimise V/Q in the right lung and encourage left lung expansion). Manual hyperinflation (MHI) (to encourage left lung expansion).
   - Potential for secretion retention – suction ± saline, consider humidification and introduction of saline nebulisers.
   - Potential for soft tissue shortening – passive movements to all four limbs.

7. 
   - Due to the increase in intrathoracic pressure during MHI, blood pressure and cardiac output can be compromised (Singer et al

1994). Given the current blood pressure of the patient and the noradrenaline requirements, MHI may not be tolerated well from a cardiovascular perspective. If MHI is indicated, close monitoring throughout treatment is essential as additional inotropic support may be required.

- As a result of the pneumonia, gas exchange and oxygenation is compromised in this patient. Positive expiratory end pressure (PEEP) is incorporated into the ventilation settings in an attempt to splint airways open at end expiration and facilitate gas exchange. As PEEP will be lost on disconnection of the patient from the ventilator, desaturation may occur as alveoli and small airways collapse. This can be minimised by inclusion of a PEEP valve in the bagging circuit. However, PEEP does take time to be restored once reconnected to the ventilator therefore breaks in the circuit should be kept to a minimum.
- MHI may enhance secretion clearance but only if there is presence of an effective cough. For coughing to be effective gas must be able to flow through airways therefore restoration of lung volume may play role in secretion clearance during MHI (Maxwell & Ellis 1998). However, in this patient, actual clearance of secretions will be by suctioning which may be hindered by the uncut ETT.

8. - Normalise breath sounds at left lower zone (2 days)
   - Affect lung volume on CXR (3–4 days)
   - Maintain joint range of movement (ongoing).



## Case Study 12

1. Acute respiratory distress syndrome develops as a consequence of an insult either involving the lungs directly (e.g. aspiration or smoke inhalation) or indirectly (e.g. sepsis or trauma). There are more than 60 recognised conditions associated with the development of this condition but, the mechanisms by which a wide variety of insults can lead to ARDS are not clear (Villar 2002). ARDS is caused by the alveolar-capillary membrane becoming disrupted due to the arrival of inflammatory mediators to the area. In the acute phase (first 1–3 days), pulmonary oedema develops and surfactant action is disrupted compromising gas exchange and reducing lung compliance. In the later stages (7–10 days later), repair processes start to take place and a degree of lung fibrosis develops as the alveolar endothelium begins to regenerate. Clinical diagnosis of ARDS is based on a combination of criteria – presence of a clinical risk factor, compromised oxygenation (despite high $FiO_2$, altered lung compliance), normal pulmonary artery wedge pressure (because the pulmonary oedema is not due to cardiac insufficiency) and

radiographic changes (bilateral pulmonary infiltrates on CXR). Medical management of these patients is predominantly supportive.

2. - To secure and clear an airway in upper respiratory tract obstruction.
   - To facilitate the removal of bronchial secretions.
   - To protect/minimise aspiration in the absence of laryngeal reflexes.
   - To obtain an airway in patients with injuries, or following surgery to, the head and neck (St George's Healthcare NHS Trust 2006).

3. - Secretions can adhere to the internal lumen of a tracheostomy tube and severely reduce the inner lumen diameter, increasing the work of breathing and possibly obstructing the patient's airway.
   - An inner cannulae is a removable tube which fits inside the tracheostomy tube. It can be removed, cleaned and replaced to ensure the patency of the tracheostomy tube.
   - As the inner tube will reduce the overall inner diameter of the tracheostomy the resistance to airflow through the tracheostomy can be increased, particularly with smaller diameter tubes (less than 7.0 mm) (St George's Healthcare NHS Trust 2006).

4. - Continuous positive airway pressure (CPAP) provides a continuous positive pressure throughout both inspiration and expiration for spontaneously breathing patients. The patient breathes at his or her own respiratory rate and tidal volume but at an elevated pressure above atmospheric, increasing functional residual capacity. This positive pressure splints open the airways and alveoli, facilitating gas exchange and oxygenation. It is therefore an appropriate treatment for hypoxic patients, i.e. type I respiratory failure. As CPAP is a continuous pressure, it does not increase tidal volume or aid $CO_2$ clearance so is not appropriate for patients in type II respiratory failure.
   - CPAP can be delivered externally by facemask or hood, or invasively such as via tracheostomy or endotracheal tube.

5. With the tracheostomy tube in place and the cuff inflated, all air/gas will pass directly in and out of the tube to the lungs, by-passing the upper respiratory tract. As no air/gas moves through the upper airway no vocalisation can be achieved. However, with the cuff deflated, air/gas can pass up through the larynx on expiration and a voice can be generated. A speaking valve is essentially a one-way valve positioned on the end of the tracheostomy tube. On inspiration it will allow air/gas to move into the airway but on expiration, it is closed redirecting flow up through the larynx giving the patient the opportunity to generate sound.

6. • Background – previous mobility and exercise tolerance.
   • Cardiovascular system:

   *Heart rate and rhythm* – if it is already within training range (50–60% of maximal heart rate, i.e. 220 minus age) there may not be sufficient reserve to tolerate the increase caused during mobilisation. May be possible to maintain ECG monitoring if mobilising short distances, e.g. into chair.

   *Blood pressure* – patient will most likely have an arterial line in situ so beat-to-beat measurements will be available. Recent changes should be considered and mobilisation delayed if significant.

   *Temperature* – an increase in temperature is associated with increased oxygen consumption therefore mobilisation may need to be postponed.

   • Oxygenation – both $FiO_2$ and $PaO_2$ should be considered. A $PaO_2/FiO_2$ ratio >300 (indicator of acute lung injury) may be an objective measure to assess adequacy of oxygenation. $SpO_2$ monitoring should continue throughout mobilisation if possible, aiming for >90%. Portable oxygen may be required.
   • Patient observation – colour, breathing pattern, pain, conscious level, emotional state and patient appearance are all subjective factors which should be considered.
   • Attachments – the patient may have numerous attachments which need to be considered as far as potential for disconnection or as to management while mobile, e.g. tracheostomy tube, arterial/central lines, urinary catheter).
   • Assistance – appropriately experienced staff (physiotherapy/nursing) will need to be available to assist with mobilising the patient
   (Stiller & Phillips 2003).

7. Assuming sufficient staff available to assist and no other contraindications:
   • Bed edge sit to assess sitting balance.
   • If appropriate attempt sit to stand.
   • If safe to do so, attempt stepping on spot initially.
   • May need to consider use of a walking aid or hoist.
   • Could also introduce individualised exercise programme for the patient to carry out independently.

8. • Maintain clear chest on auscultation (ongoing).
   • Sitting out of bed daily for minimum 1 hour (immediately).
   • Effective independent secretion clearance (2 days).
   • Independent sitting balance for 10–15 minutes (3 days).
   • Sit to stand with minimal assist of 2 (3–4 days).

CHAPTER FIVE

## Case Study 13

1. - The major physiotherapy problem is that of reduced lung volume. Every patient will have some reduced lung volume but the degree will vary. The effect of a prolonged anaesthetic and a median sternotomy give a reduced functional residual capacity and tidal volumes that are close to closing volumes. If the patient was a smoker until recently they will frequently retain secretions. The mucociliary escalator is stopped during anaesthesia and combined with pain on coughing post-operatively patients have difficulty clearing secretions.
   - All patients will have a reduced exercise tolerance due to the effects of major surgery but this can be worsened by a reduced exercise tolerance pre-operatively.

2. For many years the main conduit used was the saphenous vein from the leg via a median incision. Depending on how far up the leg this extends some patients experience stiffness and pain on mobilisation and many have some swelling of the ankle and on occasion leg. Mammary artery grafts are now commonplace and provide longer patencey rates. There is an increased rate of pleural effusion and pain reported on the side used. Radial artery harvesting is also now commonplace with patient often not reporting many complications. It is wise to keep the arm slightly elevated during the first few days post-operatively and patients should be encouraged to actively move the arm.

3. The intercostal chest drain (ICD) is placed into the pleural space to either remove fluid or air. They are routinely inserted in theatre during coronary artery bypass grafting and are usually removed during the first few post-operative days. They can also be inserted if a patient develops pneumothorax or pleural effusions in the ward/ICU setting. The tube from the patient is connected to an underwater seal drain and the tubing should not be raised above the height of the chest. The drain may be connected to low-grade suction to aid removal of air/fluid. Patients report some increase in pain with an ICD so adequate analgesia is vital. Patients can mobilise with the drain providing it is kept below the height of the chest.

4. The patient has reduced lung volume and reduced exercise tolerance. Reduced lung volume is identified due to the fact they have undergone coronary artery bypass grafting, are in a poor position, have mildly reduced oxygenation, raised hemi-diaphragms on X-ray and reduced breath sounds on auscultation plus reduced expansion on palpation. They have a reduced exercise tolerance due to the

effects of major surgery coupled with a reduced exercise tolerance pre-operatively.

5. • Normal breath sounds in all areas in 3/7
   • Oxygen saturations 95% or above on room air in 3/7
   • Independent mobilisation 25 m in 2/7.

6. • Positioning to high sitting
   • Mobilisation to chair during first post-operative day
   • Advised on supported coughing
   • Progressive mobilisation regime from second post-operative day.

   The current literature indicates that the routine use of breathing exercises post coronary artery bypass surgery is not warranted. This patient shows only mild lung volume loss with no areas of lung collapse or significantly reduced oxygenation. Good positioning and early mobilisation are the cornerstones of treatment. In the majority of units patients would sit out of bed first post-operative day and commence mobilisation on the second. This is only possible if the patient has adequate analgesia.

7. • Thoracic expansion exercises with inspiratory hold. If the patient has shown signs of significant lung volume loss initially or their condition deteriorated then the therapist could instruct the patient in thoracic expansion exercises with an inspiratory hold to improve collateral ventilation.
   • Incentive spirometer – provides visual feedback and can help improve technique. If the patient continued to deteriorate then adding positive pressure to augment the patient's own respiratory effort may be necessary.
   • Positive pressure techniques (IPPB/CPAP) – Intermittent positive pressure breathing increases tidal volumes while continuous positive airway pressure helps splint the alveoli open.

8. Length of stay is reducing for cardiac surgery patients with a large proportion of patients being discharged straight home with follow-up rehabilitation. In the initial discharge period patients are encouraged to mobilise daily, gradually building up their exercise tolerance. Most will have had stair practice prior to discharge and climbing stairs should not be avoided. The sternum takes 6 weeks to unite so forceful activities with the upper limbs are to be avoided but gentle upper limb movements are encouraged as often patients complain of shoulder stiffness. The majority of patients will then progress on to formal cardiac rehabilitation. Early detection of respiratory problems is also useful for patients in the unlikely event this occurs.

## Case Study 14

1. - Cardiac output is dependent on stroke volume and heart rate. Stroke volume is dependent on myocardial contractility and filling (more stretch more contraction). Patients therefore require a satisfactory circulating volume. Too much, however, will cause backpressure into the lungs.
   - Blood pressure is dependent on the cardiac output and peripheral vascular resistance. If a patient is peripherally vasodilated the peripheral vascular resistance is reduced and hence so is their blood pressure. If a patient has a reduced cardiac output they will also have a reduced blood pressure.

2. The central venous pressure provides information on circulating volume, the pulmonary artery catheter (Swann-Ganz catheter) provides reading of cardiac output, peripheral vascular resistance, the pulmonary artery pressure and pulmonary capillary wedge pressure. Patients will also undergo 12-lead electrocardiographs to look at the electrical activity of the heart. Patients may also undergo ultrasound to look at ventricular function.

3. The IABP can be used with patients with unstable angina or following cardiac surgery. This is a balloon that is usually inserted via the femoral artery. It is positioned in the thoracic aorta. The balloon inflates during diastole and deflates during systole. When it is inflated it pushes blood into the coronary arteries, the renal arteries and empties the aorta. This makes ejection during systole easier therefore reducing the afterload. It is synchronised using a set of ECG leads, therefore care is required when handling the patient. Due to its insertion site there can be restrictions on hip flexion, which has implications for positioning.

4. Adrenaline and noradrenaline are positive inotropic drugs and have major effects on the cardiovascular system. They are used to support the heart. Adrenaline has the action of increasing the force of contraction and can also increase heart rate. This results in an improved cardiac output. Noradrenaline is a potent peripheral vasoconstrictor and therefore will help raise blood pressure. Use of both drugs requires close monitoring. They are usually given as an infusion and must be weaned off.

5. Patients who have compromised cardiovascular systems will often not cope with the demands of cardiorespiratory physiotherapy. A majority of cardiorespiratory physiotherapy techniques increase oxygen demand and the compromised patient may well not be able to cope with this. Due to the increased intrathoracic pressure caused by manual hyperinflation there is the potential to reduce venous return and hence cardiac output. Therefore techniques

including manual hyperinflation should be used with caution and, if used, the patient should be monitored closely.

6. • Retention of secretions
   • Volume loss
   • Reduced exercise tolerance.

   The patient's main problem is with retention of secretions. They have a history of smoking and the effect of a general anaesthetic would be reduced mucociliary clearance. The coarse crackles on auscultation and small amount of thick secretions confirms this.

7. • Expectoration with maximal assistance within 1 day.
   • Breath sounds all areas within 2 days.

8. • Ensure that the patient has humidified ventilation circuit. To further aid humidification and secretion clearance there may be the need for saline nebulisers.
   • Endotracheal suction. The use of closed suction may be appropriate.
   • Positioning to side lying if tolerated.
   • Manual hyperinflation providing the cardiovascular system remains stable. It would need to be carried out with close cardiovascular monitoring.



## Case Study 15

1. • Acts as past medical history in assessing young baby.
   • Important to know what gestation the baby was at birth as it indicates the maturity of the lungs.
   • No neonatal problems so neurologically and respiratory normal baby. No previous ventilation so no damage to developing lungs.

2. • Nasal cannulae at 4 L will generate a flow that is difficult for a small baby to breathe out against.
   • Babies are obligatory nose breathers. Changing oxygen delivery will remove nasal cannulae obstruction to nasal airflow.
   • Could change to oxygen delivered via a head box. This also means with an oxygen analyser you can be certain of the exact percentage of oxygen being delivered and ensure the developing lung will not be damaged by delivery of too much oxygen.

3. • Position – baby is flat and in supine. Relatively large abdomen, floppy rib cage means supine is hardest position for breathing. Cot base should be tilted head up. Could be turned prone or into side lying. If in prone, saturation monitor must be used because of the risk of sudden infant death syndrome.

- Tipping head up will relieve pressure on the diaphragm. Because of horizontal rib configuration, babies cannot utilise intercostals and accessory muscles and are totally dependent on diaphragm for respiration.
- Infants are obligatory nose breathers therefore nasal flaring is a sign of trying to increase respiratory interface, nasal secretions can compromise respiration. These are removed by nasopharyngeal suction.
- Nasogastric tube is also blocking nasal airway and is relatively large in comparison to airway size. You may consider discussing with medical and nursing staff changing to intravenous fluids.

4.
- Parents have 24-hour access and should not be asked to leave during physiotherapy treatment sessions.
- Careful and sensitive explanation of what you are doing and why you are doing it should be given.
- Obtaining consent for treatment is a legal requirement.

5.
- Normal respiratory rate is 40–60 for this age group. This patient's respiratory rate is 60–80 and the baby is therefore working hard.
- Baby is having apnoeas and is reaching the limit of being able to cope with increased work of breathing.
- ABGs indicate respiratory acidosis with $CO_2$ retention.
- Careful monitoring is needed with perhaps referral to High Dependency Unit for more intensive monitoring. Infant's conditions deteriorate quickly and this baby is tiring.
- Minimal handling and stress is indicated.

6.
- Positioning in left side lying to preferentially ventilate right lower lobe and get air behind secretions.
- Percussion and vibrations to move secretions.
- Nasal suction to stimulate cough and clear secretions.

7.
- Continue frequent position changes to ventilate all areas of the lungs.
- Consider prone positioning to decrease work of breathing. This stabilises the relatively floppy anterior portion of the chest wall against the mattress and gives the diaphragm a more fixed spinal attachment to work against.
- Nasopharangeal suction as required to keep nasal passages clear.

8.
- Patient is working hard and will tolerate short treatments frequently.
- Depending on further assessment you may treat the patient four times over the working day.

## Case Study 16

1. - May be due to poor oral intake and vomiting prior to admission.
   - IV fluids will hydrate.
   - Removal of hyoscine patches. These are used to dry up troublesome secretions and may need to be removed if infection is present. This patient is using them long term at home for secretion management.

2. - Respiratory problems may get worse due to acidic vomit in the airways. High risk of developing acute respiratory distress syndrome (ARDS) requiring increased ventilatory support.
   - Retention of secretions due to poor cough and decreased mobility.
   - Neurological condition means he may lose muscle power quickly during acute illness and therefore be difficult to wean from ventilator.

3. - This is called synchronised intermittent mandatory ventilation (SIMV). Ventilator is delivering a set (mandatory) number of breaths timed (synchronised) with any effort the patient may make. Patient is sedated and not taking any breaths in between at the moment (BPM 25 RR 25). If taking his own breaths the machine would top up pressure if patient did not achieve set pressure.
   - The ventilator is delivering a positive end expiratory pressure (PEEP) which keeps alveoli slightly inflated and decreases work of breathing.
   - Peak airway pressure (pressure delivered on mandatory breath), is 25, PEEP is 6.
   - When the ventilator delivers a set pressure expired minute volume can be used as an outcome of airway clearance as improved compliance with a set pressure will allow a larger volume to be delivered.

4. - As child develops and grows, weak low toned muscles may mean a mechanical disadvantage for breathing.
   - Postural muscles are also respiratory muscles and respiration will always dominate so posture may become worse.
   - Developing scoliosis due to low tone will also cause mechanical disadvantage. Neither stretched lung nor squashed lung will work well.
   - Due to increased demands of growing, swallowing and coughing are deteriorating.

5. - Turn into left side lying. In ventilated patients and self ventilating children under 12 years ventilation is best to upper lung.
   - Although ventilator settings allow patient to breathe spontaneously he is not taking breaths above the set rate. May use manual

hyperinflation to increase volume and recruit collateral ventilation to get air behind secretions, will also increase expiratory flow and move secretions.
- Percussion and vibrations to mobilise secretions.
- May also consider using autogenic drainage holds on hyperinflated left side to ventilate right lung.
- Endotracheal suction to clear secretions.

6. 
- As discussed in question 2 this patient is at high risk of losing muscle power and being unable to wean from ventilation. He may also have a weak cough and be unable to maintain gas exchange and clearing secretions off the ventilator. Secretion clearance needs adequate volume and flow.
- Positioning in his own supportive wheelchair during weaning may give him a good postural base to breathe from.
- Weaning onto non-invasive ventilation may help work of breathing and increase volumes to allow secretion clearance. Teaching the patient to stack breaths by not breathing out completely before coughing will also increase flow.
- Manual techniques such as manual cough assist or using a mechanical cough assist machine (insufflator/exsufflator) would be considered.

7. 
- Community staff should be informed of admission.
- Long-term management needs discussed with family and patient. This is a sensitive area and may be best done either by the intensivist who is not involved in long-term care or community consultant who knows the family best.
- Appropriateness of further ventilation in future needs to be discussed because of the risks of being unable to wean.
- Further escalating of long-term interventions requires the family wishes to be clarified such as overnight non-invasive ventilation, chest physiotherapy, antibiotic treatment.



### References


Blanchard M 2006 Pre-operative risk assessment to predict post-operative pulmonary complications in upper abdominal surgery. Journal of the Association of Chartered Physiotherapists in Respiratory Care 38:32–40.

British National Formulary 2006 British National Formulary home page Available: http://www.bnf.org 18 Feb 2007.

Chartered Society of Physiotherapy 2002 PA 53 Emergency respiratory on call working: guidance for physiotherapists. Chartered Society of Physiotherapy, London Available: http://www.csp.org.uk/uploads/documents/csp_physioprac_pa53.pdf 28 Feb 2007.

Desborough J P 2000 The stress response to trauma and surgery. British Journal of Anaesthesia 85:109–117.

Donald K J, Robertson V J, Tsebelis K 2000 Setting safe and effective suction pressure: the effect of using a manometer in the suction circuit. Intensive Care Medicine 26:15–19.
Fiorentini A 1992 Potential hazards of tracheobronchial suctioning. Intensive and Critical Care Nursing 8:217–226.
Hickey J 1992 The Clinical Practice of Neurological and Neurosurgical Nursing, 4th edn. Lippincott, Philadelphia, p 138–139.
Hinds C J, Watson D 1996 Intensive Care – a Concise Textbook, 2nd edn. Saunders, London, p 183.
Hough A 2001 Physiotherapy in Respiratory Care – an Evidence-based Approach to Respiratory and Cardiac Management, 3rd edn. Nelson Thornes, Surrey UK.
Jackson V L C 2006 Normal saline instillation as an adjunct to endotracheal suctioning – a review of the literature. Journal of the Association of Chartered Physiotherapists in Respiratory Care 38:41–46.
Maxwell L, Ellis E 1998 Secretion clearance by manual hyperinflation: possible mechanisms. Physiotherapy Theory & Practice 14:189–197.
Odell A, Allder A, Bayne R, Everett C, Scott S, Still B, West S 1993 Endotracheal suction for adult, non-head-injured patients. A review of the literature. Intensive and Critical Care Nursing 9:274–278.
Orfanos P, Ellis E, Johnston C 1999 Effects of deep breathing and ambulation on pattern of ventilation in post-operative patients. Australian Journal of Physiotherapy 45:173–182.
St George's Healthcare NHS Trust 2006 Guidelines for the Care of Patients with Tracheostomy Tubes. Smiths Medical International, Herts UK.
Scottish Intercollegiate Guidelines Network 2004 SIGN 77 Postoperative management in adults: a practical guide to postoperative care for clinical staff. SIGN, Edinburgh Available: http://www.sign.ac.uk/pdf/sign77.pdf 20 Feb 2007.
Singer M, Vermaat J, Hall G 1994 Haemodynamic effects of manual hyperinflation in critically ill mechanically ventilated patients. Chest 106(4):1182–1187.
Stiller K, Phillips A 2003 Safety aspects of mobilising acutely ill inpatients. Physiotherapy Theory and Practice 19:239–257.
Villar J 2002 Acute respiratory distress syndrome: searching for a satisfactory definition in the new millennium. International Journal of Intensive Care Spring:45–48.

## Further reading

### General

Hodgkinson D W, O'Driscoll B R, Driscoll P A et al 1993 ABC of emergency radiology: chest radiographs 1. British Medical Journal 307 (6913):1202–1206.

Hough A 2001 Physiotherapy in Respiratory Care – an Evidence-based Approach to Respiratory and Cardiac Management, 3rd edn. Nelson Thornes, Surrey UK.

Pryor J A, Prasad S A (eds) 2002 Physiotherapy for Respiratory and Cardiac Problems, 3rd edn. Churchill Livingstone, Edinburgh.

Simpson H 2004 Interpretation of arterial blood gases: a clinical guide for nurses. British Journal of Nursing 13(9):522–528.

### Medical Respiratory

British Lung Foundation 2005 The British Lung Foundation home page Available: http://www.lunguk.org 18 Feb 2007.

Cystic Fibrosis Trust 2002 Clinical guidelines for the physiotherapy management of cystic fibrosis. Cystic Fibrosis Trust, Bromley Available: http://www.cftrust.org.uk/aboutcf/publications/consensusdoc/C_3400physiotherapy.pdf 18 Feb 2007.

Hodson M E, Geddes D M (eds) 2000 Cystic Fibrosis, 2nd edn. Arnold, London.

National Collaborating Centre for Chronic Conditions 2004 Chronic obstructive pulmonary disease: management of chronic obstructive pulmonary disease in adults in primary and secondary care clinical guideline 12. Thorax 59(suppl 1):S1-S232 Available: http://www.nice.org.uk/pdf/CG012_niceguideline.pdf 18 Feb 2007.

Scottish Intercollegiate Guidelines Network 2005 SIGN 80 Management of patients with lung cancer: a national clinical guideline. SIGN, Edinburgh Available: http://www.sign.ac.uk/pdf/sign80.pdf 18 Feb 2007.

### *Paediatrics*

Harden B 2004 Emergency Physiotherapy: An On Call Survival Guide. Churchill Livingstone, Edinburgh.

Prasad S A, Hussey J 1995 Paediatric Respiratory Care: a Guide for Physiotherapists and Health Professionals. Chapman and Hall, London.

### *Cardiothoracic surgery*

Allibone L 2003 Nursing management of chest drains. Nursing Standard 17(22):45–56.

Brasher P A, McClelland K H, Denehy L et al 2003 Does removal of breathing exercises from a physiotherapy program including pre-operative education and early mobilization after cardiac surgery alter patient outcomes? Australian Journal of Physiotherapy 49(3):165–173.

Little C 2004 Your guide to the intra-aortic balloon pump. Nursing 34(12):32cc1–32cc2.

Pasquina P, Tramer M R, Walder B 2003 Prophylactic respiratory physiotherapy after cardiac surgery: systematic review. British Medical Journal 327(7428):1379–1381.

CHAPTER SIX

# Case studies in neurological physiotherapy

*Mandy Dunbar*



## INTRODUCTION

Neurological physiotherapy covers a broad area of practice spanning intensive care, acute, rehabilitative and community services. New ways of working have seen an increase in physiotherapists working in community and primary care settings, a number of case studies presented touch upon the differences experienced when working in these areas. The case studies based in acute settings highlight transferable skills which may impact on the approach to treatment of the patient with neurological impairment.

Physiotherapy practice in neurology can be focussed on prevention, maintenance, restoration, prevention or in palliative care. The case studies presented in this chapter aim to touch upon each of these areas, highlighting the role of the physiotherapist, the need to develop an underpinning knowledge of the pathophysiology of a condition in order to set appropriate goals and the need to work as part of a multi/inter disciplinary team.

In neurological physiotherapy the evidence base for treatment interventions is a developing one (Pomeroy & Tallis 2002). Moves have been made by a number of researchers to identify what constitutes neurological physiotherapy. Studies by Ballinger et al (1999), Davidson & Waters (2000), Lennon & Ashburn (2000) and Lennon (2003), have begun to address this issue mainly in the form of surveys and focus groups. These studies have sought to isolate the components of neurological physiotherapy treatment and what concept of treatment physiotherapist's professed to use. Previous studies by Nilsson & Nordholm (1992), Carr et al (1994), and Sackley & Lincoln (1996) as cited in Davidson & Waters (2000), identified that the main approach used by physiotherapists in the United Kingdom, although eclectic in nature, was based on the Bobath concept. This was supported by Davidson & Waters (2000) who reported that the majority of physiotherapists questioned (88%), professed to use the Bobath approach, although the majority of these also used other approaches in the treatment of their clients. The second most popular approach was identified as the Motor Re-learning Programme (MRP), though this was practised by only 4% of the respondents.

Much of the evidence available informing neurological physiotherapy practice supports the MRP as an effective treatment approach in the management of neurological conditions. However, given the low numbers of physiotherapists reported to be practising MRP in the UK and the eclectic approach reported, a similar approach has been taken when compiling this chapter. It is therefore suggested that any preparation for a new area of clinical practice should include familiarisation with the approach adopted in that area.



## CASE STUDY 1 ACUTE STROKE

### Subjective assessment

| | |
|---|---|
| PC | 68-year-old male admitted via A&E following collapse at home<br>CT scan shows infarct of right middle cerebral artery<br>Chest X-ray (CXR) – patchy shadowing right base |
| HPC | Found in garden at home by wife – drowsy, uncommunicative and had vomited. Thought to have suffered collapse several hours previously<br>Ambulance called and patient transferred to A&E<br>On arrival to A&E patient was drowsy but appeared to be able to respond to basic commands, though was not recognizing stimuli from the left<br>Left sided weakness, reduced tone and reduced reflexes<br>Temp 38.9°C |
| PMH | Non-smoker<br>Atherosclerosis<br>Bilateral OA knees |

| | |
|---|---|
| DH | Simvastatin – for atherosclerosis<br>Commenced on IV antibiotics and IV fluids in A&E along with 300 mg aspirin |
| SH | Lives with wife in a semi-detached house with bedroom and bathroom upstairs<br>Retired plumber<br>Keen gardener |

## Objective assessment

Referred by ward staff to assess chest and initial bed mobility.

| | |
|---|---|
| **Observation** | Positioned in bed with IVs *in situ* in right upper limb<br>Falling to the left with left upper limb hanging over the edge of the bed<br>Conscious and responsive, but drowsy, appears to recognise basic commands<br>No attempts to communicate, making eye contact only<br>Facing to right and unresponsive to attempts to gain attention from the left – attempts made both verbally and when repositioning left upper limb<br>Long-leg compression stockings in situ. Left lower limb externally rotated with retraction of left pelvis evident in lying<br>Pressure-relieving mattress *in situ* |
| **Bed mobility** | Patient unable to participate in attempts to alter position, due to level of consciousness. Dense low tone noted throughout left upper and lower limbs<br>No subluxation evident at left glenohumeral joint |
| **Respiratory** | RR 10 breaths per minute<br>Oxygen saturation – 94% on 28% oxygen via face mask<br>Palpation – reduced basal expansion bilaterally<br>On auscultation – reduced air entry with bronchial breath sounds in right basal lobe |

## Questions

1. How is stroke (CVA) defined?
2. What are the recognised risk factors for stroke?
3. What symptoms could be associated with occlusion of the right middle cerebral artery?
4. Thrombolytic treatment was not administered in this instance – why was this the case?
5. Why is aspiration pneumonia associated with the right basal lobe?

6. What are the treatment priorities in the acute phase of stroke management for this gentleman?
7. What positions are favourable in terms of maintaining oxygen saturations in acute stroke management?

## CASE STUDY 2 STROKE REHABILITATION, UPPER LIMB HYPOTONICITY

### Subjective assessment

| | |
|---|---|
| PC | 72-year-old female with right-sided hemiplegia primarily affecting the upper limb following CVA 6/52<br>Low tone in upper limb proximally with subluxation of glenohumeral joint<br>Increased tone in right wrist, fingers and elbow, with moderate associated reaction evident on activity |
| HPC | Complained of severe headache immediately prior to collapse at local bingo hall<br>CT scan showed extensive haemorrhagic stroke affecting the thalamus. Intracranial pressure was monitored closely in the acute stages, though surgical intervention was not indicated<br>Transferred to stroke rehabilitation unit after 2/52 once medically stable, where significant improvements have been made |
| PMH | Smoker – 30 per day<br>Hypertension<br>Previous myocardial infarction × 3 in past 5 years |
| DH | Lisinopril |
| SH | Lives alone in ground floor flat in sheltered accommodation<br>Retired cleaner<br>Goes to bingo twice weekly |

### Objective assessment

Independently mobile on ward, returned to previous level of function with regard to mobility.

**Sitting** Kyphotic posture which can be minimally corrected. Patient reports having adopted this posture for a number of years.
Stiffness in lower back preventing movement beyond patients 'normal' range
Left scapula protracted, but can align with verbal prompting
Right scapula – reduced tone evident with scapula protracted and medially rotated
Right humerus medially rotated with significant subluxation evident

CHAPTER SIX

Unable to recruit activity at shoulder girdle or glenohumeral joint
Increased tone noted at elbow flexors with associated reaction evident on activity
Increased tone of right wrist and finger flexors – increasing with any activity
Some soft tissue adaptation noted in right wrist and fingers, unable to achieve full extension nor accept a base of support through palmar aspect of the hand

## Questions

1. Why is hypertension in particular associated with haemorrhagic strokes?
2. Initial prognosis following haemorrhagic stroke is poor; however, recovery after the acute episode can be significant. Why is this the case?
3. What is meant by the term glenohumeral joint subluxation?
4. What treatment options are available in the management of this problem?
5. Considering your role in the multidisciplinary team (MDT), what educational role might you adopt with other staff members with regard to this patient?
6. What other members of the multi/interdisciplinary team might be involved in the care of this patient?
7. What psychosocial issues might this lady have to address as part of her rehabilitation process?



# CASE STUDY 3 STROKE REHABILITATION, GAIT DISTURBANCE

## Subjective assessment

**PC** 55-year-old male admitted via A&E following collapse
CT scan showed sub-arachnoid haemorrhage (SAH) of the left anterior cerebral artery (ACA)
Current problems relate to standing balance, unable to stand unaided. Mobilising few steps in therapy sessions only
Keen to return home, but unable to do so while balance remains problematic as wife works away from home for periods of time during the week

**HPC** Complained of sudden intense headache while doing DIY at home
Collapsed and ambulance called – transferred to A&E
On arrival CT scan conducted which showed extensive SAH
Angiogram completed which showed ruptured berry aneurysm on the ACA

| | |
|---|---|
| | Transferred to regional neurosurgical unit, where urgent coiling procedure was completed<br>Following surgery transferred to ICU (3 days) followed by Neurosurgical HDU (6 days)<br>Transferred to neurological rehabilitation unit 3/52 post surgery<br>Continues to be closely monitored due to high risk of re-bleed in sub-acute phase |
| **PMH** | Chronic low back pain, attributed to driving as part of job, manages with medication<br>Nil else of note |
| **DH** | Ibuprofen prn for back pain |
| **SH** | Lives with wife in a terraced house with bedroom and bathroom upstairs. Toilet facilities available downstairs<br>Alcohol consumption 40+ units per week<br>Sales representative for engineering company<br>Two children – both live away from home |



## Objective assessment

| | |
|---|---|
| **Sitting** | Kyphotic posture in sitting with decreased lumbar lordosis. With verbal prompting, able to anteriorly tilt pelvis and increase lumber lordosis<br>Static sitting balance good – able to withstand challenges to balance and effectively recruit equilibrium reactions<br>Dynamic sitting balance – difficulty recruiting activity at right hip when reaching outside base of support on the right. Able to correct with verbal prompting, though fatigues quickly<br>No evidence of increased tone in sitting, though tendency to overuse left lower limb to assist with weight transfer to right<br>Slight weakness in right upper limb though no tonal change |
| **Sit to stand** | Sit to stand – independent<br>Weight bearing left > right with overuse of left upper limb evident<br>Retraction of right hip and hyperextension of right knee during extension into full stand minimal weight bearing through right lower limb<br>Decreased activity tibialis anterior with ankle remaining in plantarflexion throughout transfer |

| | |
|---|---|
| Standing | Weight bearing left > right with retraction at right hip, hyperextension of right knee and right ankle in plantarflexion<br>With facilitation to extend right hip, able to transfer weight to the right, though complains of fear of falling |

## Questions

1. What symptoms could be associated with damage to the ACA?
2. What is a sub-arachnoid haemorrhage?
3. This patient had a surgical intervention to treat the underlying cause of his condition, what factors indicate that surgical intervention is appropriate?
4. This gentleman has a coiling procedure performed as opposed to clipping – what is the benefit of this procedure?
5. Orthoses can be used in the treatment of neurological conditions. What advantages might the use of an AFO have for this gentleman?
6. This gentleman presents with some weakness of the right upper limb, can exercise be used to increase muscle strength in this patient?

## CASE STUDY 4 HEAD INJURY, ACUTE PHASE

The following patient is on intensive care following admission via A&E 2 weeks ago.

### Subjective assessment

| | |
|---|---|
| PC | 28-year-old male, admitted to ICU with extensive head injury following an assault<br>Ventilated and sedated, though sedation is being reduced as ventilator weaning commences<br>Evidence of increasing tone once sedation began to be reduced, which has caused concern for staff involved in nursing interventions |
| HPC | Admitted via A&E 2/52 ago after being found in local town centre unconscious with bruising and lacerations consistent with assault<br>On admission GCS = 5, with some respiratory distress evident<br>Decision taken to sedate and ventilate<br>CT scan showed diffuse injury with development of oedema. No repeat CT scan conducted as yet<br>Initially medically unstable with physiotherapy input focussed in positioning and respiratory monitoring. Treatment sessions minimal due to risks associated with increasing intra-cranial pressure<br>Now medically stable and sedation is being reduced and ventilator weaning commencing |

| | |
|---|---|
| PMH | Fractured pelvis and right femur 2 years ago in motorbike accident<br>Nil else of note |
| Family history | Parents and sister live nearby, close family network |
| DH | Extensive medications at present |
| SH | Self-employed electrician<br>Lives with a friend in a rented two-bedroom terraced house, all bedroom and bathroom facilities upstairs<br>Parents live nearby and are concerned at meeting rental payments on their son's home<br>Previously very fit and active, enjoyed socialising with friends, motorbiking and surfing |



## Objective assessment

Lying in supine

Increased tone in upper limbs bilaterally, with upper limbs demonstrating severe flexor patterns

Flexion at wrists, fingers and elbows with adduction and internal rotation at shoulder joints

Attempts to lower tone in order to move upper limbs prove difficult. Movement of the upper limbs away from the chest wall is possible with slow stretching and tissue mobilisation though cannot be maintained with positioning

Increased tone into extensor pattern in the lower limbs. Severe increase in tone which prevents any movement into flexion at the hips and knees. Ankle joints are held in plantarflexion. Unable to affect level of tone within the lower limbs with handling

On repositioning to assist with nursing care, rolling performed via a log-rolling technique due to difficulties with increased tone in the lower limbs. On rolling increased tone within the neck and trunk extensors evident

Further assessment postponed due to patient agitation

## Questions

1. What would the primary problem list be for this gentleman on admission to ICU?
2. What would the initial goals of physiotherapy management be for this gentleman?
3. Prior to weaning commencing physiotherapy intervention was kept to a minimum due to concerns with increasing intra-cranial pressure. Why was this a concern for physiotherapy interventions in particular?

4. Why has an increase in tone become evident once weaning has commenced?
5. How might these increases in tone be described?
6. What difficulties could increased tone at this stage pose for long-term rehabilitation goals?
7. How might increased tone be managed from a physiotherapy perspective?

## CASE STUDY 5 HEAD INJURY, LONG-TERM REHABILITATION

You have been asked to see the following patient in the community. She suffered a head injury 4 years ago and is seeking advice on exercise and social activity, having previously been discharged from physiotherapy 2 years ago.

### Subjective assessment

| | |
|---|---|
| PC | 22-year-old female, suffered a head injury 4 years ago following an RTA in which she was a passenger<br>With rehabilitation made a good recovery and has now been in part-time paid employment for 6/12 as an administrative assistant<br>On starting work, complained of high levels of fatigue. This has now settled<br>Keen to focus on physical performance as mobility levels have decreased over the past few months which the patient attributes to a lack of exercise<br>Complains of right leg feeling weak, with a fear of her knee giving way if walking any distance |
| HPC | RTA 4 years ago, in which the patient sustained a head injury, fractured left tibia and fibula and facial fractures<br>MRI scan showed damage to the temporal and parietal lobes on the left due to a blunt piercing trauma<br>Underwent extensive surgery and rehabilitation at the time of injury<br>Discharged home 8/12 post injury using a powered wheelchair for mobility, transferring with the assistance of one to step round, with mild increased tone in the right upper limb and lack of selective control of movement<br>Rehabilitation commenced on an out-patient basis, on discharge 2 years ago mobilising independently with a walking stick to aid balance. Walking approximately 50 m both indoors and outdoors. Good upper limb function, able to carry out most functional tasks, with just fine control affected<br>Unable to drive on discharge due to epilepsy following head injury, though has now returned to driving |

| | |
|---|---|
| PMH | ORIF left tibia and fibula following RTA<br>Nil else of note |
| DH | Coproxamol prn |
| SH | Lives alone in a one-bedroom ground floor flat<br>On discharge from hospital, lived with parents, moved to own accommodation 1 year ago and has lived independently since<br>Parents are supportive, but now only call when needed as daughter has worked hard to achieve her independence following her RTA<br>Works part-time as an administrative assistant at a local architects, looking to increase hours to full-time once she feels physically able<br>Returning to a more active social life – enjoys going out with friends, bingo and cinema |



## Objective assessment

Mobilising independently indoors at time of visit. Reports using stick at work as works in an open-plan office and doesn't feel safe. Mobilises without stick only in familiar environments, such as home and parent's home

Gait indoors – reduced stance phase on right, with an increased base of support throughout gait cycle. Reduced heel-strike on right, with decreased eccentric control of plantarflexion to achieve foot-flat

Outdoor mobility – using walking stick in left upper limb. Overusing when weight bearing on right, with elevation and abduction of left shoulder evident during stance on right. All other observation as indoor mobility

Lower limb strength – all lower limb muscles tested using Oxford Scale. All major muscle groups – grade 5, except right quadriceps, hip extensors and dorsiflexors, which were assessed as Oxford Scale grade 4

Berg balance scale – 38 out of a maximum 56. Patient reported that fear of falling meant that she often 'gave up' rather than having to stop due to physical factors

## Questions

1. What problem list would you establish for this patient?
2. What goals may be appropriate?
3. The patient scored 38 on the Berg Balance scale – why might this outcome measure have been selected to complete as part of her assessment?
4. What other outcome measures may have been used in your assessment of this lady?

5. What treatment options may be available to you in order to address the goals identified?
6. Are there any other services which you may access to continue treatment for this patient?

## CASE STUDY 6 SPINAL CORD INJURY AT C3

The following gentleman was discharged 4/52 ago from a regional spinal unit. He has 24-hour care provided at home by a dedicated nursing team. You have been asked to see him by the lead nurse in the team due to difficulties with positioning.

### Subjective assessment

| | |
|---|---|
| PC | 45-year-old man who suffered an incomplete disruption of C3/4 following a motorbike accident<br>Recently discharged home, ventilated and has a 24-hour package of care provided by a dedicated nursing team who all undertook an extensive training package at the regional spinal unit once appointed to their post<br>Contracted a chest infection 2/52 ago. Has had a full course of antibiotics but was unwell at the time and nursed in bed<br>Nursing staff report difficulties in achieving a good sitting posture in attendant powered wheelchair since chest infection. This has prevented participation in social activities and restricted engagement with family members |
| HPC | Sustained an incomplete disruption of C3 15/12 ago following a motorbike accident<br>Requires full ventilatory support and regular suctioning to clear excess secretions. Staff are trained in respiratory management and provide manual hyperinflation and suctioning at regular intervals<br>Paraplegic; reports being able to feel pain though unable to localise. No other recognised sensation present or motor control<br>During chest infection did not require hospital admission and was managed at home with antibiotics and increased respiratory management<br>Chest is now clear and staff are happy with respiratory procedures in place. Suctioning technique reviewed by senior nursing staff for all team members to ensure correct sterile technique adhered to during procedure<br>Passive movements usually performed twice daily to all joints of upper and lower limbs through range. During chest infection unable to perform all movements fully due to positioning and marked increase in tone |

| | |
|---|---|
| | Tracheostomy tube changed during chest infection, communicates effectively by staff lip reading |
| PMH | Mild asthmatic – controlled well with inhalers<br>Nil else of note |
| DH | Extensive medications<br>Of note – Baclofen |
| SH | Lives in a four-bedroom detached home. This has recently been extensively adapted to accommodate needs. A large ground floor extension has been built which includes: ramped access, bedroom for the patient, bathroom with level access shower and sluice, a generator (to provide power for the ventilator in the event of a power cut) and accommodation for nursing staff<br>Lives with wife who works full time as a teacher and two boys aged 8 and 10<br>Previously worked as a pharmacist at local chemists<br>Previous social activities included motorbike holidays with friends, hill walking and helping out with son's football team |

## Objective assessment

You are asked to focus your attention on seating and positioning difficulties.

| | |
|---|---|
| **Observation** | Patient positioned in powered adjustable bed, upper limbs supported on pillows maintaining alignment throughout<br>End of bed raised to position lower limbs with hips in approximately 70° flexion and knees at approximately 30° flexion<br>Ankles plantarflexed and inverted |
| **Passive movement** | Passive movements performed to all upper limb joints<br>Shoulder extension difficult to assess due to positioning in bed<br>Full range of movement available at shoulders and elbows, though distal increase in tone noted toward end of range. Patient complained of pain on movement, though unable to localise<br>Full range pronation available, marked increase in tone noted at approximately neutral when moving toward supination, with wrist and fingers developing flexor pattern |

Nursing staff present report that this has become an increasing problem since chest infection and they are concerned about skin integrity. Patient reports hand position causing concern though wants to be able to sit out in wheelchair so that he can spend more time with his sons

Once blood pressure stabilised, patient hoisted into wheelchair to enable assessment of lower limb alignment and sitting position

---

**Sitting posture**

Tilt in space wheelchair, with rear wheels set back to accommodate the weight of the portable ventilator

Gutter arms to provide support for upper limbs, which can be positioned into pronation with wrists and fingers in neutral position after approximately 5 minutes to allow tone to settle following hoisting

Head support in situ though able to maintain alignment of head independently

**TABLE 6.1 UPPER LIMB ROM**

| Joint | Movement | Right | Left |
|---|---|---|---|
| Wrist | Flexion | FROM - ↑tone | FROM - ↑tone |
| | Extension | Unable to move beyond neutral due to ↑tone<br>R = L | Unable to move beyond neutral due to ↑tone<br>R = L |
| | Radial Deviation | Unable to move beyond neutral due to ↑tone<br>R = L | Unable to move beyond neutral due to ↑tone<br>R = L |
| | Ulnar Deviation | FROM - ↑tone | FROM - ↑tone |
| Thumb | Flexion | Assessment of proximal upper limb range of movement increased tone in distal upper limbs significantly, with patient complaining of increased pain.<br>Increased tone into flexion noted throughout – detailed assessment abandoned until further session due to increasing blood pressure. Patient suffers from autonomic dysreflexia. To be assessed in future treatment session. | |
| | Extension | | |
| | Abduction | | |
| | Adduction | | |
| Fingers | Flexion | | |
| | Extension | | |
| | Abduction | | |
| | Adduction | | |

Lateral trunk support maintaining trunk position

Hips at 90°, positioning aided by gravity as hoisted into wheelchair in tilted position

Increased tone at knees into extensor pattern, unable to flex knees passively beyond 140° on right and 130° on left to place feet on footplates

Increased tone at both ankles, held in plantarflexion and inversion. Unable to achieve neutral position at ankles to place feet onto footplates

Patient complained of pain and fatigue after approximately 10 minutes in wheelchair and returned to bed

---

### Questions

1. Why does this patient require full ventilatory support?
2. Detailed assessment had to be postponed due to concerns with increasing blood pressure. Why is this a concern for this gentleman?
3. What implication does autonomic dysreflexia have for planning treatment interventions?
4. Why is this gentleman experiencing an increase in tone at the present time?
5. What would your goals for treatment be?
6. How might these be addressed in collaboration with nursing team members who work with this gentleman?



## CASE STUDY 7 SPINAL CORD INJURY AT T5

The following patient has recently been transferred to a rehabilitation unit following a period of care for a spinal fracture at T5. Surgical intervention was required to stabilise the fracture site and decompress the spinal cord. The patient is now wearing a brace, which is due to be reviewed in the next few weeks.

### Subjective assessment

PC

19-year-old female who suffered a crush fracture with spinal cord compression at T5 following a fall while rock climbing 4/52 ago

Wearing brace which needs to be worn for 3/12 to maintain alignment at fracture site

Recently transferred to rehabilitation unit for intensive rehabilitation

Wheelchair has been prescribed. Having difficulty self-propelling due to poor sitting balance and atrophy of all upper limb muscles

Transferring with assistance of one or two with banana board

| | |
|---|---|
| | Anxious to be discharged – university course recommences in 2 months time and wants to return<br>Has made enquiries at local university about the possibility of transferring studies so that she can live with parents |
| **HPC** | Sustained a complete disruption of spinal cord at T5<br>No sensory function or motor function present below nipple line<br>Surgical intervention required to stablise anteriorly and posteriorly following injury<br>Provided with a self-propelling wheelchair 2/52 ago with pressure relieving cushion in situ. Difficulty in self-propelling due to poor sitting balance<br>Becoming increasingly frustrated with lack of independence<br>Recently had catheter removed, now intermittent self-catheterisation with assistance from nursing staff with a view to full independence. Currently hampered by poor sitting balance<br>Treated initially at regional spinal unit. Requested transfer to local rehabilitation unit to be closer to family and friends |
| **PM** | Nil of note |
| **DH** | Nil of note |
| **SH** | Lives with parents in terraced house. All facilities upstairs. Parents have converted second reception room on ground floor into bedroom which is separate to main living areas<br>Occupational therapists have undertaken an initial home assessment and temporary ramps and a commode have been provided. Referral to social services occupational therapy for assessment for home adaptations has been arranged<br>Keen to commence weekend leave from the rehabilitation unit<br>Student at university studying law. Lives in halls of residence, but was due to move into shared housing with friends at start of next academic year<br>Has been in contact with local university about the possibility of transferring her studies to allow her to live at home. Agreement has been reached re: transferring studies. New academic year starts in 2/12 time, though can delay starting second year of studies for a year to allow further time for recovery<br>Both parents work full-time, younger brother who also lives at home is due to start college in 1/12<br>Active sportswoman enjoys rock-climbing, netball and hockey and represented university sports teams in the previous year |

## Objective assessment

Brace in situ throughout assessment.

| | |
|---|---|
| **Lying** | Supine<br>Full range of movement both upper limbs (within limits of position)<br>Patient reports decreased muscle strength throughout upper limbs (Grade 4+ Oxford Scale) and atrophy<br>Previously had good upper-limb strength due to rock climbing<br>Full passive range of movement available in both lower limbs, low tone throughout. No active movement or sensory discrimination evident on full assessment |
| **Lying to sitting** | With assistance from one, able to push through upper limbs to move into long sitting<br>Requires assistance from one to move lower limbs over edge of bed to achieve sitting. Able to adjust sitting position by pushing through upper limbs to lift trunk. Facilitation from one required to maintain balance during transfer |
| **Unsupported sitting** | Able to maintain sitting posture through overuse of upper limbs to increase base of support<br>Overuse of thoracic and cervical extension to maintain sitting posture<br>Unable to move within base of support in sitting or release upper limbs to enable function |
| **Transfers** | Requires maximum assistance of two to transfer weight laterally and place banana board<br>Able to initiate movement along banana board by pushing through upper limbs though requires facilitation to maintain balance and reposition lower limbs during transfer |



## Questions

1. What problems can be associated with spinal cord injury at T5?
2. This patient has a complete disruption of the spinal cord, what pattern of dysfunction might you see had she sustained an incomplete disruption?
3. What would your problem list be for this patient?
4. How would you prioritise these goals and why?
5. What long-term goals are relevant for this patient?

## CASE STUDY 8 MULTIPLE SCLEROSIS, RELAPSING–REMITTING

You have been asked to see the following lady in an out-patient setting by the multiple sclerosis (MS) specialist nurse following a recent relapse.

### Subjective assessment

| | |
|---|---|
| PC | 35-year-old lady complaining of difficulties maintaining balance in standing, particularly when carrying out ADLs<br>Has tripped several times and feels unsafe when mobilising outdoors. Currently not leaving the house without someone to accompany her<br>Recent relapse mainly affected right lower limb, recovery slower than with previous relapses<br>Confidence affected considerably<br>Unable to drive at present as patient 'does not trust' right leg when braking |
| HPC | Diagnosed with MS 4 years ago following three incidents of illness accompanied by loss of movement in lower limbs. Has previously returned to full normal functional levels following these incidents<br>GP referred to consultant neurologist, who diagnosed MS following a number of investigations<br>Reviewed 6 monthly by Consultant and 3 monthly by MS nurse<br>5/52 ago complained of feeling unwell with associated loss of movement in right lower limb. Contacted MS specialist nurse who arranged for admission to day unit for intravenous methyl-prednisolone<br>Good recovery initially, though remaining symptoms have persisted |
| PMH | Caesarean section × 2 for youngest two children<br>Nil else of note |
| FH | Sister has MS now uses a wheelchair for mobility |
| DH | Betainterferon |
| SH | Lives with husband and three young children aged 3, 5 and 7<br>Housewife, previously worked as a personal assistant before giving up work to care for children full-time<br>Active member of Parent Teachers Association, helps at children's school three times weekly<br>Goes to gym four times a week, enjoys cooking and family days out |

CHAPTER SIX

### Objective assessment

Arrives for therapy session mobilising with husband, reports 'linking' as feels unsafe mobilising outside own home independently. Husband reports that his wife has been maintaining her balance by holding on to furniture while walking around the home.

| | |
|---|---|
| **Standing posture** | Large base of support, with knees pushed back into full extension to adopt close-packed position of the joint<br>Pelvis – anterior tilt, with increased lumbar lordosis<br>Centre of gravity falling posterior to the knee joint<br>Shoulders elevated bilaterally, unable to release upper limbs to 'relax' into standing posture |
| **Standing balance** | Balance assessed in standing by applying small forces anteriorly, posteriorly and laterally to central key point. Patient asked to push against the pressure to maintain midline standing<br>Unable to activate postural control mechanisms at the ankles to correct for postural threat. Equlibrium reactions evident immediately. Correction achieved by movement of upper limbs or by stepping left leg to increase base of support<br>No attempts to increase BOS by stepping right lower limb<br>Further progression of balance assessment abandoned due to patient confidence and health and safety concerns |
| **Gait** | Increased BOS<br>Decreased step length evident, with decreased heel strike on left and no heel strike on right<br>Decreased stance phase on right lower limb<br>Circumduction of right lower limb during swing phase, with decreased dorsiflexion during swing<br>Elevated shoulder girdles bilaterally, unable to release upper limbs to achieve reciprocal arm swing<br>No trunk rotation evident during observation |

### Questions

1. What is the pathophysiology of multiple sclerosis?
2. What is meant by the term relapsing–remitting?
3. How is multiple sclerosis diagnosed?
4. What is meant by the term righting reaction?
5. How might you address re-education of these reactions?
6. How will you progress to re-education of dynamic standing balance?
7. What other services could be involved in this lady's care?

## CASE STUDY 9 MULTIPLE SCLEROSIS, SECONDARY PROGRESSIVE

You have been asked to see the following gentleman at home by the home care team, who have reported increasing difficulty with transfers on visits to assist with personal care.

| | |
|---|---|
| **PC** | Uses a powered wheelchair for indoor and outdoor mobility<br>Currently using a banana board with the assistance of one for all transfers<br>Home care staff have reported increased difficulties with transfers, with one member of staff having injured her back during transfer from bed to shower chair<br>Sacral pressure sore – district nurse visits three times weekly for dressing. Recently provided with higher pressure relief mattress and wheelchair cushion<br>District nurses have expressed concerns about the shearing forces experienced during banana board transfers which they feel may be a contributing factor to pressure sore development and healing |
| **HPC** | 56-year-old gentleman, diagnosed with MS 20 years ago<br>Initially presented with relapsing–remitting clinical presentation. Began to deteriorate physically 3 years ago without any acute periods. Consultant Neurologist diagnosed with secondary progressive MS<br>Reported recurrent UTIs 5 years ago. Continence specialist nurse diagnosed detruso-sphincter dyssernygia. Initially managed with medication and self-catheterisation to address retention. Upper limb function deterioration led to increasing difficulty with self-catheterisation, has therefore been catheterised for previous 2 years<br>Reported difficulties with fatigue, with increasing difficulty with transfers and carrying out functional tasks as the day progresses<br>Under the care of the speech and language therapist for swallowing difficulties, currently on a modified diet including syrup thick fluids and soft diet |
| **PMH** | Angina |
| **DH** | GTN spray<br>Amantadine<br>Baclofen |
| **SH** | Previously worked as a solicitor. Retired 10 years ago due to deteriorating health |

Lives alone in a large detached bungalow, adapted to allow wheelchair access throughout. Level access shower and ramped access in situ

Divorced 12 years ago, two grown children live locally and are very supportive of their father

Active role in local church, though this has decreased in recent years and now plays a largely administrative role

## Objective assessment

| | |
|---|---|
| **Posture in sitting** | Uses powered wheelchair for mobility indoors and outdoors<br>Seated in power-chair for 11 hours per day on average<br>Postural management system to provide lateral trunk support at ribcage<br>Retraction at right hip and increased tone throughout lower limbs<br>Pelvis in posterior tilt, increased tone in abdominals – unable to release to achieve anterior tilt<br>Shoulders protracted, increased flexor tone in both upper limbs and hands. Soft tissue adaptation evident at elbows and all digits but index fingers bilaterally<br>Unable to passively move through range |
| **Transfers** | Currently transferring with banana board with the assistance of one<br>Assessed with two due to moving and handling safety concerns raised by home care staff<br>Lateral trunk support removed to allow movement of trunk in sitting<br>Assisted to flex left hip to remove wheelchair footrest<br>Significant increase in tone into hip flexion and knee extension on movement – facilitation provided to accept base of support and decrease tone – took some time to settle. Assistance required to reposition right lower limb, though no significant change in tone noted<br>Maximum assistance from two to transfer weight laterally and step each hip forward to achieve perch sitting with both feet in contact with the floor. Extreme difficulty in moving to perch sitting with minimal participation achieved by patient<br>Transfer attempt abandoned due to risks perceived to staff members |

Patient reported that transfers were much more difficult later in the day due to levels of fatigue, though at time of assessment, participation not affected

## Questions

1. Secondary progressive MS is one form of the condition. What forms of MS are there, and how can these be classified?
2. What risk assessment needs to take place when evaluating moving and handling intervention?
3. Beta-interferon is a disease-modifying drug recognised as providing benefit to some people who have MS. Why is this gentleman not prescribed this drug?
4. What would your advice be with regard to moving and handling in the short term?
5. What might the possible psychosocial implication of your advice be for this gentleman?
6. Noticeable soft tissue adaptation and increase in tone in the upper limbs may lead to difficulties for this gentleman in using the powered wheelchair. What treatment interventions might you access in order to manage this problem?
7. If banana board transfers are no longer possible, access to a car will be difficult. What other options are available?



## CASE STUDY 10 PARKINSON'S DISEASE

You are asked to see the following gentleman at his home by the Parkinson's disease specialist nurse who reviewed him at her clinic 1 week ago. He has been finding transfers increasingly difficult. His medication has been changed, but increasingly difficult home circumstances have triggered an urgent referral.

### Subjective assessment

| | |
|---|---|
| PC | 83-year-old gentleman diagnosed with Parkinson's disease 10 years ago<br>2/12 ago, started to experience difficulties with transfers – particularly sit to stand and getting out of bed<br>Wife has been finding it difficult to cope. They are both extremely worried and feel that they may need to move into residential care but don't want to leave their home |
| HPC | Diagnosed 10 years ago, following a number of falls outdoors<br>Independently mobile around the home environment. Uses two hand rails to aid balance on stairs. Uses an attendant pushed wheelchair outdoors<br>Rarely leaves the house as no ramped access and wife cannot manage the wheelchair and daughter lives a considerable distance away |

| | |
|---|---|
| | Monitored primarily by Parkinson's disease specialist nurse 6 monthly at clinic. Appointments are arranged to coincide with daughters visits<br>Reports difficulty getting in and out of daughter's car when attending last clinic appointment<br>Complains of dry mouth due to diuretic treatment<br>Taking frequent sips of water through a straw<br>Experienced a number of episodes of coughing during subjective assessment |
| **PMH** | Osteoarthritis right hip<br>Left ventricular failure<br>Recurrent chest infections over past 12 months |
| **DH** | Sinemet (CR) – controlled release – medications are released over a 4–6-hour period to prevent fluctuations of levadopa levels<br>Ropinirole – dopamine agonist – just commenced as symptoms worsening. On low dose currently being closely monitored by specialist nurse, who is visiting at home every 2 weeks<br>Furosemide – diuretic used to treat heart failure<br>Coproxamol – to control pain from OA hip |
| **SH** | Lives in a two-storey house with bathroom and bedroom upstairs. Two hand rails fitted to stairs – reports no difficulties<br>No other aids/adaptations in situ<br>Lives with wife who has RA and osteoporosis, she is finding it increasingly difficult to support her husband<br>Retired HGV driver<br>No regular social activities due to difficulties experienced when leaving the house |

## Objective assessment

| | |
|---|---|
| **General** | Atrophy of quadriceps and gastroc's evident. Able to achieve knee extension in sitting, but with difficulty<br>Quads strength 4/5 on Oxford Scale |
| **Supported sitting** | Kyphotic sitting posture, with protracted and depressed shoulder girdles<br>Mask-like face and considerable pill rolling tremor. No other added movements noted<br>Sitting in deep armchair, with low seat height – feet raised on stool to prevent ankles swelling |

| | |
|---|---|
| | Difficulty adjusting position in sitting. Unable to initiate weight transfer to alter base of support. Chair cushion very soft contributing to difficulties |
| **Sit to stand** | Attempts made to stand independently, though unable to adjust position in chair to move forward to stand. Using upper limbs to push on arms of chair, while extending within trunk. Unable to bring centre of gravity forward over changing base of support to achieve stand<br>With facilitation and verbal prompts able to 'slide' forward in chair using upper limbs to initiate movement. Unable to achieve anterior pelvic tilt independently to allow lateral weight transfer to move forward in chair |
| **Mobility** | Mobilising independently, with festinant gait and slouched posture evident. Freezing noted at doorways. Patient reports this has been a difficulty for a number of years, which he overcomes by imagining a ticking clock, then transferring weight laterally in time with the clock<br>Climbs stairs independently with reciprocal gait pattern using stair rails for balance only. No apparent difficulties noted |
| **Bed mobility** | Experiencing marked difficulty rolling – initiates movement by reaching forward with right upper limb. Dining chair placed by the side of the bed, which patient reports he uses to pull on to assist with roll. No movement initiated at head or lower limbs<br>With verbal prompting able to move lower limbs into crook lying, turn head in direction of movement and reach upper limb across the body in the direction of movement. With light facilitation at the knees able to roll to left without difficulty. Patient reports concerns that his wife would be unable to offer this degree of support as she is in increasing levels of pain<br>In side lying able to drop feet over side of bed, though required assistance to push upper body into sitting position. Mattress very soft, offering little resistance to downward force needed to achieve this movement |

## Questions

1. What problems can be identified for this gentleman?
2. What treatment priorities would you establish?
3. Why does he not experience difficulties when climbing stairs?

4. What outcome measures may be appropriate to evaluate treatment intervention?
5. The gentleman experiences a number of episodes of coughing on taking drinks from a straw, along with a history of recurrent chest infections. What may this indicate and what action should you take?
6. Multidisciplinary/inter-professional management may be beneficial for this gentleman. What referrals might you make?
7. Are there any immediate actions you can take to address this family's current situation?

## CASE STUDY 11 GUILLAIN–BARRÉ SYNDROME

The following lady has been transferred to the rehabilitation unit for rehabilitation and discharge planning. She was diagnosed with Guillain–Barré syndrome (GBS) 8 weeks ago following giving birth to her daughter by caesarean section.

| | |
|---|---|
| PC | 34-year-old lady gave birth 8/52 ago by caesarean section<br>Good progress with recovery to date, transferring by stepping round with the assistance of two to maintain balance<br>Using a self-propelled wheelchair to increase independence in mobility on the ward<br>Keen to commence walking as soon as possible and to be discharged home to care for her daughter |
| HPC | On recovering from epidural complaining of tingling and weakness in both lower limbs, which progressed over the next few days<br>Weakness progressed to encompass all motor function in lower limbs and trunk, upper limbs were unaffected<br>Diagnosed with GBS 1 week later and due to decreased vital capacity transferred to the intensive care unit and ventilated<br>Weaned off ventilator support after 2/52 and transferred to medical ward<br>Physiotherapy initially focussed on respiratory care and maintaining range of movement in lower limbs as pain allowed<br>On medical ward regained sitting balance and began working in standing with therapists 1/52 ago |
| PMH | Normal pregnancy with no complications reported<br>In last 2/12 of pregnancy complained of low back pain and was receiving physiotherapy treatment at local health centre<br>Nil else of note |
| DH | Gabapentin |
| SH | Lives in a three-bedroom, semi-detached home with bedroom and bathroom upstairs. Toilet facilities are available downstairs |

Full-time housewife and mother to her two children (aged 3 and 8 weeks), husband works full-time

Husband currently off work and caring for the children, having support from family members to look after newborn daughter

Family have been very supportive and bring children in twice daily to spend time with their mother. They have been particularly concerned that lack of time spent with the newborn may affect bonding and have taken advice from the midwife

Previously fit and active, ran three times weekly with friends

## Objective assessment

| | |
|---|---|
| **Sitting** | Independent sitting balance in supported and unsupported sitting<br>Able to move outside base of support recruiting normal balance reactions<br>Carrying out personal care activities independently in sitting with support from occupational therapist for supervision only |
| **Lying to sitting** | Moving from lying to sitting independently utilising normal movement patterns, reports that occasionally requires some assistance towards the latter part of the day when fatigued, though this is becoming less frequent<br>Complains of discomfort at caesarean incision |
| **Sitting to standing** | Requires assistance from one<br>Positions self appropriately, pushing through upper limbs to initiate weight transfer forward over feet<br>Normal movement pattern displayed, needing assistance to maintain balance only |
| **Standing** | Able to transfer weight laterally with support from two to maintain balance<br>Able to step with support to maintain balance, no abnormal movement patterns noted |
| **Transfers** | Stepping round with assistance of two<br>Placing feet appropriately with verbal prompting<br>Reports limited sensation in lower limbs distal to the knee joint<br>Some weakness noted in hip extensors bilaterally, minimal facilitation and verbal prompting required to maintain hip extension in stance on weight-bearing leg |

| | |
|---|---|
| Gait | Has not yet attempted walking in treatment<br>Treatment sessions have been limited by pain in both lower limbs |
| Mobility | Using self-propelled wheelchair on ward |

### Questions

1. What is Guillain–Barré syndrome, what are the disease characteristics and causes?
2. How is Guillain–Barré syndrome diagnosed?
3. Why was the decision taken to ventilate this lady?
4. Why is she prescribed gabapentin?
5. What are the main problems identified at this time?
6. What would your treatment goals be?
7. How might these be addressed?
8. What psychological and sociological problems might present for this lady?

## CASE STUDY 12 MOTOR NEURONE DISEASE

The following lady has been referred by the consultant neurologist. She has recently been diagnosed with motor neurone disease (MND).



### Subjective assessment

| | |
|---|---|
| PC | 62-year-old lady recently complained of increased clumsiness. History of dropping objects and tripping leading to a number of falls<br>Wasting of intrinsic muscles, thenar and hypothenar eminences of the hands right > left<br>Noticeable foot drop on the right<br>Numerous neurological investigations completed<br>Consultant diagnosed MND 1/52 ago<br>Asked to see urgently due to deterioration in functional ability and a high number of falls |
| HPC | 6/12 history of tripping and falling, initially unreported to GP. Fall outdoors 4/12 ago – sustained a left colles fracture<br>While attending A&E, falls risk assessment completed – highlighted high number of falls<br>Full neurological assessment completed which identified deterioration of motor neurons<br>Referred to consultant neurologist for investigations and discharged home with plaster of paris in situ<br>While left upper limb immobilised, noticed increasing difficulty grasping objects with right hand. Realised that had been using both hands to grip objects more recently<br>Neurological investigations carried out have confirmed MND |

| | |
|---|---|
| | Due to initial presentation, the consultant has suggested the type of MND presenting is likely to be amyotrophic lateral sclerosis (ALS) with life expectancy suggested to be 2 years |
| **PMH** | MI – 4 years ago<br>CABG × 2–3 years ago |
| **DH** | No current drug management – has an appointment with consultant in 3/7 time to discuss medical management |
| **SH** | Lives alone in a large semi-detached home. Bedroom and bathroom facilities, with level access shower downstairs<br>Adaptations completed some years ago for use by husband who had suffered a CVA<br>Widowed 2 years ago<br>Two sons who live locally with their wives and children, sees on a regular basis<br>Member of local Women's Institute and local bowling club |

## Objective assessment

| | |
|---|---|
| **Gait** | Mobilising independently, reaching for furniture to provide support when walking – reports that this is since falling and sustaining colles fracture<br>High stepping gait<br>Increased base of support<br>No heel strike bilaterally<br>Decreased stride length<br>Not using stairs has moved to downstairs accommodation since fall 4/12 ago at the insistence of her sons<br>Not mobilising outdoors without the support of a family member. Family carries out all shopping |
| **Lower limbs** | All movements full range<br>Decreased strength dorsiflexors (Grade 4 Oxford Scale) right > left<br>Atrophy noted right tibialis anterior |
| **Upper limbs** | *Elbow*<br>■ Noticeable atrophy of biceps and triceps bilaterally<br>■ Full range flexion and extension available<br>■ Oxford Scale 4 right and left for flexion and extension<br>■ Fasciculation noted in right biceps<br>*Wrist*<br>■ Decreased active range of right wrist extension, full range passive movement available – good alignment noted in radius and ulnar |

CHAPTER SIX

**TABLE 6.2 GLENOHUMERAL JOINT ROM (√ = FULL RANGE OF MOVEMENT)**

| | Range of movement | | Muscle strength (Oxford Scale) | |
|---|---|---|---|---|
| **Glenohumeral Joint** | **L** | **R** | **L** | **R** |
| Flexion | 110° | 90° | 4 | 4 |
| Extension | √ | √ | 4 | 4 |
| Abduction | 90° | 80° | 4 | 4 |
| Adduction | √ | √ | 4 | 4 |
| Medial Rotation | √ | √ | 4 | 4 |
| Lateral Rotation | √ | √ | 4 | 4 |



**TABLE 6.3 SHOULDER GIRDLE ROM (√ = FULL RANGE OF MOVEMENT)**

| | Range of movement | | Muscle strength (Oxford Scale) | |
|---|---|---|---|---|
| **Shoulder girdle** | **L** | **R** | **L** | **R** |
| Protraction | √ | √ | 4 | 4 |
| Retraction | √ | √ | 4 | 4 |
| Elevation | ½ range | ½ range | 4 | 4 |
| Depression | √ | √ | 4 | 4 |

- All other wrist movements full range actively and passively, muscle strength decreased to Grade 4 Oxford Scale throughout

*Hands*

- Full range of movement available throughout – right and left
- Significant decrease in grip strength bilaterally – hand dynamometer not available at time of assessment
- Notable wasting of intrinics, thenar and hypothenar eminences bilaterally.

Functional assessment not completed as patient became very distressed and tearful. Further assessments to be completed on future appointments.

## Questions

1. What is MND and what is its clinical presentation?
2. What diagnostic tests may have been completed to aid the diagnosis of MND?
3. This lady has been diagnosed with amyotrophic lateral sclerosis (ALS) which is one form of the disease. Name each type and its characteristics. What leads to the diagnosis of each form of the disease?
4. What problem list would you formulate for this lady based on the assessment completed?
5. How would you prioritise these problems and why?
6. What other health professionals may be involved in the support of this lady?
7. An appointment has been made with the consultant to consider drug management. What is the likely drug regime which will be introduced for this lady?

## CASE STUDY 13 CEREBRAL PALSY

You have been asked to see this child by the speech and language therapist who is working with him. He has recently been experiencing increased difficulties with swallowing which the speech and language therapist feels are being influenced by poor postural control in sitting.



### Subjective assessment

**PC**
12-year-old boy, diagnosed with cerebral palsy (CP) at birth
Spastic quadriplegia with a mixture of spasticity and dyskinesia
Uses powered wheelchair for mobility
Parents and carers have had increasing difficulty in helping him to achieve a good sitting position for last 4/52
Windswept deformity of hips and pelvis appears more prevalent
Recent chest infection due to aspiration
Speech and language therapist currently monitoring swallowing difficulties and is concerned about posture in sitting and the effect of this on swallowing capability

---

**HPC**
Born prematurely at 32 weeks weighing 4 lb 6 oz
Transferred to a neonatal unit where he was ventilated for 4 days
Diagnosed with CP 4/52 after birth when concerns raised at failure to thrive
Physiotherapy involvement initially focussed on parental advice on handling to promote normal motor development
Modular seating was prescribed at 12 months of age, due to difficulties maintaining sitting. Has used adapted seating from

| | |
|---|---|
| | then onwards to promote upper limb function and social engagement<br>Difficulties experienced with feeding since birth, with prolonged mealtimes and high calorie supplements prescribed<br>Scoliosis evident in the lumbar region, with windswept hips and pelvis to the right<br>No dislocation or subluxation of hip experienced |
| PMH | Epilepsy |
| DH | Baclofen<br>Carbamazepine<br>Melatonin |
| SH | Lives with parents and older sister in a four-bedroom, semi-detached house. Extensive adaptations have been completed, including a ground-floor extension with bathroom and bedroom facilities. A ceiling track hoist is in situ and all doors have been widened to allow wheelchair access<br>Father works full-time as a dentist and mother returned to work part-time at a bank 5 years ago, having initially given up work to care for her son<br>Family are heavily involved with their son's care and carry out a stretching programme on a daily basis<br>Attends a mainstream high school, with a special educational needs unit and has a full-time learning support assistant (LSA)<br>Engages in schoolwork with the assistance of the LSA and is able to access the majority of the curriculum |

## Objective assessment

| | |
|---|---|
| Sitting | Seated in powered wheelchair with moulded seating<br>Poor alignment of hips and pelvis, with pelvis shifted forward in seat leading to sacral sitting<br>Attempts to reposition unsuccessful – unable to accept the base of support of the wheelchair<br>Ankle–foot orthoses in situ – maintaining good alignment and length in tendo-achilles<br>Windswept hips and pelvis to right<br>Slumped within trunk with difficulty maintaining extension at neck<br>Increased dyskinesia within upper limbs – patient reports that he has had some difficulty controlling powered wheelchair |

CHAPTER SIX

and has had to ask LSA to push his wheelchair at school for the past week

Further detailed assessment not conducted at this time – urgent appointment made at wheelchair service for review of moulded seating

Due to present difficulties noted with current special seating, a second appointment arranged for tomorrow to assess with standard power chair. Postural support to be trialled with cushioning until moulded seating review completed

Outcome of assessment and subsequent treatment plans discussed with mum, who agreed and will attend appointment tomorrow to ensure that seating arrangements are appropriate for family to implement

---

### Questions

1. What is cerebral palsy?
2. What is meant by the term spastic quadriplegia?
3. Why does the speech and language therapist feel that there is a link between poor sitting position and swallowing difficulty?
4. Modular seating was introduced at an early age for this child – what are the possible reasons for implementing specialist seating?
5. This patient's family play an active role in his treatment, implementing a daily stretching regime. Which muscle groups are most likely to be affected?
6. It is noted that the patient exhibits a windswept pelvis – special seating has been implemented to try to address this – are there any other forms of postural management available?



## ANSWERS TO CHAPTER 6: CASE STUDIES IN NEUROLOGICAL PHYSIOTHERAPY

### Case Study 1

1. The World Health Organization definition of stroke is 'a rapidly developed clinical sign of focal disturbance of cerebral function of presumed vascular origin and of more than 24 hours' duration' (Aho et al 1980).

2. Risk factors can be classified as major or minor (see Table 6.4). As a health care professional it constitutes professional responsibility to be mindful of risk factors, which may be evident in patient groups in contact with physiotherapy services for a range of conditions. Health promotion strategies should be implemented where appropriate to reduce risks of developing CVA.

| TABLE 6.4 RISK FACTORS FOR STROKE (WEINER & GOETZ 1994) | |
|---|---|
| **Major** | **Minor** |
| Hypertension<br>Raised cholesterol<br>Atherosclerosis<br>Diabetes mellitus<br>Cardiac disease<br>Smoking | Contraceptive pill<br>Excessive alcohol consumption<br>Physical inactivity<br>Obesity |



3. The middle cerebral artery supplies nearly all of the outer brain surface and most of the basal ganglia, along with the posterior and inferior internal capsule via the cortical and penetrating branches. Clinical features will depend on the size and severity of the lesion but could include:
   - Cortical sensory loss – basic modalities of pain sensation remain intact such as pain and light touch, but more complex mechanisms which require more extensive cortical processing such as texture and two-point discrimination can be affected
   - Dense contralateral hemiplegia – affecting upper and lower limbs, the trunk and face
   - Contralateral hemianopia – optic radiation can be affected
   - Visuospatial disturbances
   - Left sided neglect – patient perceives stimulus only from the unaffected side
   - Denial of symptoms.

   (Stokes 2004)

4. Thrombolytic treatment should be administered within 3 hours of onset of symptoms of CVA and only if the patient is within a specialist centre (National Clinical Guidelines for Stroke 2000). As the patient had been collapsed for a number of hours prior to discovery by his wife, treatment was not indicated. However, as haemorrhagic stroke was deemed unlikely due to clinical presentation and patient history. 300 mg aspirin was administered on admission to A&E in accordance with National Clinical Guideline for Stroke (2000).

5. The anatomy of the lung is such that the right bronchiole is oriented in a vertical position which allows a less restricted passage of substances into the right base than other lobes of the lung (Drake et al 2004). Aspiration following acute stroke is common and has been estimated to occur in one-third of acute stroke patients.

Decreased level of consciousness is recognised as one of the most important contributing clinical features leading to:

- a decrease in protective reflexes
- impaired functioning of the lower oesophageal sphincter and delayed gastric emptying
- worsening of the coordination of breathing and swallowing.

These three factors combine to predispose the individual to aspiration independent of the underlying disease (Dziewas et al 2003).

6. Acute phase stroke management should focus on three priorities:
   - Chest clearance and maintenance of respiration. Modified postural drainage positions for the right base should be employed as tolerated. During the acute phase of stroke care a primary aim of treatment is to minimise cerebral damage by avoiding hypoxia (Tyson & Nightingale 2004). Respiratory management is therefore of the highest priority in the acute phase of stroke management.
   - Positioning strategies to maximise recognition of left side and to avoid soft tissue adaptation (joints maintained in mid-range) – working in conjunction with nursing staff taking BP and oxygen saturations into account. In order to maximise the potential of rehabilitation interventions in the long term, prevention of soft tissue adaptation requires careful consideration in the acute phase. Poor management at this stage of recovery can lead to increased periods of rehabilitation as joint range of movement is recovered.
   - Passive/assisted limb movements to maintain joint range of movement.

7. A recent systematic review focussed on the effect of positioning in stroke patients. This suggested that there was strong evidence that body position did not affect oxygen saturations in patents without co-morbid respiratory problems. There was limited evidence to suggest that sitting upright had a beneficial effect, and lying had a negative effect on oxygen saturations in patients with co-morbid respiratory problems (Tyson & Nightingale 2004). Therefore for this gentleman it could be argued that due to the aspiration pneumonia present, he should primarily be positioned as upright as possible.

## Case Study 2

1. Hypertension can lead to a particular type of degeneration known as lipohyalinosis. This can result in necrotic lesions in the small arteries of the brain. As a result, the arterial walls weaken and collagen is laid down, thickening the walls of the arteries and therefore reducing the size of the lumen, increasing local pressure. It is suggested that this leads to the creation of micro aneurysms (MacDonald 2005).

2. The haematoma and surrounding oedema are reabsorbed. It is thought that recovery can be so significant as fewer neurones are destroyed than in severe ischaemic strokes (Stokes 2004).

3. Glenohumeral joint subluxation refers to the displacement of the humeral head from its alignment with the glenoid cavity (Edwards 2002).

4. Post stroke shoulder subluxation is a common complication that is thought to be irreversible without intervention (Zorowitz 2001). Physiotherapeutic intervention in the management of the subluxed shoulder is a subject which has undergone considerable research, with treatments ranging from supportive devices and strapping to electrical stimulation; trialled to try to restore alignment at the shoulder and ultimately functional ability. A number of reviews have been conducted to evaluate the increasing evidence base on this subject. A recent Cochrane review by Ada et al (2004) concluded that there is insufficient evidence to support the use of supportive devices such as wheelchair supports, slings and orthoses, however there was some evidence that strapping applied to the shoulder had some influence in delaying the onset of pain.

   Evaluation of the use of electrical stimulation (ES) has indicated that there may be some positive benefits, with reviews concluding that, although the evidence available from randomised controlled trials does not confirm or refute that ES reduces pain at the shoulder, there is some evidence to suggest improvements in passive humeral lateral rotation. It has been suggested that this could be due to the reduction of glenohumeral subluxation (Price & Pandyan 2000), suggesting the need for further research in this area. In a 6-month study evaluating recovery patterns of subluxed shoulders, authors concluded that reductions in shoulder subluxation may occur spontaneously only when significant motor recovery of the affected upper limb occurs (Zorowitz 2001).

   While a number of different treatment interventions are available, the most effective treatment option remains under debate. In clinical practice an eclectic approach is often adopted dependant on the resources and clinical skills available. Prevention of pain provides the main focus of intervention in the majority of cases with treatment interventions focussed on supporting the upper limb and maintaining alignment at the glenohumeral joint. This is most frequently achieved by positioning with the upper limb supported in sitting and lying through the use of pillows and/or supportive devices and by strapping applied to the glenohumeral joint.

5. As the main problem experienced for this patient is with regard to subluxation of the shoulder with increased tone distally, it is likely that there are some difficulties experienced with maintaining high

levels of personal hygiene in the hand. This could lead to deterioration in the condition of the skin in the palmar aspect of the hand. Nursing staff will often be involved in monitoring hygiene of this area. Joint working to address this issue could prove beneficial for the patient, with physiotherapy staff working with nursing team members to decrease tone in the upper limb to allow thorough hand hygiene while discussing the need for careful handling of the affected upper limb to avoid damaging structures at the glenohumeral joint. In this situation, considering how to convey important handling issues to the entire nursing team deserves some consideration. The most effective way of ensuring that all staff are familiar with appropriate handling and positioning may be to spend time with each of the team members reviewing handling and explaining the importance of good alignment. However, due to time constraints and large numbers of staff, alternative approaches may need to be considered, for example, positioning diagrams, photographs of the correct position, targeting key-workers and writing in the nursing notes. The most appropriate and successful method of establishing a cohesive approach to positioning and handling should be considered carefully in each individual care setting.



6. The importance of a collaborative approach to rehabilitation is a common theme within literature relating to neurological rehabilitation (Edwards 2002, Fawcus 2000, Plum & Morissey 2002, Stokes 2004). It is important to recognise the role of each member of the team in contributing to a patient's recovery:
   - *Occupational therapist* – assessment and management of participation in function, working with different model/frameworks of rehabilitation to maximise independence.
   - *Consultant* – neurosurgeon to monitor the initial haemorrhage.
   - *Consultant* – rehabilitation involved in the overall management of the patient, focussing on prevention of further complications. May consider botulinum toxin injections to treat increased tone at the wrist and hand should tissue viability become threatened.
   - *Orthotist* – splinting of the wrist and hand to prevent complications with tissue viability.

7. Motivational levels and attitude have been recognised as contributory factors in the process of recovery (Stokes 2004). It will therefore be important to consider collaborative goal setting with the patient appropriate to previous activities. There may be a sense of loss or grieving may be experienced, and involvement in ADL can have a significant impact on the motivation of patients to participate in therapy.

## Case Study 3

1. The ACA supplies the anterior three-quarters of the medial aspect of the frontal lobe, a parasagittal strip of cortex extending as far back as the occipital lobe and most of the corpus callosum.

   Clinical features of damage to the left ACA could include:

   - *Right monoplegia* – affecting the lower limb. The ACA supplies blood to the area of the motor homunculus responsible for the control of lower limb movement.
   - *Cortical sensory loss* – basic modalities of pain sensation remain intact such as pain and light touch, but more complex mechanisms which require more extensive cortical processing, such as texture and two-point discrimination, can be affected.
   - *Behavioural disturbance* – the frontal lobe contributes to many aspects of behaviour. Damage to the frontal lobe can result in complex behavioural difficulties which can have a significant impact on rehabilitation interventions. The frontal lobe can be associated with the following functions; impulse control, judgment, language production, working memory, motor function, problem solving, sexual behaviour, socialisation and spontaneity. This area also has an assistive role in planning, coordinating and controlling and in executing behaviour.
   - *Urinary incontinence.*

   (Stokes 2004)

2. A SAH is a type of haemorrhagic stroke characterised by bleeding into the subarachnoid space around the brain. The subarachnoid space is the space between the pia mater which covers the outer surface of the brain and the arachnoid mater. These two cerebral meninges form a protective covering around the brain which contains cerebrospinal fluid. A hemiplegia may be evident initially if blood erupts into the deep parts of the brain, though further neurological signs may become evident over the subsequent 2 weeks as blood vessels can go into spasm leading to secondary ischaemic brain damage (Stokes 2004). Seventy per cent of SAHs are as a result of a rupture of a cerebral aneurysm. A further 10% of cases are due to arteriovenous malformation. Traumatic head injury can also lead to SAH. The incidence of SAH in the UK is approximately 8 per 100 000 population (RCSE 2006). SAHs account for less than 5% of all strokes. It is estimated that up to 50% of patients suffering an aneurysmal SAH will either die or be left with serious disability. Without treatment approximately 25–30% of patients would rebleed within the first 4 weeks of the haemorrhage. Of these, approximately 70% would die (RCSE 2006).

3. As the risk of rebleed for aneurysmal haemorrhages has been established as a significant cause of concern (Hidjra et al 1988), with

25–30% of patients identified as re-bleeding within the first 4 weeks of haemorrhage and the high risk of death identified as a result of a re-bleed (RCSE 2006), surgical intervention is now the most common course of management for patient presenting with SAH.

4. Surgical treatment of SAH usually involves occlusion of the aneurysm by either surgical clipping or endovascular coiling to prevent re-bleeding. Clipping involves a craniotomy, locating and dissecting out the aneurysm neck and occluding this with a clip. With the endovascular coiling, a catheter is inserted into a blood vessel in the patient's groin and guided up within the blood vessels to the aneurysm fundus. Platinum coils are then packed into the aneurysm fundus through the catheter, until the aneurysm is obliterated (RCSE 2006). An international study published in 2002 evaluating the two different methods of surgical intervention concluded that for the types of patients in with ruptured intracranial aneurysms suitable for both treatments, endovascular coil treatment was significantly more likely to result in survival free of disability 1 year after the subarachnoid haemorrhage than surgical clipping (Molyneux et al 2002). Indeed, the results were so significant that patient recruitment for the trail was halted early in order for dissemination of results to take place as soon as possible.

5. An AFO would have some advantageous effects for this gentleman. It should be noted, however, that long-term use could hinder the recovery of dynamic stability at the ankle joint and therefore re-education of dynamic balance should be included as part of the rehabilitation programme. As this gentleman has decreased activity of tibialis anterior he has significant difficult in achieving a neutral position of the ankle joint during standing with the ankle maintaining plantarflexion during stance. This alters the ground reaction forces applied through the lower limb during standing and walking. Ground reaction forces without an AFO increase the tendancy of the knee to move toward hyperextension and the hip to maintain the retracted alignment. Provision of an ankle foot orthoses for stroke patients has been widely researched from a biomechanical perspective with patients reporting increased confidence while walking (de Witt et al 2004), decreased energy expenditure while walking (Danielsson & Sunnerhagen 2004) and increased speed in timed up and go test, stairs test and walking speed (de Witt et al 2004). However, no studies could be located that evaluated the effectiveness of AFOs on the rehabilitation of normal alignment in the lower limb when AFOs were used in the short term as an adjunct to treatment. It could be suggested that re-education of normal movement using an AFO could provide normal sensory feedback necessary for neuroplastic changes.

6. Resisted muscle strengthening in neurological rehabilitation has been avoided for a number of years due to the belief that it could lead to an increase in spasticity, increase associated reactions and adversely affect functional ability (Bobath 1990). However, research now suggests that resisted exercise does not worsen spasticity (Miller & Light 1997, Fowler et al 2001) for patients with mild to moderate spasticity when participating in short bursts of resisted muscle work. Further studies have supported this presentation when longer periods of resisted exercise were used (Sharp & Brouwer 1997). These findings would therefore support the argument for including specific strengthening exercises into this gentleman's rehabilitation programme. It may also be prudent to include a strengthening programme targeted specifically at the lower limb muscles which are found to be less active during stance, i.e. tibialis anterior, hamstrings and quadriceps, and the hip extensors.

## Case Study 4

1. On admission, presenting problems for this gentleman would be:
   a. compromised respiratory status, requiring ventilation. Risk of developing complications as a result of ventilation
   b. risk of increasing intra-cranial pressure
   c. risk of soft tissue adaptation.



2. Initial goals for this gentleman would be to monitor his respiratory status and prevent complications arising as a result of ventilation. Elective ventilation is sometimes undertaken with patients suffering from head injury to prevent secondary complications. Cell damage caused by injury to the skull causes the release of excitotoxic neurotransmitters. This leads to an excess of calcium in the cells of the brain causing cell death. Although damage caused by the initial injury and resultant cell death cannot be reversed, maintenance of oxygenation, blood pressure and intracranial pressure within normal limits can prevent secondary damage (Critchley 2004). NICE Clinical guidelines have been established for the management of head injuries and state that intubation and ventilation should be undertaken when a GCS of less than 8 is identified (NICE 2003). Ventilation allows the patients intracranial pressure to be controlled more effectively preventing further damage due to displacement of the structures of the brain.

   While respiratory management is of utmost importance, the risks associated with increased intracranial pressure dictate that any interventions with the patient must take this into account. Physiotherapists must therefore work closely with ICU nursing and medical staff to ensure that any treatments undertaken do not raise intracranial pressure. Physiotherapy management of the respiratory system may therefore be less aggressive than with other patients and may be more frequent, with short durations of input.

While in ICU the physiotherapist should also focus on the long-term rehabilitation needs of the patient. Prolonged periods of immobility and reduced muscle tone as a result of sedation can lead to significant changes in muscle length and joint range of movement. Maintenance of range of movement through effective positioning and moving limbs through passive ranges of movement is an important aspect of care. This may involve working alongside nursing staff to ensure positioning is appropriate over the 24-hour period and splinting may be introduced with the occupational therapist.

3. Passive movements are performed in order to reduce the risk of soft tissue adaptation and contractures occurring. However, certain positions may need to be avoided or implemented with care to avoid increasing intracranial pressure. Neck flexion and a dependent head position should be avoided. Passive movements of the lower limbs, particularly hip flexion can result in an increase in intra-thoracic pressure. This can lead to an increasing intracranial pressure and should therefore be implemented with care (Stokes 2004).

4. In the early stages of recovery from head injury, a significant increase in tone is often noted. This is often noted as weaning commences from a ventilator as sedation is reduced. A reduction in sedation allows the function of the brain to be demonstrated in motor terms (Stokes 2004).

5. In head injury, and with this patient in particular, there is marked increase to resistance across both extensor and flexor muscle groups. This arises when passive movements are performed slowly and presents throughout the range of movement. This type of resistance is known as 'lead-pipe'.

   Due to the distinct positions adopted by patients with rigidity as a result of damage to the brain, these are described by two specific terms, which can be associated with the area of damage in the brain causing the resultant increase in tone:

   - Decerebrate posturing – opisthotonus (increased tone, where head, neck and spine extend severely), clenched jaws, extended limbs. Occurs in acute and subacute brainstem disorders.
   - Decorticate posturing – flexion of the upper limbs and extension of the lower limbs. Occurs with lesions of the midbrain or above (Stokes 2004).

   Therefore the gentleman in the case study could be described as displaying decorticate posturing, which would indicate a lesion of the midbrain or above.

6. Increased tone could potentially lead to severe soft tissue adaptation and contractures which could restrict the rehabilitation potential of the patient. This gentleman is demonstrating decorticate posturing,

which includes plantarflexion at the ankles. This could lead to difficulties in achieving a suitable sitting position and impact on attempts to transfer and stand at a later date. It is therefore of high importance that focussed attempts to manage tone and maintain range of movement are implemented to maximise the potential of long-term rehabilitation.

7. It has been noted that the overall pattern of recovery of the head injured patient often leads to an overall pattern of low tone, with the initial high tone subsiding. Interventions should therefore be of short-term duration or be reversible to prevent further hindrance to a patient's rehabilitation (Stokes 2004).

   Suggested interventions may therefore focus on drug management, positioning and stretches where achievable. It has been argued that preventative casting can be used to prior to the development of rigid postures seen in head injured patients to maintain alignment and prevent development of postures which can lead to severe soft tissue adaptation (Edwards 2002). It is advisable to seek support of a colleague familiar with this intervention prior to implementation due to the risks to skin integrity associated with casting.



## Case Study 5

1. The problem list for this patient should include:
   a. Fear of falling
   b. Reduced muscle strength in right quadriceps, hip extensors and dorsiflexors
   c. Reduced stance phase on right lower limb
   d. Reduced balance mechanisms
   e. Self-reported general deconditioning.

2. All goals are largely inter-dependent for this lady, as they all rely on increasing strength and control of lower limb muscle groups to allow progression in other areas. Goals should always be negotiated with and agreed with the patient. In order to establish objective measures, it may be appropriate to establish goals in three distinct areas:
   a. To achieve 48 on Berg Balance scale in 6 weeks – this would reflect changes in fear of falling, ability to weight bear on right lower limb and balance mechanisms. As a raw score is achieved it may be appropriate to break this down further and select certain points on the Berg Balance where improvement should be achieved, for example turning 360° to right and left, where the patient displays highest levels of difficulty.
   b. To achieve Grade 5 Oxford Scale in right quadriceps, hip extensors and ankle dorsiflexors. It could be argued that, as the patient reports deconditioning generally and the Oxford Scale is largely

subjective in its measurement, a more objective measure should be used. If detailed assessment of strength were performed utilising specified weights and repetitions, more objective goals could be established using assessment data as a baseline.

c. To improve general fitness. General fitness was not measured at the time of assessment, it may be appropriate to consider formally assessing fitness to again provide a baseline. Determining levels of fitness may be difficult to establish without equipment and due to the presenting limitations in strength and balance demonstrated on assessment. It may be appropriate to utilise an outcome measure related to ability to perform daily activities; however, due to the significant recovery of this patient, a sensitive measure would have to be used to reflect her abilities. The Nottingham Health Profile (NHP) may be an appropriate measure to use with this lady, due to its wide-ranging focus which may also serve to identify other areas of concern. The NHP has been found to be reliable (Gompertz et al 1993) and valid in a number of different patient groups (Bowling 1997, Ebrahim et al 1986, Hilding et al 1997) and is widely used in health care.

3. The Berg Balance Scale was selected for use with this lady for a number of reasons. It takes approximately 5 minutes to complete, and covers a wide variety of balance tasks, therefore assisting the physiotherapist in identifying areas that need addressing during treatment. It has been found to be reliable (Berg et al 1995) and valid (Usuda et al 1998, Whitney et al 2003) and can be used at no cost to the site implementing it into its assessment battery. Copies can be downloaded at http://www.physicaltherapy.utoronto.ca/assetfactory.aspx?did=126

4. Measures of lower limb strength and general fitness are discussed in the answer to question two, though there are a number of different outcome measures which can be used to assess balance. Thorough evaluation of the available outcome measures is beyond the scope of this book; however, balance outcome measures that you may wish to research further include:
   a. Timed up and go test
   b. Rhomberg and Sharpened Rhomberg
   c. Elderly Mobility Scale
   d. Rivermead Mobility Index
   e. Falls Efficiency Scale
   f. Standing Balance Test.

5. Given the high level of recovery of this patient and her focus being one of exercise it would seem appropriate to introduce specific exercises to target strength, balance and general fitness. Initially a home programme of strengthening exercises designed to strengthen

both type I and type II muscle fibres, along with general fitness, would establish a level of ability whereby the patient will be able to participate in balance retraining exercises during treatment sessions more safely (for examples of treatment interventions for balance see case study 8: Multiple Sclerosis, Relapsing – Remitting).

6. Given the age of the patient, her recovery to date and the desire to return to social activities, it would seem prudent to suggest that rather than pursue a home-based exercise programme, involvement with the local exercise on prescription scheme may serve a more realistic means of maintaining long-term fitness and strength. Working alongside a local provision may allow a comprehensive staged programme to be established, which would also allow more objective measurement of strength and cardiovascular fitness. Returning to normal activities and promoting involvement in the community has been associated with the physiotherapists role in the rehabilitation of patients with head injury (Stokes 2004). It is important to recognise that rehabilitation is not just focussed on physical recovery but also on supporting patients to adjust to their impairments in long-term rehabilitation (Stokes 2004).



## Case Study 6

1. In a complete injury, functional outcome is more straightforward to predict than for incomplete lesions. This gentleman has a complete lesion to the spinal cord at C3, which would indicate that functional control below this level is not present, complete lesions are always bilateral, with both sides of the body affected equally. Nerve supply to the diaphragm originates from the cervical plexus, with origins from C3–C5 combining to form the phrenic nerve. Damage to the spinal cord above the origin of the phrenic nerve results in paralysis of the diaphragm, as nerve impulses can no longer be sent along this nerve (Drake et al 2004). As this gentleman has sustained damage above the origins of the phrenic nerve, there is no nerve supply to the diaphragm, therefore ventilatory support is indicated.

   Phrenic pacing can also be considered for patients with this level of injury. Diaphragm pacing is conducted with low frequency electrical stimulation at a slow repetition rate (mimicking respiratory rate) to condition the diaphragm muscle against fatigue and maintain it fatigue-free. Retrospective studies have suggested that response to phrenic nerve pacing can occur up to 1 year after initial injury and testing for suitability for treatment should be conducted at 3-monthly intervals (Oo et al 1999).

2. Patients with spinal cord injury can present with autonomic dysreflexia. This has been described as a dysfunction of the sympathetic nervous system, with symptoms including

bradycardia, hypertension, headache and sweating above the level of the lesion. These symptoms can arise as a result of any noxious stimulus including pain, bladder or rectal distension (Stokes 2004). This gentleman has presented with an episode of increasing blood pressure during assessment which could be associated with pain caused by moving joints which have been restricted due to increased tone and possible soft tissue adaptation. Hypertension as a result of autonomic dysreflexia can rise considerably, with cerebral haemorrhage identified as a risk (Stokes 2004), immediate treatment is indicated which includes sitting the patient upright, administering appropriate medications and identifying and treating the underlying cause (Consortium for spinal cord medicine 2001). When treating any patient with a spinal cord injury attention should be focussed on the possibility of autonomic dysreflexia and knowledge of the appropriate management strategy for the patient should be maintained.

3. As this gentleman presented with an episode of increasing blood pressure during assessment of joint range, care should be taken during treatment sessions to avoid interventions which induce noxious stimuli due to the risks associated with autonomic dysreflexia. Liaison with the nursing care team with regard to administration of pain medication prior to treatment intervention and with the GP or consultant with regard to baclofen treatment could contribute to minimising the noxious stimuli induced by treatment. Treatment should be progressed with caution with small movement working to slowly increase range of movement at end of available range. Treatment sessions should be short in duration and regular enough to ensure carryover of treatment between each session. Progress should be monitored regularly and treatment sessions modified as a result. Although an episode of increased blood pressure was experienced on this occasion, it should be noted that other causes could be identified therefore treatment could potentially be more aggressive, though caution should be applied at all times.

4. This patient has presented with increased tone following a period of illness and bed rest. While muscle tone is an integral part of movement and function, abnormally increased tone which negatively impacts on function must be addressed. Tone can increase as a result of noxious stimuli to the nervous system. As the patient has been unwell for a period of time and suffered an acute infection, it could be argued that this has had the resultant effect of increasing tone.

   It should be noted, however, that this may be incidental and plastic changes within the nervous system itself may have led to the increase in tone.

5. Goals for this gentleman should be focussed around functional aims. At present the main problems presenting are related to inability to adopt an appropriate sitting position which is interfering with social interaction and increased flexor tone with the upper limbs which could potentially cause problems in the long term with maintaining skin integrity. Short-term goals should address seating, for example: 'To be able to maintain an aligned posture in sitting for 30 minutes within 1 month' with more long-term goals focussed on achieving neutral alignment of the wrists and hands.

6. Due to the nature of care this gentleman is receiving a 24-hour approach to rehabilitation can be adopted. Goals should be addressed in collaboration with the nursing team by introducing a seating programme which may involve review by the wheelchair service. Once review of the seating has been completed it may be appropriate to introduce a seating programme, whereby the patient should be enabled to adopt a sitting posture for short periods before being hoisted back into bed. This should take place throughout the day and may begin with 15-minute periods, increasing as tolerance allows. Alignment of the upper limbs may be addressed through a similar programme whereby nursing staff implement a programme of stretching and, possibly, splinting supervised by the therapists involved. It may be appropriate to work alongside an occupational therapist to introduce a splinting programme. Should high tone persist despite these interventions, it may be appropriate to request a medication review by the patient's consultant in view of increasing anti-spasticity medication.



## Case Study 7

1. Spinal nerves T2–T11 are known as intercostal nerves as they do not enter into plexuses. These nerves are distributed directly to the structures which they innervate and pass in the intercostal spaces, therefore the effects of disruption of the spinal cord between T2 and T11 are more straightforward to establish than might be the case for levels where spinal nerves enter into plexuses.

   Dermatome distribution for T5 is at approximately the nipple line, therefore for this patient's sensation below this line is lost (Drake et al 2004). It is possible that motor control will remain in the back extensors (Stokes 2004), which would indicate that full wheelchair independence should be achieved. No motor control will be evident within the lower limbs.

2. Spinal cord injuries are classified as complete or incomplete based on assessment with the American Spinal Injuries Association (ASIA) Impairment scale (ASIA 1992) (an assessment document can be found at: http://www.asia-spinalinjury.org/publications/

2006_Classif_worksheet.pdf). Lesions are classed as incomplete if sensory or motor functions are detectable in the sacral segment S4–S5. (Sacral sensation includes perianal and deep anal sensation. Voluntary contraction of the anal sphincter muscle is used to demonstrate preserved muscle function.) Preservation of sacral sensation or motor activity can be a positive indicator of neurological recovery as it suggests that long tracts have been preserved through the level of the spinal cord injury.

Incomplete lesions are referred to clinically as syndromes or injuries, as patterns of symptoms present dependent on the anatomical area of the spinal cord injured. The five identified clinical syndromes are outlined briefly below:

*Central cord syndrome* – Occurs almost exclusively in the cervical region. Central cord syndrome indicates there is an injury to the central grey structures of the spinal cord and is most commonly seen in older patients with cervical spondylosis. Osteophytes, possible disc bulges and spondylitic joint changes and thickening of the ligamentum flavum all combine to compress the cord in the canal and can lead to compression of the cord. Central cervical tracts are predominantly affected. There is greater weakness in the upper limbs than in the lower limbs with preservation of sacral sensation.

*Brown–Sequard syndrome* – Caused by an injury to only half of the spinal cord. This results in motor loss on the same side as the lesion and sensory loss on the opposite side due to the crossing of the spinothalamic tract. This syndrome is very often associated with fairly normal bowel and bladder function and has a good prognosis in terms of return of ambulatory function (Johnston 2001).

*Anterior cord syndrome* – Also known as anterior spinal artery syndrome, refers to damage to the anterior spinal artery which originates from the vertebral arteries and basal artery at the base of the brain. It supplies the anterior two-thirds of the spinal cord to the upper thoracic region. There is complete loss of motor control below the lesion and loss of pain and temperature sensation due to the anatomical position of these tracts in the spinal cord. As the posterior columns are unaffected proprioception and vibration are unaffected.

*Conus medullaris syndrome* – Injury of the sacral cord and lumbar nerve roots within the neural canal. Bladder and bowel dysfunctions are usually present with bilateral lower limb impairment, though the extent of involvement of the lower limbs is variable.

*Cauda equina syndrome* – Flaccid paralysis of the lower limbs. The type of bladder and bowel impairment that results from such an injury depends on the level of the injury and can be problematic, particularly for women, who may have difficulty with urinary drainage and incontinence (Stokes 2004).

3. Problems identified for this patient are:
   - poor sitting balance
   - dependence in wheelchair mobility
   - dependence on one to two with transfers
   - requirement of assistance from one to self-catheterise
   - decreased strength in upper limbs
   - eagerness to be discharged
   - university course commencement in 2/12 time
   - decreased social activity.

4. Prioritisation should be given to improving sitting balance for this patient as all other goals are dependant on improvement in this area. While focus should be maintained on sitting balance, treatment programmes directed at achieving increased upper limb strength, independence in transfers and wheelchair mobility could also be structured to address the goal of improved sitting balance.

5. Long-term goals for this patient should focus on full independence within personal and domestic activities of daily living, vocational and social activities. The National Service Framework for Long Term Conditions (DoH 2005) sets out eleven standards with the aim of supporting people with long-term conditions to live as independently as possible. While all quality requirements need to be taken account of during this patient's rehabilitation, long-term rehabilitation in particular needs to reflect Quality Requirement 6, which aims to ensure that people with a long-term neurological condition are enabled to work or engage in alternative occupations (DoH 2005). For this patient this would include active efforts to support her in returning to university studies. As the patient has a desire to return home as soon as possible, long-term rehabilitation in the community would also have to be a focus of long-term treatment planning. This is in line with Quality Requirement 5 of the NSF for Long Term Conditions which aims to enable and support people with long-term neurological conditions to lead a full life in the community. Early liaison with community rehabilitation services to ensure continuity of care following discharge would be advised.



## Case Study 8

1. Multiple sclerosis is a chronic, inflammatory, demyelinating disease that affects the central nervous system (CNS). In the CNS some nerves are surrounded by oligodendrocytes known schwann cells. These organelles are known as myelin.

   Myelin is arranged along the length of a 'myelinated nerve' at regular intervals, with an exposed gap between each sheath known as the node of Ranvier. When an action potential is conducted along a myelinated axon the transfer of ions associated with conduction occurs primarily at the nodes of Ranvier, with the myelin sheath acting as an insulator to transfer of ions. This allows for 'saltatory' conduction, which allows the signal to spread rapidly from one node of Ranvier to the next.

MS is a disease in which the myelin degenerates. When myelin is lost, the insulation fails resulting in a loss of normal functioning of the axon. Myelin degeneration affects not only the myelin along nerve routes, but also demyelination in the cortex and deep grey matter nuclei, as well as diffuse injury of the normal-appearing white matter (Lassmann et al 2007). Grey matter atrophy is independent of the MS lesions and is associated with physical disability, fatigue and cognitive impairment in MS (Pirko et al 2007).

The cause of demyelination is largely unknown, though a greater understanding of the specific pathology has been described. It is understood that T cells (lymphocytes) play a key role in the development of MS. In a person with MS, T cells recognise healthy parts of the central nervous system as foreign and attack them as if they were an invading virus, triggering inflammatory processes. Normally the blood–brain barrier prevents the passage of antibodies through it, but in MS patients this is deficient, the inflammatory processes triggered by the T cells creates leaks in the blood–brain barrier activating macrophages and cytokines. This results in a perivascular inflammatory lesion that leads to tissue damage with the final result of demyelination. The intensity and duration of the attack determines the overall extent of the damage (Stokes 2004).

The oligodendrocytes that originally formed a myelin sheath cannot completely rebuild one destroyed by an acute episode of the disease. However, the brain can recruit stem cells, which migrate from other regions of the brain. These stem cells differentiate into mature oligodendrocytes, and rebuild the myelin sheath. New myelin sheaths are often not as effective as the original ones. Repeated attacks lead to successively fewer effective remyelinations, until a scar-like plaque is built up around the damaged axons.

2. Relapsing–remitting MS is characterised by a number of discreet attacks, followed by periods of remission, when the disease is not active. Recovery during these periods of remission is either complete or partial (Stokes 2004).

3. Diagnosis of MS can be difficult, with two clinically separate incidents of demyelination occurring at least 30 days apart usually required to determine the presence of the disease process (McDonald et al 2001).

Recent efforts to standardise the diagnosis of MS have been established with the publication of the McDonald criteria (McDonald et al 2001), which utilise a number of different procedures to establish the diagnosis:

- Clinically definite MS – Two separate episodes of neurologic symptoms characteristic of MS, with consistent abnormalities on physical examination.
- MRI of the brain and spine shows areas of demyelination as bright lesions. MRI can reveal lesions which occurred previously but produced no clinical symptoms and can therefore provide the evidence of chronicity needed for a definite diagnosis of MS.
- Cerebrospinal fluid (CSF) testing can provide evidence of chronic inflammation of the central nervous system. The CSF is tested for oligoclonal bands, which are immunoglobulins found in 85–95% of people with definite MS. Combined with MRI and clinical data, the presence of oligoclonal bands can help make a definite diagnosis of MS. CSF is collected by lumbar puncture.
- Visual evoked potentials (VEPs) and somatosensory evoked potentials (SEPs) can also be used to assist with diagnosis as stimulation of the optic nerves and sensory nerves can elicit a less active response in those with MS. Decreased activity on either test can reveal demyelination which may be otherwise asymptomatic. Along with other data, these exams can help find the widespread nerve involvement required for a definite diagnosis of MS.



4. Righting reactions are defined as 'automatic reactions that enable a person to assume the normal standing position and maintain stability when changing positions' (Barnes et al 1978 as cited in Shumway-Cook & Woollacott 2001). These can be further broken down into five discreet reactions that take place in order to maintain the orientation of the head in space and the orientation of the body in relation to the head and ground.

   The three righting reactions which interact to maintain orientation of the head in space are:

   - *optical righting reaction* – reflex orientation of the head using visual inputs
   - *labyrinthine righting reaction* – orientates the head into the vertical position in response to input from the vestibular system
   - *body-on-head righting reaction* – orientates the head in response to proprioceptive and tactile signals from the body in contact with a supporting surface.

   Two further reactions have been identified which keep the body orientated with respect to the head and the supporting surface, these are:

- *neck on body righting reaction* – orientated the body in response to sensory feedback from the cervical region of the spine
- *body-on-body righting reaction* – maintains orientation of the body with the supporting surface regardless of the position of the head.

The presence of these reactions is paramount in maintaining alignment and preventing disturbances in balance and ensuring that the body can adapt to challenges on balance without having to employ equilbrium reaction to 'save oneself'.

5. A rehabilitation programme addressing loss of righting reactions should aim to challenge those aspects of balance which pose a threat to maintenance of posture within activities of daily living. It can be argued that balance retraining should be focused on performance of ADLs to ensure performance is affected and that goals are concrete rather than abstract (Carr & Shepherd 1998).

   It has been suggested that initial treatment focus should remain on small excursions of the body mass, which can include:
   - Looking up at the ceiling
   - Turning to look behind
   - Reaching for objects – forwards, backwards and to either side – gradually moving objects further away as performance allows
   - Reaching down to the floor and differing heights (Carr & Shepherd 1998).

6. Progression of balance rehabilitation can include:
   - Changing the shape, size and texture of the base of support
   - Tasks to include increased flexion and extension of the lower limbs
   - Increasing the objects distance from the body
   - Increasing the objects weight
   - Increasing the size of the object so that both hands must be used
   - Increasing speed demands
   - Requiring a quick response – e.g. catching a ball (Carr & Shepherd 1998).

7. By law, patients are required to inform the DVLA of any medical conditions which may affect their ability to drive safely (DVLA 2006).

   A number of mobility centres are available nationwide which offer assessment and advice for people who have a medical condition or are recovering from illness or injury and are having difficulties driving, accessing or exiting a vehicle. They can provide assessment and advice on adaptation to overcome difficulties with vehicle control and advice on driving safely; details of nationwide centres can be found at www.mobility-centres.org.uk

## Case Study 9

1. There are four definable classifications of MS:

   *Benign MS*. One or two relapses, with a considerable period of time between them. Full recovery occurs with no continuing neurological deficit.

   *Relapsing–remitting MS*. This is characterised by a number of discrete attacks, followed by periods of remission, when the disease is not active. Recovery during these periods of remission is either complete or partial.

   *Secondary progressive MS*. This follows relapsing–remitting. Having begun with phases of remission, the disease enters a phase of progressive deterioration, with or without relapses. Deterioration continues even when no relapse has been identified.

   *Primary progressive MS*. No remission or noticeable exacerbation are evident, yet progressive neurological deficit occurs (Stokes 2004).

2. Each Trust will have its own moving and handling policy in place, assessments should follow the guidance outlined in these policies. Work-related musculoskeletal disorders in physiotherapists have recently been identified as a significant problem, with newly qualified staff identified as most at risk (Glover et al 2005). It is therefore imperative that full risk assessments are carried out in order to reduce the risk of injury.

   One frequently used risk assessment acronym used is TILE:

   T – Task – The individual task to be performed should be considered. It is important to note that transfers between different supporting surfaces can have a significant impact on ability to perform a transfer. For example, if a patient is moving from a soft, supportive surface, their tone may have been lowered by acceptance of this base of support. More energy and effort will therefore be required to recruit activity and raise the base level of tone in order to perform a task.

   I – Individual – The abilities of all those involved in a transfer should be taken into consideration. This includes the patient, and all staff members involved. Consideration may also need to be taken of different heights of those involved and transfers modified accordingly.

   L – Load – In this case the patient. It is important to recognise factors such as increased tone and ability of the patient alongside the more obvious weight of the patient. Lifting should not occur under any circumstances.

   E – Environment – This is of particular importance when working within a patient's home. In hospital environments, beds and other equipment is usually height adjustable, this is not often the case in the home environment. Due recognition of the height of surfaces, available space and floor coverings should be taken into account (Adapted from HSE 1992).

Moving and handling training is a mandatory component of employment within health care environments. It is always advisable to seek support from a more experienced member of staff if in any doubt with regard to moving and handling risk assessments.

3. 'Clinical trials have shown that all three interferon products reduce relapse frequency and severity in patients with relapsing–remitting MS and may also influence duration of relapse. The reduction in frequency amounts to about 30% on average, and is equivalent to approximately one relapse avoided every 2.5 years in people with relapsing–remitting MS. This reduction has been demonstrated for the first 2 years of therapy.

   The proposition that the beta-interferons have a positive effect beyond 2 years is supported by open-label studies. These longer-term studies have assessed the effectiveness of beta-interferon by comparing observed with expected levels of disease activity. For people who have taken the drug in studies for approximately 4 years, disease activity appears to be lower than might otherwise be expected from studies of the natural history of MS.

   One of the interferon products (Betaferon) has also been shown to reduce relapse frequency and severity in secondary progressive MS (SPMS). In a clinical trial in SPMS of another interferon product there was a difference from placebo in reduction of relapse frequency but this effect did not reach formal statistical significance' (NICE 2004).

   As this gentleman has secondary progressive MS, the evidence does not support its use in prevention of the progression of the disease process. NICE did not support its use with patients with MS; however, those patients who had been using the drug with positive benefit before publication of the initial guidance in 2002 were supported to continue its use.

4. Given the risks to staff members in terms of injury, banana board transfers can not be considered a safe form of moving and handling for this gentleman. The risks posed are not only to staff members however. Due to the difficulties experienced with this type of transfer, it could be argued that the patient is at risk of injury, particularly when fatigue levels are at their highest. Given these concerns it would be advisable to introduce a hoist into the home environment to allow safer transfers for both the patient and staff involved with assisting him.

   It is important to recognise, however, that considerable difficulty was noted in achieving lateral weight transfer in sitting. Ability to perform this movement, would allow for easier and safer positioning of a hoist sling. It may therefore be appropriate to commence a period of treatment aimed at addressing difficulties in trunk mobility, particularly lateral weight transfer in sitting.

5. The role of the physiotherapist in the care of a patient with MS will undoubtedly also involve providing psychological support. The decision to move to hoist transfers, removes a degree of independence for the patient and can signify for some a significant deterioration of functional ability. Consideration of the implication of recommending hoist transfers must be taken, working in partnership with the patient to identify the most appropriate and safe approach to adopt.

6. Botulinum toxin (Botox) has been used to treat focal spasticity in patients with MS, with positive effects identified (Simpson 1997). The use of this drug is becoming more widespread and its use may be considered with this patient, alongside a treatment programme to maximise the effects, which may include soft tissue mobilisations, stretching and splinting.

   It is worth noting, however, that the evidence base underpinning the use of Botox with patients with MS is a developing one, with a recent Cochrane review investigating the effects of a number of anti-spasticity agents in MS concluding that 'The absolute and comparative efficacy and tolerability of anti-spasticity agents in multiple sclerosis is poorly documented and no recommendations can be made to guide prescribing. The rationale for treating features of the upper motor neurone syndrome must be better understood and sensitive, validated spasticity measures need to be developed' (Shakespeare et al 2003).

7. Assessment of different transport options may be an important consideration for some patients. Advice with regard to contacting a local mobility centres may be appropriate in this case. They can provide assessment and advice on adaptation to overcome difficulties with vehicle control and advice on driving safely, details of nationwide centres can be found at www.mobility-centres.org.uk



## Case Study 10

1. • Reduced social activity as unable to access outdoor environments
   • Recurrent chest infections
   • Difficulties with transfers – sit to stand, bed mobility and lying to sitting
   • Reduced trunk mobility
   • Reduced strength in quadriceps
   • Kyphotic posture
   • Reduced independence in activities of daily living.

2. This gentleman has marked difficulties in carrying out transfers independently. As his wife and sole carer has medical problems of her own it would be of utmost importance that the primary aim of treatment would be to increase independence in transfers to reduce the strain placed upon her. Exercise to increase range of movement and flexibility have been identified as promoting increased flexibility and preventing secondary complications (Partridge 2002). For this gentleman exercise specifically focussed at increasing trunk flexibility should address a number of issues identified as problematic when attempting transfers independently. Specific strengthening exercises for the lower and upper limbs may also assist with the compensatory approaches he has adopted.

   Progression of the disease would indicate that the introduction of compensatory strategies to promote independence would be prudent (KNGF 2005).

3. The performance of automatic and repetitive movements in patients with Parkinsons disease is disturbed as a result of problems of internal control. This patient reports the use of cues to assist with overcoming problems experienced with 'freezing' when approaching doorways. Cues are stimuli either from the environment or generated by the patient which increase the patient's attention and facilitate automatic movement. It is suggested that cues allow a movement to be directly controlled by the cortex, with little or no involvement of basal ganglia (KNGF 2005). In some patients with Parkinson's disease it appears that the presence of stairs acts as an external cue which increases concentration and promotes automatic movement.

4. A number of outcome measures may be appropriate to evaluate the effectiveness of treatment intervention and provide some feedback to the patient to aid motivation:
   - Checklist for rating turning in bed (Ashburn et al 2001)
   - Timed up and go test (Podsilado & Richardson 1991)
   - Parkinson's Activity Scale (Nieuwboer et al 2000).

5. Urgent referral to a speech and language therapist should be made. Recurrent chest infections and coughing on drinking could indicate swallowing difficulties with possible aspiration. Discussion of your clinical reasoning underpinning this decision should be held with the patient to ensure permission is given to pursue a referral.

6. Referrals should be considered to:
   - speech and language therapy for assessment of swallowing function
   - occupational therapy for consideration of provision of aids to increase functional independence in activities of daily living, for example a bed lever to aid with rolling and chair raisers. Further

assessment of independence in activities of daily living may also be considered for example bathing
- wheelchair services for assessment of wheelchairs which may promote independence.

7. Due to the potential 'crisis' situation which the family are experiencing, it may be appropriate to discuss referral to a social worker for assessment for home care support. This may reduce anxieties faced by the family and reduce the pressure placed upon the patient's wife.

## Case Study 11

1. Guillain–Barré syndrome (GBS) or acute inflammatory demyelinating polyneuropathy is an acute, autoimmune disease that affects the peripheral nervous system and is usually triggered by an acute infectious process. Demyelination is the primary pathological process in GBS due to an immune response to foreign antigens (such as infectious agents or vaccines). The autoimmune response is directed to the tissues of the nervous system. This results in inflammation of myelin resulting in a decrease in nerve cell conduction (Stokes 2004). GBS predominantly affects the motor system, though sensory disturbance is reported in 42–75% of patients (Pentland & Donald 1994 as cited in Stokes 2004).

   The disease is characterised by weakness which initially affects the lower limbs progressing proximally. Initial symptoms are reported as weakness in the lower limbs often with associated numbness or tingling. Progression of the disease can occur, encompassing all muscle groups of the trunk, upper limbs and face. This is not always the case, however, with some patients experiencing weakness of the lower limbs only. Progression to 'peak disability' or nadir is within 4 weeks of onset to be classified as GBS, though deterioration can be rapid with some patients requiring ventilatory support within 48 hours (Pritchard 2006).

   Causes of GBS are the subject of considerable research. Two-thirds of cases are associated with an infection a few weeks before the onset of neurological symptoms. Suggestions of a causal link with medications, vaccines and malignancy have also been suggested, though these have not been supported in the literature (Pritchard 2006).

   Recovery generally begins within 1 month of nadir with the potential for full recovery high (Stokes 2004).

2. GBS, like many other neurological diseases, remains a clinical diagnosis with testing helping to exclude other causes and support the clinical diagnosis. Diagnosis is based upon a clinical presentation of flaccid paresis and areflexia (absence of reflexes), with nadir

reached within 4 weeks of onset. It can therefore be more difficult to diagnose GBS in the very early stages (Pritchard 2006).

3. 25% of GBS patients require ventilatory support during their illness. Progression of paralysis to include muscles of the trunk can affect respiratory muscles, therefore monitoring of vital capacity is crucial in patients presenting with progressive weakness. A decrease in vital capacity to <15 mL/kg or which is rapidly dropping is critical and therefore ventilatory support is required (Pritchard 2006). In these cases physiotherapy will focus on chest physiotherapy and maintenance of joint range of movement. Periarticular contractures have been reported as a major cause of residual disability (Soryal et al 1992 as cited in Stokes 2004). Focus on prevention in the acute phase is therefore imperative.

4. Pain is a significant feature of GBS, which can often pose a barrier to rehabilitation. It has been suggested that pain in GBS can be neuropathic as well as nociceptive in origin. Medications prescribed are often therefore focussed on treatment of pain of a neuropathic origin where traditional analgesics would have no effect. Gabapentin has been found to be effective in the management of neuropathic pain in patients with GBS with minimal side effects (Pandey et al 2002).

5. The main problems identified for this lady at the time of assessment are:
   - reduced distal sensation
   - pain
   - weakness in lower limbs bilaterally
   - reduced mobility
   - reduced balance in standing.

6. Goals for treatment should be agreed with the patient:
   - To be able to mobilise independently
   - To be able to reach outside base of support in standing, and react appropriately to threats to balance
   - To be able to perform all activities of daily living without restriction from pain
   - To be able to perform Grade 5 (Oxford Scale) muscle contractions in all muscle groups within the lower limbs bilaterally.

7. Within the limits of pain, a treatment programme should be established which can be followed over a 24-hour period to maximise the benefits of the rehabilitation process.

   An exercise programme focusing on lower limb strength should be introduced, with consideration taken of exercises to be performed with support/supervision of staff members and exercises to be performed independently.

As progress has been swift to date, assessment of mobility with assistance of the therapists should be undertaken as soon as possible, with the possibility of introducing a walking aid to maximise independence. Participation of all staff members should be sought to promote mobility wherever possible and reduce dependence on the wheelchair when mobilising on the ward. Monitoring of progress should be conducted on a regular basis to ensure walking aids are reviewed to support progress.

As pain has limited participation in rehabilitation to date, liaison with medical staff should take place with regard to medications. Treatment interventions should be organised to ensure they take place when pain medications have taken effect to maximise the potential of treatment interventions. Discussion with the patient with regard to practising mobility and strength exercises throughout the day as pain allows should ensure that progress can be made despite difficulties experienced with levels of pain.

Balance retraining will be an important aspect of treatment for this lady as she progresses. As she has two small children, the ability to respond to threats to balance and to maintain balance while picking up her children will be of utmost importance. Further discussion of the treatment interventions which may be appropriate can be found in the case study entitled 'Multiple Sclerosis – Relapsing–Remitting'.



8. Discharge planning for this lady will be complex due to the need for good physical recovery to enable her to fulfil her role as a housewife and mother to two small children. As she was unwell immediately following the birth of her baby she has been unable to care for her baby and fully develop the initial bond with her child. As she has been unwell she may also be concerned that her older child may have felt neglected. It will be important to discuss and recognise these issues as part of the rehabilitation process, encouraging the twice daily visits and planning treatment interventions around them. It may be appropriate to suggest a period of counselling or discussion of any problems encountered with the midwife who may be able to offer support.

## Case Study 12

1. MND is a progressive neurodegenerative disease that affects the motor neurones and can affect those in the brain, brain stem or spinal cord. It leads to progressive weakness and wasting of the muscles causing loss of mobility in the limbs and can also affect speech, swallowing and breathing.

Clinical presentation is dependent on the location of the lesions in each individual but can include spasticity, muscle wasting and fasciculation of the muscle. Reflexes may be diminished or brisk and weakness may be either flaccid or spastic. Sensory neurones remain intact, which means that those with MND continue to have full sensation throughout the course of their disease:

- The disease is more common in people over 40
- Those between 50 and 70 most likely to be affected
- Men are affected twice as often as women
- 100 000 people develop MND each year
- 7 in every 100 000 people are living with MND at any one time (Stokes 2004, NICE 2001).

2. Diagnosis of MND can prove difficult as there is no specific test which confirms the presence of the disease. This can lead to delays in diagnosis, which has been reported as taking more than 16 months from the initial presentation of symptoms in some cases (NICE 2001). Diagnosis is based upon clinical signs and symptoms originating from lesions in the brain and spinal cord at different levels (Brook et al 1988 as cited in Stokes 2004).

   Extensive investigations are commonly carried out in order to exclude other neurological causes for the presenting signs and symptoms (Stokes 2004).

3. There are three main types of motor neurone disease: amyotrophic lateral sclerosis (ALS), progressive bulbar palsy and progressive muscular atrophy:

   *ALS* – The most common of the three types of MND, accounting for approximately 65–85% of patients. Involvement of both the upper and lower motor neurone is noted. There may also be bulbar signs (which refers to speech and swallowing difficulties) along with emotional lability. Common upper motor neurone symptoms include spasticity and weakness, while lower motor neurone damage can present as muscle fasciculation, weakness and a reduction in tone.

   Initial presentation of ALS is insidious and can be associated with weakness in the hands, clumsiness and wasting of the thenar eminences or stumbling and foot drop (Stokes 2004, NICE 2001). Respiratory failure is the usual cause of death due to progressive wasting of the respiratory and bulbar muscles and occurs within 3 years of the onset of symptoms (NICE 2001).

   *Progressive bulbar palsy* – As the name suggests, this form of the disease mainly affects the bulbar muscles, with patients presenting with speech and swallowing difficulties. When the upper motor neurone is affected, patients present with spasticity of the tongue causing dysarthria. Nasal speech along with fasciculation, atrophy and reduced mobility of the tongue indicated lower motor neurone involvement (Stokes 2004). The limbs can show symptoms of weakness at later stages of the disease process, though due to the severity of symptoms of the bulbar region, respiratory failure often occurs early in the disease process. Life expectancy is between 6 months and 3 years from the onset of symptoms (MND association 2007). Affects approximately 25% of patients with MND (MND association 2007, Stokes 2004).

*Progressive muscular atrophy* – Affects approximately 10% of patients with MND and has a slower rate of progression with life expectancy of between 5 and 10 years and beyond (Stokes 2004). This form of the disease presents as affecting mainly the lower motor neurones initially, with symptoms within the upper limbs. Lower limb involvement can be noted, though bulbar symptoms are rare until the later stages of the disease process. Initial symptoms of this form of the disease present most frequently in men under the age of 50 (Stokes 2004).

Diagnosis is based upon clinical presentation, with no specific test available to confirm which form of the disease is active in each individual. A thorough case history can aid diagnosis, though it is important to note that symptoms rarely conform to those predominantly associated with one form of the disease.



4. The following problems can be identified from the initial assessment carried out with this lady:
   - Wasting of intrinsic muscles, thenar and hypothenar eminences of the hands right > left
   - Decreased grip strength
   - Noticeable foot drop on the right
   - Frequent falls
   - 'Furniture' walking
   - Reduced outdoor mobility
   - Reduced independence in domestic activities of daily living
   - Reduced muscle strength in upper and lower limbs (globally Grade 4 Oxford Scale)
   - Reduced active ROM; shoulder – flexion, abduction and elevation bilaterally and wrist extension on the right.

5. In collaboration with the patient, prioritisation of problems should occur. Due to the risk of injury due to falls, this should form the highest priority. This problem has close associated links with bilateral drop foot, indoor mobility issues and dependence in outdoor mobility.

As the lady lives alone, indoor mobility should be addressed as a high priority, though this may be concurrent with addressing the bilateral foot drop.

Decreased grip strength, wasting of muscles of the hand, decreased range of movement and dependence in domestic ADLs would form a second category of priority with a view to increasing independence once the risk of falls has been addressed. This would form the second grouping again due to the patient living alone. Difficulties with upper limb function could lead to injury when carrying out activities around the home environment.

Final consideration should be given to outdoor mobility as risks have been reduced in this area by increasing dependence on family members. It is likely that the most appropriate intervention in this instance would be to consider wheelchair provision. At such an early stage of diagnosis, introducing wheelchair use may not be advisable as it may cause some distress.

6. It is likely that a number of health professionals may be involved with this patient therefore a co-ordinated approach is imperative to ensure that the patient's wishes are taken into account and the patient remains at the core of all care interventions:

*Occupational therapist* – The patient has reported difficulties with activities of daily living. Dependent on her wishes focus may be initially on maximising independence to ensure changes to role are minimised. As the disease progresses alternative strategies may be considered in order to preserve strength and energy for social activities to ensure maximum quality of life throughout the disease. Regular reviews should take place working in collaboration with the OT to ensure that any strategies implemented in terms of mobility, movement and physical functioning work in conjunction with functional strategies' employed by the occupational therapist.

*Speech and language therapist* – If bulbar signs present, urgent involvement of the speech and language therapist is imperative. Collaboration may focus around ensuring familiarity with communication difficulties and strategies employed to ensure both consistency in approach and postural management which may be required to support interventions focussed on swallowing difficulties.

*Consultant* – Regular liaison with the medical professionals involved will ensure that the whole team is familiar with disease progression and any difficulties faced. If communication difficulties are experienced this may also reduce pressure on the patient when attending appointments with their consultant.

*GP* – regular review of medication and focus on monitoring disease progression and the involvement of other health professionals.

*MND association* – Family support workers supported by the MND association provide regular support and a point of contact for both the patient and their carers and the health professionals involved. Can also provide sources of funding for small pieces of equipment, equipment loan and education.

7. Guidelines published by NICE in 2001, and later reviewed in 2004 supported the use of Riluzole (rilutek) for the treatment of patients with ALS. This is the only drug currently licensed in the UK for the treatment of MND and is only recommended for the treatment of ALS. Riluzole works by inhibiting the release of glutamate which is thought to play an important role in the destruction of motor neurones in MND, thus reducing the progression of the disease process and extending life expectancy (NICE 2001).



## Case Study 13

1. CP has been defined as 'a persistent but not unchanging disorder of posture and movement, caused by damage to the developing nervous system, before or during birth or in the early months of infancy' (Griffiths & Clegg 1988). The term encompasses a wide number of clinical presentations where a non-progressing pathology of the immature brain results in disorders of motor function.

   The causes of CP are still open to debate, with the term cerebral palsy encompassing a wide-range of causative factors. Postnatally CP usually develops as a result of cerebral infection or infantile spasms. Causative factors before and during birth are more difficult to categorise. There has been a considerable increase in the rates of CP in infants of low and very low birth weight (Stokes 2004), with low birth weight accounting for nearly half of all cases of CP in industrial nations (Hagberg & Hagberg 1996, Pharoah & Cooke 1996 as cited in Stokes 2004).

   The risk of CP increases with multiple pregnancies. Stanley et al (2000) reported an increase in the risk of developing CP by 4.5 times for a twin and 18.2 times for triplets as compared to single pregnancies. Other causes have been recorded as birth asphyxia, damage prior to birth as a result of hypoxia, trauma, toxicity or infection.

2. As the term CP encompasses a wide range of clinical presentations, further classification is used to describe the type, severity and distribution of symptoms.

   The type of CP is described dependant on the most prevalent symptom and is classified as ataxic, dyskinetic, spastic or hypotonic. As with other neurological conditions, distribution is described using the terms hemiplegia, diplegia and quadriplegia. Severity is classified according to the Gross Motor Function Scale (GMSC) (Stokes 2004, Griffiths & Clegg 1988, Robinson & Robertson, 1998) a downloadable copy of the GMSC can be found at http://www.canchild.ca/Default.aspx?tabid=195

The patient described presents with spastic quadriplegia, he therefore has symptoms affecting all four limbs, with the most prevalent symptom of spasticity, though high levels of dyskinesia are also found within this classification. Patients with spastic quadriplegia are often at the severe end of disability, scoring 4 or 5 on the GMSC, requiring support to maintain seating postures and having difficulty with co-ordinated movement of the upper and lower limbs.

3. Children with CP often have decreased postural control which can have a considerable effect on their ability to swallow effectively. Abnormal muscle tone and dyskinesia influences control of the facial and bulbar muscles which can compromise chewing and swallowing. This can increase the risk of aspiration and subsequent chest infections (Redstone & West 2004).

   It has been noted that control of the facial and bulbar muscles is influenced by head control, which in turn is dependent upon trunk control. Pelvic stability is essential in achieving and maintaining alignment of the head and trunk. It is therefore suggested that any change in swallowing ability should be addressed from a holistic viewpoint, with all influencing factors addressed. Improvements in sitting posture should impact on swallowing ability as improvements are noted in head and trunk alignment.

4. A child with CP will not achieve normal development milestones, it is therefore important for the therapist to recognise when adaptive approaches are appropriate to ensure that a child continues development in as 'normal' a way as possible. This child was unable to achieve independent sitting balance at age 12 months, therefore interaction with the external world was limited. Encouraging engagement and sensory feedback are important aspects of neural development and adopting an aligned sitting posture enabled use of the upper limbs and social interaction. The use of the upper limb is essential for many functional tasks including reaching and grasping. Such movements can be difficult for children with CP (Gordon & Duff 1999), due to difficulty in co-ordinating muscular contractions to enable postural control, joint stabilisation and initiation of upper limb movement (Robinson & Robertson 1998). Correct postural alignment and stability have been associated with

improvements in the quality of voluntary arm movements (Hadders-Aldra et al 1999).

5. Musculoskeletal deformities are common to each type of CP the following problems have been identified as being widely associated with children with spastic quadriplegia: contractures of the hip flexors, hip adductors, hamstrings, internal rotators of the hip and tendo-achilles (Stokes 2004). Treatments to decrease tone and stretch these affected groups will aim to prevent deterioration in postural alignment.

6. A 24-hour approach to postural management has been recognised as an important aspect of care. Sleep systems can be used to aid postural alignment, though their implementation can prove complex due to the aggravation of co-morbid conditions (Stokes 2004). Research evaluating the effects of sleep systems to reduce hip subluxation highlighted the complexities of introducing a system, with just seven of the fourteen children completing the trial. However, results in those children were favourable (Hankinson & Morton 2002). Extensive discussion is beyond the scope of this case study, and it is suggested that further reading and training should be sought before trialling this intervention.



### References

Ada L, Foongchomcheay A, Canning C 2004 Supportive devices for preventing and treating shoulder subluxation after stroke. The Cochrane Database of Systematic Reviews 2007 Issue 2.

Aho K, Harmsen P, Hatono S 1980 Cerebrovascular disease in the community: results of a WHO collaborative study. Bull WHO 58:113–130.

American Spinal Injuries Association (ASIA) 1992 International Standards for Neurological and Functional Classification of Spinal Cord Injury. Chicago.

Ashburn A, Stack E, Dobson J 2001 Strategies used by people with Parkinson's disease when turning over in bed: associations with disease severity, fatigue, function and mood. Southampton Health and Rehabilitation Research Unit. University of Southampton.

Ballinger C, Ashburn A, Low J, Roderick P 1999 Unpacking the black box of therapy – a pilot study to describe occupational therapy and physiotherapy interventions for people with stroke. Clinical Rehabilitation 13:301–309.

Berg K Wood-Dauphine S, Williams J I 1995 The Balance Scale: reliability assessment for elderly residents and patients with an acute stroke. Scandinavian Journal of Rehabilitation Medicine 27:27-36.

Bobath B 1990 Adult Hemiplegia. Evaluation and Treatment, 3rd edn. Elsevier, London.

Bowling A 1997 Measuring health – a review of quality of life measurement scales. Open University Press.

Carr J, Shepherd R 1998 Neurological Rehabilitation. Optimizing Motor Performance. Butterworth Heinemann, Edinburgh.
Consortium for spinal cord medicine 2001 Acute Management of Autonomic Dysreflexia: Individuals with spinal cord injury presenting to healthcare facilities, 2nd edn. Available at http://www.pva.org/site/PageServer?pagename=pubs_generalpubs
Critchley G 2004 Assessment and Management of Head Injuries. Surgery 22(3):54–56.
Danielsson A, Sunnerhagen K S 2004 Energy expenditure in stroke subjects walking with carbon composite ankle foot orthosis. Journal of Rehabilitation Medicine 36(4):165–168.
Davidson I, Waters K 2000 Physiotherapists working with stroke patients. A national survey. Physiotherapy 86(2):69–80.
Department of Health (DoH) (2005) National Service Framework for Long Term Conditions. London: Crown Publcations. Available at http://www.dh.gov.uk/en/Publicationsandstatistics/Publications/PublicationsPolicyAndGuidance/DH_4105361
de Witt DCM, Buurke JH, Nijlant JMM et al 2004 The effect of an ankle-foot orthosis on walking ability in chronic stroke patients: a randomised controlled trial. Clinical Rehabilitation 18(5):550–557.
Drake R, Vogl W, Mitchell A 2004 Gray's Anatomy for Students. Churchill Livingstone, Edinburgh.
DVLA 2006 Medical Rules for Drivers available at www.dvla.gov.uk/medical.aspx
Dziewas P, Stögbauer F, Lüdemann P 2003 Risk Factors for Pneumonia in Patients With Acute Stroke. Stroke 34:38.
Ebrahim S, Barer D, Nouri F 1986 Use of the Nottingham Health Profile with patients after stroke. Journal of Epidemiology & Community Health 40:166–169.
Edwards S (ed) 2002 Neurological Physiotherapy: A Problem Solving Approach, 2nd edn. Churchill Livingstone, London.
Fawcus R (ed) 2000 Stroke Rehabilitation: A Collaborative Approach. Blackwell Scientific, Oxford.
Fowler E G, Ho T W, Nwinge A I 2001 The effects of quadriceps femoris muscle strengthening exercises on spasticity in children with cerebral palsy. Physical Therapy 81:1215–1223.
Glover W, McGregor A, Sullivan C, Hague J 2005 Work-related musculoskeletal disorders affecting members of the Chartered Society of Physiotherapy. Physiotherapy 91:138–147.
Gompertz P, Pound P, Ebrahim S 1993 The reliability of stroke outcomes measures. Clinical Rehabilitation 7:290–296.
Gordon A M, Duff S V 1999 Relation between clinical measures and fine manipulative control in children with hemiplegic cerebral palsy. Developmental Medicine & Child Neurology 41:486–591.
Griffiths M, Clegg M 1998 Cerebral Palsy: Problems and Practice. Souvenir Press, London.

Hadders-Algra M V, Fits I B M, Stremmelaar E F, Touwen B C L 1999 Development of postural adjustments during reaching of infants with CP. Developmental Medicine and Child Neurology 41:766–776.
Hankinson J, Morton R E 2002 Use of lying hip abduction system in children with cerebral palsy: a pilot study. Developmental Medicine and Child Neurology 44:77–180.
Health & Safety Executive (HSE) 1992 The Manual Handling Operations Regulations available at www.hse.gov.uk
Hidjra A, van Gijn J, Nagelkerke N, Vermeulen M, van Gevel H 1988 Prediction of delayed cerebral ischaemia, rebleeding and outcome after aneurismal subarachnoid haemorrhage. Stroke 19:1250–1256.
Hilding M B, Backbro B, Ryd L 1997 Quality of life after knee arthroplasty: a randomized study of 3 designs in 42 patients, compared after 4 years. Acta Orthopeadica Scandanavica 68(2):156–160.
Johnston L 2001 Human spinal cord injury: new and emerging approaches to treatment. Spinal Cord 39:609–613.
Koninklijk Nederlands Genootschap voor Fysiotherapie 2005 Guidelines for physical therapy in patients with Parkinson's disease available from http://www.cebp.nl/?NODE=69 date accessed 14/9/07.
Lassmann H, Bruck W, Lucchinetti CF 2007 The immunopathology of multiple sclerosis: an overview. Brain Pathology 17(2):210–218.
Lennon S 2003 Physiotherapy practice in stroke rehabilitation: a survey. Disability and Rehabilitation. 25(9):455–461.
Lennon S, Ashburn A 2000 The bobath concept in stroke rehabilitation: a focus group study of the experienced physiotherapists' perspective. Disability and Rehabilitation 22(15):665–674.
MacDonald R L 2005 Molecular Mediators of Haemorrhagic stroke. In: Freese A, Simeone F A, Leone P, Janson C (eds) Principles of Molecular Neurosurgery. Progress in Neurological Surgery. 18:377–412.
McDonald W I, Compston A, Edan G et al 2001 Recommended diagnostic criteria for multiple sclerosis: guidelines from the International Panel on the diagnosis of multiple sclerosis. Annals Neurology 50(1):121–127.
Miller G J T, Light K E 1997 Strength training in spastic hemiparesis: should it be avoided? Neurorehabilitation 9:17–28.
Molyneux A, Kerr R, Stratton I et al 2002 International Subarachnoid Aneurysm Trial (ISAT) of neurosurgical clipping versus endovascular coiling in 2143 patients with ruptured intracranial aneurysms: a randomised trial. Lancet 360(9342):1267–1274.
Motor Neurone Disease Association (2004). Standards of care. [online]. Available from: http://www.mndassociation.org/life_with_mnd/getting_more_information/publications/publications_1.html.
National Clinical Guidelines for Stroke 2000 Royal College of Physicians/ Chartered Society of Physiotherapy intercollegiate working party.
NICE (National Institute for Clinical Excellence) 2001 Guidance on the use of Riluzole (Rilutek) for the treatment of Motor Neurone Disease. London:NICE.

NICE (National Institute for Clinical Excellence) 2003 Head Injury Triage, assessment, investigation and early management of head injury in infants, children and adults. Oaktree Press, London.
NICE (National Institute for Clinical Excellence) 2004 Beta interferon and Glatiramer acetate for the treatment of multiple sclerosis. Oaktree Press, London.
Nieuwboer A., de Weerdt W, Dom R et al 2000 Development of an activity scale for individuals with advanced parkinson disease: reliability 'on-off' variability. Physical Therapy 80(11):1087–1096.
Oo T, Watt J W H, Soni B M, Sett P K 1999 Delayed diaphragm recovery in 12 patients afterhigh cervical spinal cord injury. A retrospective study of the diaphragm staus of 107 patients ventilate dafter acute spinal cord injury. Spinal Cord 37(2):117–122.
Pandey C K, Bose N, Garg G et al 2002 Gabapentin for the treatment of pain in Guillain–Barré syndrome: a double-blinded, placebo-controlled, crossover study. Anaesthesia and Analgesia 95(6):1719–1723.
Partridge C 2002 Neurological Physiotherapy: Evidence Based Case Reports. John Wiley & sons London.
Physical therapy asset factory (date unknown) Berg Balance Scale. Available at: www.physicaltherapy.utoronto.ca/assetfactory.aspx?did=126.
Pirko I, Lucchinetti C F, Sriram S, Bakshi R 2007 Gray matter involvement in multiple sclerosis. Neurology 68(9):628–629.
Plum H, Morissey D 2002 Cross-speciality collaboration. Physiotherapy 88:530–533.
Podsilado D, Richardson S 1991 The timed 'up and go': a test of basic functional ability for the frail elderly persons. Journal of the American Geriatrics Society 39:142–148.
Pomeroy V, Tallis R C 2002 Restoring movement and functional ability after stoke. Now and the future. Physiotherapy 88(1):3–17.
Price C I M, Pandyan A D 2000 Electrical stimulation for preventing and treating post stroke shoulder pain. The Cochrane Database of Systematic Reviews 2007 Issue 2.
Pritchard J 2006 What's new in Guillain-Barre syndrome? Practical Neurology 6:208–217.
Redstone F, West J 2004 The importance of postural control for feeding. Paediatric Nursing 30(2):97–100.
Robinson M J, Robertson D M 1998 Practical Paediatrics, 4th edn. Churchill Livingstone, Edinburgh.
Royal College of Surgeons of England (RCSE) 2006 National Study of Subarachnoid Haemorrhage. London: Royal College of Surgeons of England.
Shakespeare D T, Boqquild M, Young C 2003 Anti-spasticity agents for multiple sclerosis. Cochrane Database Systematic Review. Available at www.cochrane.org/reviews
Sharp S A, Brouwer B J 1997 Isokinetic strength training of the hemiparetic knee: effects on function and spasticity. Archives of Physical Medicine and Rehabilitation 78:1231–1236.

Shumway-Cook A, Woollacott M H 2001 Motor Control, Theory and Applications. Lippincott, Williams & Williams, Philadelphia.
Simpson D M 1997 Clinical trials in the use of botulinum toxin. Muscle & Nerve (supplement) 6:S169–175.
Stanley F, Blair E, Alberman E 2000 Cerebral Palsies: Epidemiology & Causal Pathways. Cambridge University Press Cambridge.
Stokes M (ed) 2004 Physical Management in Neurological Physiotherapy, 2nd edn. Churchill Livingstone, London.
Tyson S F, Nightingale P 2004 The effects of positioning on oxygen saturation in acute stroke: a systematic review. Clinical Rehabilitation 18:863–871.
Usuda S, Araya K, Umehara K et al 1998 Construct validity of functional balance scale in stroke inpatients. Journal of Physical Therapy Science 10:53–56.
Weiner W J, Goetz C G 1994 Neurology for the Non-Neurologist, 3rd edn. Lippincott, Williams & Williams, Philadelphia.
Whitney S, Wrisley D, Furman J, 2003 Concurrent validity of the Berg Balance Scale and the Dynamic Gait Index in people with vestibular dysfunction. Physiotherapy Research International 8(4):178–186.
Zorowitz R D 2001 Recovery patterns of shoulder subluxation after stroke: a six-month follow-up study. Topics in Stroke Rehabilitation 8(2):1–9.

# Case studies in orthopaedics

*Anne-Marie Hassenkamp, Diane Thomson, Sophia Mavraommatis, Kaye Walls*



## INTRODUCTION

Orthopaedics is a wide area of practice for physiotherapists and one which we encounter in most settings be it in a hospital (e.g. elective surgery, trauma or disease) or a community setting (e.g. post-operative, injury, secondary issues and long-term musculoskeletal problems). Due to the wide spectrum of orthopaedics the therapist is likely to encounter patients of all ages, from all backgrounds and with various health beliefs. Each one of these factors can have a huge influence on therapy management.

Excellent communication and team working skills are essential. The orthopaedic physiotherapist is an integral member of the multidisciplinary team (MDT) and works closely with surgeons. The clinical reasoning and problem-solving approaches used are directed by the medical intervention. Clearly, a good knowledge of what is a normal change and what is a pathological one is of paramount importance. Higgs & Titchen (2000) remind us that knowledge is an essential element for reasoning and decision making, and how both of these are considered central to clinical practice. The therapist working in these settings has to have excellent anatomical, physiological and pathological background knowledge within a framework of an understanding of the psychosocial influences on rehabilitation goals. Atkinson (2005) advises the adoption of the long published movement continuum (Cott et al 1995) as a good framework for orthopaedic reasoning. The changes from the person's preferred movement capacity (PMC) to their current one (CMC) is the orthopaedic physiotherapist's frame of reference. The process of getting from one to the other engages the therapist in educational as well as treatment situations which need the collaboration of the patient. Orthopaedic therapy goals therefore have to be patient-centred and collaborative rather than following a prescribed protocol.

This makes orthopaedic physiotherapy an ideal training ground in reasoning for the starting professional. The hypothetico-deductive reasoning model (Elstein et al 1978) adopted by junior physiotherapists is particularly well suited to this surgically directed arena as it stems from research in medical reasoning and hence mirrors that of the surgeon in charge of the patient. Pattern recognition (Higgs & Jones 2000) – a sign of the more expert professional – allows for a quick integration into the clinical puzzle of many different pieces virtually simultaneously. Orthopaedic practice is an ideal setting for physiotherapists to become more aware of and more secure in their cognitive skills as well as honing them to expert level.



## CASE STUDY 1 ROTATOR CUFF REPAIR

### Subjective assessment

**PC** 50-year-old female admitted for an arthroscopic left rotator cuff repair.

The indications for surgery are:

- large rotator cuff tear demonstrated by MRI
- pain interfering with work as unable to use arm effectively above 90°
- night pain waking her 2–3 times per night
- failed course of conservative treatment including cortisone injection (twice) and physiotherapy over last 4/12

---

**HPC** Intermittent shoulder pain for about 18/12

Aggravated by reaching, particularly if sustained or repeated

Patient felt excruciating pain while hanging curtains but worked through the pain for the rest of the day

Was unable to sleep that night due to severe pain

Attended A&E where X-ray showed no abnormality

She was referred for physiotherapy which has now been ongoing for several months to no effect

GP had given cortisone injections on two occasions which didn't help

Patient was then referred to an orthopaedic surgeon who organized an MRI and diagnosed a full thickness rotator cuff repair. She was listed for surgery

---

| | |
|---|---|
| SH | Self-employed curtain maker. Has employed help for the time she will be off work<br>Lives with husband<br>Smoker |

## Objective assessment

| | |
|---|---|
| Observation | Increased thoracic kyphosis in relaxed standing/sitting but is able to actively correct this to a reasonable level<br>Mild forward head posture and protracted shoulders which she can control<br>Cervical and thoracic movements appear fine |
| Pre-operative treatment aims | Teach bed exercises for circulation<br>Teach deep breathing exercises to maintain good chest expansion<br>Explain post-operative management and introduce post-operative precautions. This is done with her husband present and it is explained that he will need to help with the exercises post operation<br>Provide any written information sheets about post-operative care and discuss |
| Post-operative treatment aims (for 0–6 week period) | Monitor respiratory and circulatory status during immediate post-operative period<br>Protect healing of soft tissues. Maximum protection phase<br>Prevent negative effects of immobilization<br>Monitor and assist in pain control<br>Re-establish scapula stability<br>Encourage good posture<br>Arrange out patient/community physiotherapy as appropriate |
| 1st day post-surgery | Breathing exercises are checked looking for basal expansion and clearance of any sputum<br>Patient is mobilised out of bed as soon as able wearing a blow-up abduction pillow<br>She is taught:<br>■ scapular setting exercises in side lying and sitting, scapula protraction/retraction for proprioception. Full range of neck movements<br>■ passive external rotation to full range minus 20° for 3/52 in lying. Passive elevation to shoulder level for 3/52. Passive movements are preferably |

| | |
|---|---|
| | done by a family member or carer. This person will need to be taught this before patient is discharged<br>■ that at 3/52 both elevation and external rotation can be encouraged into full passive range both in lying and in sitting. Aim for full passive range soon after 6/52 post operation (Gibson 2007)<br>■ good postural alignment using a mirror in sitting and standing |
| After 6/52 | Start weaning from the immobilisation device and use her arm for light use at waist level<br>Increasing ROM in all directions including behind the back<br>Isometric internal and external rotation in neutral can be started to strengthen the cuff<br>Progression to resisted and anti-gravity exercises will be as stability and pain permit<br>Correct postural positioning is important throughout<br>Pain will be monitored and addressed by her GP if necessary |



## Questions

1. What are the rotator cuff muscles and what is their function?
2. The rotator cuff is said to be part of a force couple. What does this mean?
3. The causative mechanisms for rotator cuff disease are divided into intrinsic and extrinsic factors. What are these?
4. Why are we concerned about the scapula position for this patient?
5. Why does this patient need good postural advice?
6. What are the complications of rotator cuff repair and what can be done to minimise the impact of these?
7. What will be included in the discharge planning for this patient?
8. What is the expected long-term outcome for this shoulder?

## CASE STUDY 2 DECOMPRESSION/DISCECTOMY

### Subjective assessment

| | |
|---|---|
| PC | 36-year-old male architect presents with a prolapsed intervertebral disc (PIVD) and is booked for a spinal decompression (L4/5) the next morning.<br>The aims of surgery are to:<br>■ decrease pain<br>■ decompress the spinal nerve |

| | |
|---|---|
| | ■ improve dural mobility to prevent adverse neural tension<br>■ prevent or reduce neurological damage |
| HPC | History of recurrent back pain (but no leg pain) for many months with an insidious onset<br>7/52 ago, moved house and a few days later developed severe low back pain radiating into his right buttock and then, a few days later, into his right leg all the way down to his foot<br>He was convinced that rest would alleviate this very sharp pain<br>When this didn't help, he was offered conservative treatment which also did not improve matters<br>From thinking that he had a back strain he now started to worry that something quite serious was happening<br>He also developed numbness on the outside of his lower leg<br>A review with his consultant resulted in him being booked for surgery |

## Objective assessment

| | |
|---|---|
| **Investigations** | MRI – showed clear protrusion of L4/5 intervertebral disk onto the spinal nerve root and due to the worsening nature of his signs and symptoms it has been decided to decompress his lumbar spine |
| **Observation** | Patient has marked contralateral shift (away from his painful side)<br>Can only sit for a very brief time<br>Marked decrease in straight leg raise on the affected side<br>Abnormal gait pattern of a shortened stride length on the affected side |
| **Pre-operative treatment aims** | Teach him bed exercises for circulation, breathing exercises and log rolling in bed<br>Explain post-operative management and precautions<br>Provide written information of post-operative management<br>Fit him with a temporary lumbar corset |
| **Post-operative treatment** | Read operation report and check for any special instruction by surgeon |

| | |
|---|---|
| | Check wound if appropriate<br>Reduce anxiety<br>Identify and prevent any post-operative complications<br>Monitor and restore respiratory function<br>Check for any neurological abnormalities<br>Get patient mobilised in his corset once muscular control of quadriceps and gluteus maximus has been demonstrated<br>Educate patient regarding life after discharge:<br>a. Recognition and prevention of complications<br>b. Ergonomic advice<br>c. Self-managed home exercise programme especially core stability and neural stretches (Shacklock 2005)<br>d. Advice on home activities including sitting, driving, working<br>Enhance patient's self-efficacy in his body |
| **Discharge criteria** | Usually discharged after 2–4 days depending on surgical procedure, wound state, neurological and muscular control<br>Able to get dressed independently<br>Able to use the toilet independently<br>Sit for a minimum of 10 minutes<br>Able to manage stairs |



## Questions

1. What is a slipped disc?
2. What are the classic clinical features of a prolapsed intervertebral disc?
3. What is the differential diagnosis of prolapsed discs?
4. What red flag elicited in an examination of low back pain will need immediate action by a doctor?
5. Why is postural education and exercise important for this patient?
6. What psycho-social problems might influence this patient's treatment outcome?

## CASE STUDY 3 FRACTURED NECK OF FEMUR

### Subjective assessment

| | |
|---|---|
| PC | 65-year-old very slightly built woman admitted via A&E with fractured neck of femur on the right<br>Once the diagnosis has been confirmed by X-ray she is considered for total hip replacement (THR) |

| | |
|---|---|
| | The indications for surgery are:<br>■ reduction of fracture<br>■ reduction of pain<br>■ increase of function |
| **HPC** | Patient fell on uneven paving stones in the street and immediately realised that she had 'broken something'<br>Was in severe pain, unable to weight bear and had to be admitted to hospital by ambulance |
| **SH** | Lives alone, has a daughter in another city<br>Completely independent and is a retired archivist |

## Objective assessment

| | |
|---|---|
| **Observation** | Her right leg appeared shortened and in external rotation in the A&E department |
| **X-ray** | Confirms fractured neck of femur – Garden classification stage III |
| **Pre-operative physiotherapy aims** | Introduce yourself to patient<br>Find out about her anxieties<br>Explain post-operative regime while still in bed<br>Explain post-operative regime once she has been allowed to mobilise<br>Breathing exercises<br>Explain role of MDT |
| **Post-operative physiotherapy aims (rehabilitation starts on 1st day post surgery)** | Read operation report in notes and look for specific post-operative instructions by surgeon<br>Reduce patient's anxiety<br>Check for post-operative complications<br>Respiratory check and care as appropriate<br>Start with vascular function maintenance (foot and ankle pumps)<br>Introduce joint movement and muscle tone around the hip especially abduction and flexion, quadriceps and gluteus strength<br>Bed mobility (especially bridging for toilet purposes)<br>Keep abduction wedge when patient lies supine or lies on operated side<br>Education about 'do's and don'ts (focussing on joint preservation and weight bearing) |

| | |
|---|---|
| | Confer with MDT (especially social worker) regarding possible hurdles to discharge (remember, she lives alone)<br>Start mobilising with two crutches (usually by day 2–3 but check with medical colleagues)<br>Reduce walking aid support to one stick (usually by day 4)<br>Discharge usually by day 5 by which time she will need to be able to get in and out of bed on her own, sit to stand without help and manage to walk up and down a flight of stairs<br>Overall aim: to enhance patient's self-efficacy in her body |

## Questions

1. What is the Garden classification of fractured neck of femur and how does it influence surgical management?
2. Is it typical for a fall to result in such severe injury in an elderly person?
3. What are possible post-operative complications?
4. What actions should the patient avoid until 6 weeks post operatively?
5. How would you start and then progress muscle re-education?
6. What could you do to assist this patient with her possible anxiety?



## CASE STUDY 4 TOTAL KNEE ARTHROPLASTY/ REPLACEMENT

### Subjective assessment

| | |
|---|---|
| PC | 71-year-old female admitted for an elective right total knee arthroplasty/replacement (TKR). The indications for surgery are:<br>■ patello-femoral and tibia-femoral osteoarthritis demonstrated on X-ray<br>■ pain interfering with and day-to-day activities including walking<br>■ loss of right knee extension<br>■ night pain<br>■ failed course of conservative management and physiotherapy |
| HPC | Intermittent right knee pain and stiffness for at least 10 years but managed her pain with analgesia and rest<br>Past 2 years pain has become more constant, her standing and walking tolerance has decreased and she is experiencing night pain<br>The patient had one course of physiotherapy which included exercises, manual therapy and |

| | |
|---|---|
| | hydrotherapy. Therapy improved right knee extension but had no effect on pain<br>Patient was referred by GP to an orthopaedic consultant where X-ray showed patello-femoral and tibial-femoral osteoarthritis<br>The patient was offered an elective TKR |
| **PMH** | Nil of note |
| **SH** | Lives in a house with her husband who is fit and well<br>No downstairs toilet and she does all the cooking and cleaning<br>The patient is originally from Italy and still works in the family restaurant |

## Objective assessment

| | |
|---|---|
| **Gait/ observation** | Antalgic gait, predominately weight bearing on her left lower limb<br>Uses a stick on the right side<br>There is a slight right knee varus deformity and a palpable patello-femoral joint crepitus<br>There is no evidence of joint effusion or swelling |
| **Functional level** | Transfers independently in standing, sitting and supine positions<br>Step-to pattern up and down stairs leading with left lower limb |
| **ROM** | Right knee ROM between 10° and 100° flexion<br>All other peripheral upper and lower limb joints have normal range of movement |
| **Pre-operative treatment aims** | Teach bed exercises for circulation<br>Teach deep-breathing exercises<br>Explain post-operative management and introduce post-operative precautions<br>Record right knee range of movement in the medical notes<br>Teach patient to use appropriate walking aids correctly, including stairs<br>Provide any written information sheets about post-operative care and discuss |
| **Post-operative treatment aims (day 1 and 2 post surgery)** | Read surgeon's post-operative instructions regarding mobilisation<br>Discuss with the MDT the patient's health status and pain relief |

| | |
|---|---|
| | Assess bed exercises for circulation<br>Assess deep breathing exercises to maintain good chest expansion<br>Control post-operative knee joint swelling<br>Commence knee joint passive and active range of movement according to the surgeons protocol<br>Mobilize the patient according to the surgeons protocol for TKR |
| **Post-operative treatment aims (day 3 to discharge date)** | Discuss with patient and MDT the discharge goals<br>Assess post-operative knee joint swelling<br>Safe progression of all transfers between supine, sitting and standing<br>Gait education with the appropriate use of walking aids<br>Safe progression of stair mobility<br>Progress active range of knee movement to 0–90°<br>Assess the need of post-discharge physiotherapy?<br>Education of the patient to include:<br>a. Prevention of complications<br>b. Self-managed home exercise programme<br>c. Advice on home activity and gradual return to full independence<br>Continuous passive motion machines, slings and springs and sliding boards are often used to increase the range of movement of the operative knee<br>The discharge date is agreed when the patient can mobilise independently with or without walking aids, can mobilise on stairs independently and has achieved 90° degrees knee flexion |



## Questions

1. What are the short-term and long-term goals for this patient and how can the therapist plan the post-discharge rehabilitation programme?
2. What is osteoarthritis?
3. What are the clinical features of osteoarthritis?
4. What can be considered conservative management for knee joint osteoarthritis?
5. Give examples of different types of total knee prosthesis
6. What are the post-operative complications of total knee replacement?

# CASE STUDY 5 ANTERIOR CRUCIATE LIGAMENT RECONSTRUCTION

## Subjective assessment

| | |
|---|---|
| PC | 35-year-old male is admitted to the ward for an elective left knee anterior cruciate ligament reconstruction (ACLR).<br>The indications of surgery are:<br>■ left anterior cruciate ligament (ACL) rupture<br>■ patient is self-employed and he is not responding to conservative management |
| HPC | Patient injured his left knee 10/52 ago playing rugby when he fell forwards and sideways while the left foot remained fixed on the ground<br>He felt immediate pain and was unable to continue with the game<br>Pain and swelling increased over the next 2 hours<br>X-rays taken in A&E were negative for fractures<br>He was prescribed anti-inflammatories, referred to physiotherapy, given elbow crutches and advice on ice, rest and elevation<br>A clinic appointment to see an orthopaedic consultant was arranged<br>The patient had a physiotherapy assessment within 5/7 post injury and therapy focused on reduction of swelling and gentle mobility exercises<br>1/52 post injury the knee swelling had not reduced and the patient was still unable to weight bear on his left lower limb<br>Soft tissue injury was difficult to assess and an urgent MRI scan was arranged which showed rupture of the left ACL and a medial collateral ligament tear<br>The orthopaedic surgeon discussed conservative and surgical options and the patient consented to surgery as one of his main concerns was the physical requirements of his job and that he was self-employed |
| SH | Self-employed carpenter<br>Married with two young children<br>Plays rugby twice a week with friends and he is otherwise fit and well |

## Objective assessment

| | |
|---|---|
| Observation | Patient partially weight bearing with elbow crutches |

CHAPTER SEVEN

| | |
|---|---|
| | Slight muscle wasting of the left quadriceps muscles compared to the right lower limb<br>Tenderness, heat and some swelling of the left knee joint but the patellofemoral joint is visible and palpable |
| **ROM** | The patient has lost 5° of knee extension and has 100° flexion<br>Restricted by pain and swelling<br>Knee extension is most painful movement |
| **Special tests** | Anterior drawer test in 70° knee flexion = positive (anterior tibial displacement) approximately 2 cm) was not conclusive due to pain and swelling<br>Valgus stress instability was not conclusive due to pain and swelling<br>Active Lachmans' test was not assessed due to pain and swelling<br>All other peripheral joints were documented as normal |
| **Pre-operative treatment aims** | Discuss aims and surgery procedure<br>Explain that post-operative pain and swelling is a common presentation<br>Discuss immediate post-operative plan<br>Discuss and give written information of the post-operative protocol and rehabilitation programme<br>Teach immediate post-operative knee joint exercises including patellofemoral mobilisations to maintain range of movement<br>Teach safe mobilisation with elbow crutches |
| **Post-operative treatment aims (day 1 and 2 post surgery)** | Read surgeon's post-operative instructions regarding mobilisation<br>Minimise swelling with advice on rest, ice and elevation<br>Advise patient on the importance of adequate pain relief<br>Mobilise partially or fully weight bearing according to surgeon's protocol. Encourage normal gait pattern and safe mobility on stairs. Mobilise with cricket bat splint or brace depending on surgeon's protocol<br>Commence active range of movement as instructed by surgeon's protocol. Common protocols aim to achieve 0–90° of active range of movement by week 2 post surgery<br>Encourage resting position in knee joint extension<br>Plan discharge goals |

CHAPTER SEVEN

| | |
|---|---|
| **Discharge goals** | Reiterate ACL post-operative rehabilitation protocol and graft protection<br>Discuss the importance of a graduated rehabilitation regime and good muscle control<br>Discuss return to work according to surgeons protocol<br>Review home exercise programme<br>Review safe mobilisation on elbow crutches<br>Re-assure the patient that immediate post-surgical pain and swelling will gradually reduce<br>Arrange post-discharge out-patient physiotherapy appointment |

## Questions

1. What is the role of the cruciate ligaments in knee joint stability?
2. Describe common ACL mechanisms of injury.
3. Why is reconstruction using grafts preferable to repair of torn tissue? What type of grafts can be used in ACL reconstruction?
4. Considering your patient's profession what might be a better choice of graft for his ACL reconstruction?
5. The patient has post-operative pain and swelling and this is increasing his anxiety about his return to work. How can the therapist re-assure him and address this anxiety?
6. What is the clinical reasoning behind open and closed kinetic chain exercises in ACL reconstruction?

## CASE STUDY 6 FRACTURED TIBIA AND FIBULA

### Subjective assessment

| | |
|---|---|
| PC | 36-year-old male admitted via A&E for surgery after a motorbike accident a few hours earlier which resulted in several open transverse and crush fractures of his right tibia and fibula<br>He also has deep friction burns on his left side from sliding on the road surface |
| HPC | Patient suffered massive blood loss due to the open nature of his fractures<br>He was referred for immediate surgery<br>Pedal pulses were weak but present and it was therefore decided to use an internal fixator to pin his leg<br>After the surgery he was transferred to the high-dependency unit where his medical condition resulting from the blood loss can be monitored |
| SH | Self-employed motorcycle courier and a trained motorbike mechanic |

| | |
|---|---|
| | Lives with his partner and their three young children<br>Patient and partner juggle their work schedule so that both look after their children without outside help |
| **Post-operative aims** | Read the operation report and check for any special post-operative instructions<br>Check chest and start with breathing exercises<br>Re-assure patient and advise him on process of rehabilitation<br>Pain relief<br>Check wounds (do not forget the left side with the burns) and distal pulses<br>Advise patient on vascular exercises (e.g. foot and ankle pumps) for his left leg. No muscle contractions of his right lower leg yet as this may put strain on the bone ends<br>As the patient will be non-weight bearing when he mobilises he will need to work his upper body and non-operated leg to achieve the endurance needed for this high effort walking pattern |



## Questions

1. How are fractures classified?
2. What is an internal fixation?
3. What are the possible disadvantages of an ORIF?
4. What are the classic healing times for fractures?
5. What are the complications of fractures in general?
6. What model of rehabilitation and clinical reasoning might be useful for Mike?

## CASE STUDY 7 ACHILLES TENDON REPAIR

### Subjective assessment

| | |
|---|---|
| PC | 41-year-old male has undergone an Achilles tendon (TA) repair 1/7 ago. You have been asked to ensure that he is safe to go home today on crutches |
| HPC | He ruptured his TA (the first time) 5/12 ago<br>Treatment consisted of full leg plaster for 3/12 followed by out-patient physiotherapy<br>3/7 ago he was walking on level ground when it re-ruptured<br>Previous diagnosis had been Achilles tendinopathy |
| SH | Lawyer working in city and travels in by underground<br>Single and lives alone in first floor flat |

| | |
|---|---|
| | He plays squash at club level. Until 2 years before he had also been playing rugby at club level. From then till his TA ruptured first time he was refereeing rugby at least one game each weekend |

## Objective assessment

| | |
|---|---|
| **Observation** | Strong, fit looking man despite the long period of recent inactivity, with a below knee cast, the foot position being full plantar flexion<br>Able to easily lift cast in all directions, has full mobility<br>Circulation appeared normal |
| **Post-operative instructions** | Below knee cast with ankle in full plantar flexion 4/52, non-weight bearing<br>Cast changed to reposition the foot into neutral, i.e. the ankle is at right angles, for a further 2/52, and a walking cast applied for weight bearing<br>Cast removed 6/52 post surgery and out-patient physiotherapy to commence<br>(Dandy & Edwards 2003) |
| **Post-operative treatment aims** | ■ To be clear with post-operation instructions<br>■ To ensure safety with crutch walking on the flat and on stairs<br>■ To support the patient psychologically<br>Elbow crutches were supplied and fitted. Instructions for use were discussed and he was taken to the staircase for stair practice. No problems were encountered – balance, transfers and on ascending/descending the stairs. Throughout the session he revealed what an extremely difficult time he was having adapting to this long period of inactivity. This was discussed and the patient decided with help, that regular visits to the gym to work on upper body and contralateral leg (the unaffected leg) strength would give him some means of having control on this situation. He was deemed safe to go home and was discharged |

## Questions

1. What is a tendinopathy?
2. How is a TA rupture diagnosed?
3. What muscles make up the TA and what is their function?
4. What are the stages of healing and how do they apply to this tendon?

5. Describe the progressive changes you think occur in the normal gait pattern when using crutches.
6. What are the complications of poor crutch walking?
7. What exercise therapy will likely to be incorporated into his rehabilitation once his plaster has been removed?

## CASE STUDY 8 IDIOPATHIC SCOLIOSIS

### Subjective assessment

| | |
|---|---|
| PC | 15-year-old girl admitted with idiopathic scoliosis.<br>Scoliosis is thought to be progressing (Cobb angle 40°, Risser four)<br>Booked in for a single stage anterior fusion in 2/7<br>The aim of the surgery is:<br>■ to stabilise the spine<br>■ to prevent further deterioration<br>■ to correct the deformity |
| HPC | Change in patient's spine was noticed by her mother 6/12 ago<br>GP referred to consultant<br>Pre-admission 8/52 ago – stayed overnight, met the MDT<br>Postural advice with emphasis on symmetrical weight bearing was given<br>Investigations including new spinal X-rays and chest X-ray, blood tests, ECG and sleep studies were carried out |
| SH | Sitting GCSE exams at the end of year and very worried about having time off school<br>Used to play netball but lately finds it too difficult but would like to be able to play again<br>Not involved in other sport as she feels awkward |

### Objective assessment

| | |
|---|---|
| Observation | Right rib 'hump' (thoracic right convex) with right shoulder protracted and a prominence of the right hip, i.e. the trunk has shifted to the left<br>Curves well hidden under loose clothing |
| Leg length | Indicates a shortening of right leg |
| Neurological signs | Nil |
| Single leg stance | Difficult on both sides due to asymmetrical weight distribution |

| | |
|---|---|
| **Gait** | Normal |
| **Pre-operative treatment aims** | Respiratory assessment – record lung function in medical notes to ascertain pre-operative values<br>Explain post-operative management and introduce post-operative precautions<br>Provide any written information sheets about post-operative care and discuss |
| **Post-operative treatment aims** | Identify and prevent post-operative complications<br>Restore respiratory function<br>Restore active muscle control<br>Safe, functional rehabilitation and progression of mobility<br>Education of the patient to include:<br>a. ergonomic advice<br>b. prevention of complications<br>c. care of the thoracolumbar spinal orthoses (TLSO) brace or corset if applicable<br>d. advice for home activity |
| **Post operation** | Neurological assessment reveals nothing abnormal<br>Respiratory care – basal expansion and clearance of any sputum<br>Lung function tests are started and continued until the patient reaches 75% of pre-operative value<br>Upper and lower limb movements are restricted to protect the bone grafts<br>Assisted log rolling is taught<br>A temporary corset is fitted once the chest drain is removed to allow early mobilisation<br>This begins with inclined sitting, progressing to perch sitting then a transfer from bed to chair<br>Standing with support progresses to independent standing and walking as the patient tolerates. Post-operative X-ray before discharge requires five minutes standing tolerance<br>Plaster cast is fitted. Transfers, log rolling, balance and posture, safety on stairs are all checked<br>Care of the brace is discussed and she is advised regarding sport and exercise on discharge |

| | |
|---|---|
| **Discharge criteria** | Independently move from lying to perch sitting via log rolling<br>Sit comfortably for up to 20 minutes<br>Walk safely around the ward and up/downstairs<br>Have knowledge of ADLs and precautions for 6–18/12 at surgeons discretion<br>Independent with exercise programme, posture retraining and clear on paced progression of activity |

## Questions

1. What is idiopathic scoliosis and how does it occur?
2. What type of investigations may have been done over the last few years while monitoring this girl's progression of curve?
3. What possible post-operative complications may occur?
4. Why is postural education and exercise important for this patient even though she has had a fusion? How would you educate the patient?
5. What precautions regarding activity may be expected after this type of spinal surgery?
6. Who will be the members of the MDT involved with this young patient?
7. What are the psychosocial implications for this patient?



## CASE STUDY 9 LEGG–CALVÉ–PERTHES DISEASE

### Subjective assessment

| | |
|---|---|
| PC | 10-year-old boy admitted with Legg–Calvé–Perthes disease (known as Perthes' disease) involving right hip and classified using the lateral pillar classification as grade B. Booked in for a varus femoral osteotomy (through the upper femur) in 3/7.<br>The aim of surgery is:<br>■ to produce 'cover' for the head of the femur in the right hip joint<br>■ to improve hip function (improvement of ROM)<br>■ to reduce the pain |
| HPC | Previous year Tom's parents noticed he was limping and complaining of pain in his knee and inner thigh which worsened when playing football and improved on rest<br>He complained that he couldn't move his right hip to the same extent as his left<br>An X-ray was taken and Perthes' disease was confirmed |

| | |
|---|---|
| | Conservative treatment was attempted to contain the femoral head within the acetabulum. He wore a weight-bearing abduction orthosis which held the hip in an abducted and flexed position<br>This was unsuccessful and surgical intervention was indicated |
| **Patient's perception** | Wants to play football and volleyball again and take part in all the school's physical activities<br>Was frustrated with wearing the orthosis and is glad to be rid of it |

## Objective assessment

| | |
|---|---|
| **Observation** | Walks with a limp<br>Wasting of the quadriceps is observed with the thigh circumference less on the right compared to the left<br>The right leg length is also slightly shorter as well |
| **ROM** | Limitation of abduction and internal rotation of the right hip due to muscle spasm |
| **Roll test** | Patient supine, the right leg is then rolled into external and internal rotation (with the knee bent)<br>Positive result evokes guarding or spasm especially with internal rotation |
| **Pre-operative treatment aims** | Carry out respiratory assessment to ascertain pre-operative values<br>Teach bed exercises<br>Teach breathing exercises<br>Teach how to use crutches and partial weight bear<br>Explain (probably as a reminder) that he will be in a plaster cast/hip spica for approximately 6/52, although will be allowed home after a few days partial weight bearing<br>Goal planning |
| **Post-operative treatment aims (before removal of plaster)** | Check medical notes for operation report and post-operative instructions<br>Vascular exercises for the foot and ankle<br>Upper limb exercises for strength and proprioception to prepare for crutch walking efficiency<br>Abdominal and back extensor exercises<br>Teach partial weight bearing with crutches |

| | |
|---|---|
| **Immediately post-operatively** | Patient monitored for pain relief to ensure comfort, then mobilised<br>All the exercises are tailored to a 10-year-old young boy<br>He is taken down to the paediatric gym and collaboratively you engage him in throwing and catching a ball and modified basketball and skittles (in prone)<br>He lies on the floor in supine and prone and does sit ups and back extensor exercises (with weights to make it more fun)<br>Goals are devised and together you, the patient and his parents establish a home exercise programme which is age appropriate and fun<br>Patient is gradually helped to become accustomed to his crutches<br>Patient will be helped to learn to transfer unaided from bed to wheelchair |
| **Post-operative treatment goals (once plaster has been removed)** | Gain full ROM in right hip<br>Strengthening of right lower limb muscles<br>Standing balance exercises<br>Walking re-education |
| **Treatment** | After 6/52 patient is readmitted and the plaster bivalved<br>Over next few days the patient is facilitated to be able to move without plaster cast, gaining hip and knee joint ranges and increasing power<br>Active assisted exercises can be used initially<br>It was considered easier to exercise in side lying to reduce the effect of gravity (muscle power grade II)<br>Hydrotherapy exercised his leg and his respiratory system<br>Active exercises were commenced once grade 3 strength was achieved (Skinner 2005)<br>Contact sports such as volleyball and football were gradually introduced over many months as radiological results were good (refer to case study of fractured tibia and fibula for healing times) |

## Questions

1. What is Legg–Calvé–Perthes disease, what is its incidence and are there gender variations?
2. How is Perthes' disease classified?

3. Describe the surgical intervention mentioned in this case study – a varus femoral osteotomy.
4. Prior to surgery this treatment was treated conservatively, what are the options that can be tried?
5. Devise a post-operative exercise schedule that will sustain the patients motivation during the time he is in the plaster cast.

## CASE STUDY 10 SURGICAL INTERVENTION FOR CEREBRAL PALSY

### Subjective assessment

| | |
|---|---|
| PC | 4-year-old girl referred for gastrocnemius slide surgery as significant fixed contracture has developed despite conservative modalities having been attempted.<br>The aim of surgery is:<br>■ to lengthen the gastrocnemious muscle<br>■ to increase stability of the ankle<br>■ to allow for the wearing of an ankle foot orthosis<br>■ to give an opportunity to strengthen the weak muscles as a result of the improved range |
| HPC | Patient been diagnosed with cerebral palsy which has been further classified as hemiplegia<br>Patient was assessed in the gait analysis laboratory which revealed a pattern of equinus in her right foot<br>The ankle is in the plantar flexion range through most of the stance phase and a variable degree of drop foot in the swing phase<br>A significant fixed contracture has developed despite conservative modalities having been attempted resulting in impaired function of the ankle dorsiflexors, especially in the tibialis anterior muscle<br>Patient had previously worn hinged ankle-foot orthosis to stabilise and stretch the ankle, oppose the muscular imbalance and to lessen the muscular tone of the plantarflexors<br>Gait analysis indicated a gastrocnemius slide at the musculotendinous junction would allow a controlled slide<br>'Baker' procedure chosen which would lengthen the gastrocnemius aponeurosis (Borton et al 2001)<br>During her wait of 6/12 for the surgery the patient continued to have physiotherapy to prevent any deterioration in her contracture |

| | |
|---|---|
| **Parents' perceptions** | Patient was born at full-term weighing 3.5 kg after a normal pregnancy and prolonged labour<br>The umbilical cord was wrapped around her neck and her parents feel that the doctor and midwife didn't act quickly enough in the situation and now blame them for their daughter's condition<br>They are anxious and worried about their daughter's walking and running and are hoping the operation will enable her to keep up physically with her peers<br>They have also noticed she plays 'one-handed' and dressing has become increasingly more difficult for her |

## Objective assessment

| | |
|---|---|
| **Observation** | The patient's ability to communicate is assessed and in particular how she expresses pain<br>Has a fixed contracture and impaired function of the ankle dorsiflexors, especially in the tibialis anterior muscle |
| **Pre-operative treatment aims** | Respiratory assessment carried out to ascertain pre-operative values<br>Breathing exercises<br>Bed exercises<br>Exercises for the dorsiflexors and hip extensor muscles of the right leg<br>Education about the below knee cast and what would be expected afterwards<br>Harness the involvement of the parents |
| **Post-operative aims** | ■ Identify and prevent post-operation complications<br>■ Restore respiratory function<br>■ Monitor pain relief<br>■ Restore active muscle control<br>■ Implement functional rehabilitation<br>■ Education<br>Patient's mother stayed with her throughout her stay<br>Surgery was performed under a general anaesthetic with a local epidural block for pain relief following the surgery |

| | |
|---|---|
| **1st day post surgery** | Patient monitored and made comfortable<br>Given a below-knee cast and encouraged to sit over the side of the bed and to stand and bear weight on her legs |
| **2nd day post surgery** | Walked with assistance and was taken up and down the stairs<br>Exercises were begun as soon as possible post operatively |
| **Discharge criteria** | ■ Sit over the side of the bed<br>■ Stand and weight bear on her legs<br>■ Go up and down the stairs<br>■ Understand and do exercises with the assistance of parents<br>The patient returned 4/52 after surgery and the cast was removed. She was given a hinge ankle-foot orthosis to wear for a minimum of 6/12 |



### Questions

1. What do you understand by hemiplegia? What would you expect to see?
2. How would you respond to the parents understandable desire to know what caused their daughter's condition?
3. What is gait analysis and what is its purpose in this situation? How do you think it was carried out in a gait laboratory for this patient?
4. What interventions would be the most useful ones to carry out in the pre-operative period?
5. How would you elicit the patient and her parents co-operation?
6. Give a detailed account of the exercises you would do post operatively. Suggest how you would gain the patient's co-operation in performing the exercises.
7. What evidence is available to support the use of strength training in cerebral palsy?

## ANSWERS TO CHAPTER 7: CASE STUDIES IN ORTHOPAEDICS

### Case Study 1

1. See Table 7.1.
2. A force couple is defined as two forces of equal magnitude but in opposite direction that produce rotation on a body (Donatelli 1997). In this way the rotator cuff acts to dynamically stabilize the shoulder. They steady the head of the humerus, maintaining it in suitable apposition to the glenoid cavity and checking excessive translation.

| TABLE 7.1 THE ROTATOR CUFF MUSCLES (STANDRING 2005) | | |
|---|---|---|
| **Muscle** | **Action** | **Nerve supply** |
| Supraspinatus | Initiates abduction<br>Resists downward pull of humerus in neutral | Suprascapular nerve C5,6 |
| Infraspinatus | Lateral rotation<br>Downward stabiliser | Suprascapular nerve C5,6 |
| Teres Minor | Lateral rotation<br>Downward stabiliser | Lower scapular nerve C5,6,7 |
| Subscapularis | Medial rotation<br>Downward stabiliser | Upper and lower subscapular nerves C5,6 |

During the initial stages of abduction subscapularis, infraspinatus and teres minor counteract the strong upward pull of the deltoid, which would otherwise cause the humeral head to slide up. When the unloaded limb is hanging supraspinatous resists the tendency for the humerus to translate downward in the glenoid cavity (Standring 2005).



3. Refer to Bunker (2002).
   Intrinsic factors:
   - Occurs within the tendon
   - Degeneration and/or overload of the collagen fibres which may be acute/chronic, tensile/compressive and leads to mechanical damage at the insertion of supraspinatus
   - Said to increase with age (DePalma 1973)
   - If damage occurs at faster rate than can be repaired then there is a loss of centring of the humeral head on movement

   Extrinsic factors:
   - These are often secondary (Bunker 2002)
   - Mechanical compression between the bursal side of supraspinatus and the acromion
   - Hypertrophy of the coracoacromial ligament
   - Bony spur formation on the acromion

4. The scapula has an important role as it:
   - is a site for important muscle attachment including middle and lower trapezeii, rhomboids, serratus anterior, upper trapezius, levator scapula. These produce a stable scapula base which enhances the actions of other muscles attached to the scapula, e.g. rotator cuff
   - transfers large proximal forces generated from the lower limbs and trunk to distal segments of the shoulder and arm
   - works with the humerus in a co-ordinated manner to maximise the stabilising constraints around the glenohumeral joint

- has the ability to protract and retract around the thoracic wall. It also produces acromial elevation especially through the actions of serratus anterior and lower trapezius (Kibler 2000)

5. Poor posture over time may lead to increased thoracic kyphosis. Movement of the thoracic spine contributes to, and is essential for normal elevation of the arm. Regardless of age approximately 15° of thoracic extension is required for full bilateral arm elevation (Crawford & Jull 1993). With good thoracic position optimal scapular position can be achieved thus allowing optimal shoulder function.

6. The complications of rotator cuff repair are:
   - pain, therefore check analgesia, pacing and progression of exercises
   - stiffness from secondary capsulitis. May add 6 months to rehabilitation time. A manipulation under anaesthetic (MUA) may be indicated at a later stage if it continues
   - recurrence of tear while the repair is vulnerable. It is justification for caution at every stage and for progression to next stage of rehabilitation to be milestone driven, e.g. no anti-gravity work until there is good cuff control and the humeral head is 'snugging' in the glenoid fossa, rather than protocol or time driven (Rubin & Kibler 2002)
   - secondary impingement due to rotator cuff insufficiency. Cuff not strengthening as appropriate. May need to refer back to medical team

7. Before discharge the patient will need:
   - occupational therapy assessment of needs
   - out-patient physiotherapy supervision of exercises
   - follow-up appointment with relevant X-rays on arrival unless otherwise indicated
   - wound check at 1–2 weeks by district nurse

8. A good outcome may take as much as 12–18 months to achieve fully. Patient should report a relatively pain-free shoulder that facilitates light to moderate upper limb activity between waist height and shoulder level.



## Case Study 2

1. This is really an emotive and slightly misleading term as the disc (or for that matter anything else) does not slip. The tough fibres of the outer annulus fibrosus are organised in obliquely arranged lamellae (a bit like a corkscrew) which contain the much more liquid inner nucleus pulposus. Part of its make-up consists of proteoglycans which are able to imbibe 8.8 times their molecular weight in water

(McDevitt 1988), i.e. the nucleus is very big and juicy after rest (e.g. sleep) and then loses the liquid throughout the day as weight bearing continues (creep effect). This process occurs via the porous cartilaginous endplates. Through ageing processes or poor posture the annular fibres can weaken and finally develop concentric tears which can allow some nuclear material to ooze out onto the dorsal root and the spinal nerve (Adams et al 1986). Ninety per cent of protrusions involve L4/5 and L5/S1 (Dandy & Edwards 2003). The aim of surgery is to decompress the root or spinal nerve rather than to take the whole disc out.

2. - Disc prolapses rarely cause acute back pain as, for example, in an acute strain (Dandy & Edwards 2003). The back pain often experienced prior to a prolapse can be due to a discitis or an inflammation of the posterior apophyseal joints (facet joints). It could also be caused by a bulging of the flattened annulus into the posterior structures.
   - A disc prolapse often presses on a nerve root resulting in a sciatic scoliosis as the postural reflex tries to reduce pressure on the root (Dandy & Edwards 2003).
   - Tests which stretch the nerve are positive (e.g. SLR below 70°, slump test).
   - Loss of flexion – forward flexion can put more anterior pressure onto the nucleus displacing it posteriorly even more and increase the pain.
   - Changed neurology – must be carefully examined when ever there is a suspicion of a prolapsed disc: sensation (test the dermatomes), power (test the myotomes) and reflexes. Some reflexes are supplied by several roots (e.g. the knee jerk is supplied by L3, 4, 5) and hence may only be slightly diminished while the ankle jerk is only innervated by S1 and hence is either present or absent (Dandy & Edwards 2003).

3. Any root irritation and leg pain can be a sign of other conditions:
   a. Tumours within the spinal canal
   b. Neurofibromas in the root canal
   c. Intracranial tumour
   d. Ankylosing spondylitis
   e. Intrapelvic mass
   f. Osteoarthritis of the hip
   g. Spondylosis
   h. Vertebral tumours
   i. Tuberculosis
   j. Infective discitis
   k. Intermittent claudication (Dandy & Edwards 2003).

4. Cauda equina lesion: this can occur if the disc herniates in the midline (i.e. posteriorly rather than postero-laterally) and the signs and symptoms are (Dandy & Edwards 2003):
   a. painless retention of urine
   b. saddle anaesthesia
   c. bilateral sciatica
   d. spasm
   e. bizarre neurological deficit
   f. positive extensor plantar response (Greenhalgh et al 2006).

5. The double S-shape of the spine is made for dynamic loading and hence a flexible rather than rigid posture will be the easiest for the patient. For this he must have developed an excellent corset of muscles in the back, stomach and pelvis areas as well as the legs. Good mobility in both spine and hips is of paramount importance. The body is designed for strength as well as endurance so care needs to be taken to address both components in the programme. In an open surgical approach (in contrast to the more frequently used micro-disection one) the multifidus muscles may have been cut which may mean a lengthy recovery period in this important stabilising muscle. Ostelo et al (2003) found in their Cochrane review that an intensive exercise programme started after 4–6 weeks post surgery has a greater effect on early functional status and return to work than a mild exercise programme. However, there seemed to be no difference regarding efficacy between these two approaches when looking at long-term outcome.

6. Long-term pain is often the cause for disability. The fear of movement (Vlaeyen & Linton 2006) is a major stumbling block in the rehabilitation of patients and must be addressed. Cognitive-behavioural strategies (e.g. looking for evidence for firmly held beliefs; recognising unhelpful thoughts and trying to change these; linking feelings to thoughts and activity; socratic questioning, etc.) offer a well evaluated way forwards (Gifford 2006, Pincus et al 2002). The focus should be on allowing the patient to regain confidence in their body by using carefully gauged pacing activities and addressing coping strategies.



## Case Study 3

1. Garden (1961) classified all intracapsular fractures of the neck of femur into four stages. These rely upon appearance of the hip on an anterior–posterior X-ray.
   Stage I: incomplete fracture of the neck (abducted or impacted)
   Stage II: complete fracture without displacement

Stage III: complete fracture with partial displacement: fragments are still connected by posterior retinacular attachment; there is a malalignment of the femoral traberculae
Stage IV: complete fracture with complete displacement

Patients with fractures with a Garden classification I and II are often offered a dynamic hip screw rather than a THR while those with fracture classifications III and IV are usually routinely considered for THR.

2. Yes. This patient falls into the high risk group for osteoporosis on several counts: her age and gender (Marcus et al 2003) as well as her profession which requires low activity levels (Korpelainen et al 2004). She has also been described as lean, which is a body-type more associated with osteoporosis as identified by Korpelainen and colleagues (2004).

3. 
   - Infection is a major risk for any operation. A recent study put the risk for THR at about 2.233% (Ridgeway et al 2005). These authors stated that *Staphylococcus aureus* was identified to be responsible for about 50% of the incidence of infection. The risk was positively correlated with age, female gender, body mass index, trauma, duration of surgery and pre-operative stay.
   - Deep vein thrombosis might necessitate a blood thinning medication and pulmonary embolism can occur and show itself in severe respiratory problems.
   - Bleeding can be problem after any kind of surgery resulting in either external loss of blood or a haematoma slowing down the healing processes as well as the start of rehabilitation.
   - Dislocation.
   - Respiratory complications.

4. Antero-lateral or true lateral incision – excessive extension, external rotation and adduction must be avoided and certainly a combination of all three.

   Postero-lateral incision – excessive flexion, internal rotation and adduction needs to be avoided (Coutts 2005a).

   In functional terms this means that the patient should avoid (Coutts 2005a):
   a. sitting on low chairs (<53 cm in height)
   b. bending forwards
   c. crossing legs in sitting or lying (use pillow in between legs)
   d. twisting legs in sitting or lying
   e. driving
   f. running or jumping
   g. contact sports (if that is an issue for this patient).

CHAPTER SEVEN

5. Programme should target the hip abductors, extensors, rotators, flexors, quadriceps and hamstrings:
   - Often these muscle groups will be very weak after a hip trauma resulting in a THR.
   - It is important to ensure the exercises are executed in the neutral hip position (check for compensatory movements, e.g. quadratus lumborum hitching the pelvis on the affected side or abdominal activity on the affected side).
   - Start with low-level programme as endurance is usually severely reduced.
   - Once a grade II has been achieved in the neutral hip position, isometric activity of the hip rotators, extensors and abductors can be started in some flexion.
   - Usually, improvement is quick and patients achieve grade III by the end of a few days (Coutts 2005a).
   - When exercising in standing ensure that the pelvis is level at all times to ensure that the correct muscle is being exercised.
   - Once a muscle has achieved a grade III it can be strengthened by free active exercise rather than by active-assisted ones (Everett 2005).
   - The need for intensive physical training after a fall cannot be emphasised enough (Hauer 2002) (see chapter 9, case study one for factors to consider following fall).

6. As a physiotherapist the following suggestions are part of your immediate practice:
   a. Relaxation techniques (e.g. breathing techniques or progressive muscular contractions)
   b. Collaborative goal planning
   c. Education/information giving re: pain, biomechanics, healing timetable
   d. Help patient to deal with the cause of stress.

   Assist patient in problem solving (describe problem, what are the options, evaluate alternatives, choose the best and make a plan) (Nicholas et al 2000).

## Case Study 4

1. The aim of a TKR is to enable to patient to reduce pain and improve function. Goals will include:

   *Short term* – be independent at home, be able to do the house work, cooking and walk to the local shops.

   *Long term* – return to work at the family restaurant.

   For the past 2 years the patient's activity level has decreased. Her rehabilitation should incorporate gait re-education and a graduated exercise programme so she is able to increase her level of fitness. It is important that the patient does not go back doing too much too soon and advice on pacing is very important at this stage.

2. Osteoarthritis is a chronic, degenerative disorder characterised by the gradual loss of articular cartilage. Inflammation is secondary to the disease rather than the cause. The cause of osteoarthritis is unknown and it is a heterogeneous group of diseases characterised by an adaptive response of synovial joints to a variety of environmental, genetic and biomechanical stresses (Haq et al 2000).

   Primary osteoarthritis can be localised or generalised and is commonly found in women in the Western world during the 5th and 6th decades (Murray & Lopez 1996).

   Secondary osteoarthritis has an underlying cause, such as trauma, obesity and inflammatory arthritis (Dandy & Edwards 2003).

3. 
   - Age 50 and above.
   - Pain and stiffness in the affected joints which is exacerbated with activity and relieved by rest.
   - Pain worse when the disease affects weight-bearing, lower limb joints.
   - Loss of function and joint range of movement, tenderness and crepitus on movement are common features (Haq et al 2000).
   - Joint swelling can be present and may be due to an effusion caused by synovial fluid accumulations.
   - Systemic symptoms are absent.

4. Conservative management includes:
   - Patient education on osteoarthritis and re-assurance.
   - Weight-loss and moderate exercise can improve pain and function and should be part of the patient's self-management plan (Messier et al 2004).
   - Appropriate footwear, home adaptations and walking aids can decrease the mechanical stresses on weight-bearing joints and may reduce joint pain.
   - Analgesia 'such as' paracetamol and non-steroidal anti-inflammatory medication (Courtney & Doherty 2002).
   - Intra-articular corticosteroids injections can reduce intra-articular inflammation but do not change the underlying pathology (Dandy & Edwards 2003).

5. *Uni-compartmental prosthesis* – used to replace the medial or lateral compartment when the other is healthy.

   *Total knee prostheses* – replace both the medial and lateral compartments and often involve the patellofemoral joint.

   *Unconstrained prostheses* – resurfaces joint, does not contribute to the stability of the joint and should be used when the ligaments are intact.

*Semi-constrained prostheses* – contribute to joint stability through the shape of the prostheses and replace the whole of both joint surfaces and patella.

*Fully constrained prostheses* – use a hinge to provide mechanical stability to a joint (Figure 7.1). This type of prosthesis is difficult to replace in cases of infection or loosening (Dandy & Edwards 2003).

6. • Substantial risk of developing *deep vein thrombosis* (DVT) and *pulmonary embolism* (PE) (Stulberg et al 1984). Patients with a previous medical history of thromboembolic disease and prolonged bed rest are considered high risk. Antithrombotic drugs, intermittent pneumatic compression of the foot (foot pumps) and early post-operative mobilisation reduce the risk of DVT and PE.
   • *Infection* is a serious post-operative complication. Infection prior to surgery, obesity, smoking, diabetes mellitus, poor nutrition and immunosuppressive therapy are factors that can increase the risk of infection post operatively (Peersman et al 2001). The difficulties treating infection can be considerable and the treatment must be carefully planned. Management includes antibiotic suppression, debridement with retention of the prosthesis, resection arthroplasty, arthrodesis, reimplantation of a prosthesis and amputation in rare situations (Leone & Hansen 2005).



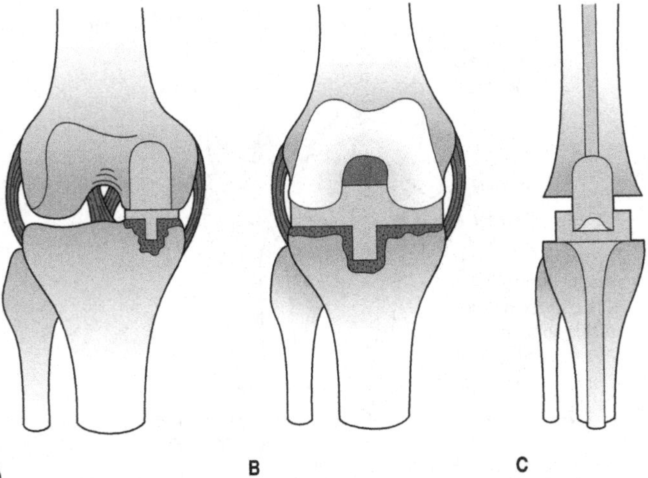


**FIGURE 7.1** Types of total knee replacement. (A) Unicompartmental. (B) Unconstraint TKR. (C) Constraint using TKR. Reproduced from Atkinson K et al (2005) with permission from the publisher.

- *Loosening* of the prosthesis can be caused by infection, faulty prosthetic design, inaccurate bone shaping and placement of the implant, poor bone quality found.

## Case Study 5

1. The anterior and posterior cruciate ligaments (PCL) ensure the anteroposterior stability of the knee by providing the restraint to anterior and posterior displacements of the tibia with respect to the femur (Figure 7.2). The ACL provides approximately 86% of the resistance to anterior displacement and the PCL about 94% of the resistance to posterior displacement of the tibia on the femur (Palastanga et al 2002). In addition to the role in an anteriorposterior direction, the cruciate ligaments also provide some mediolateral stability. The PCL provides 36% of the restraint to lateral

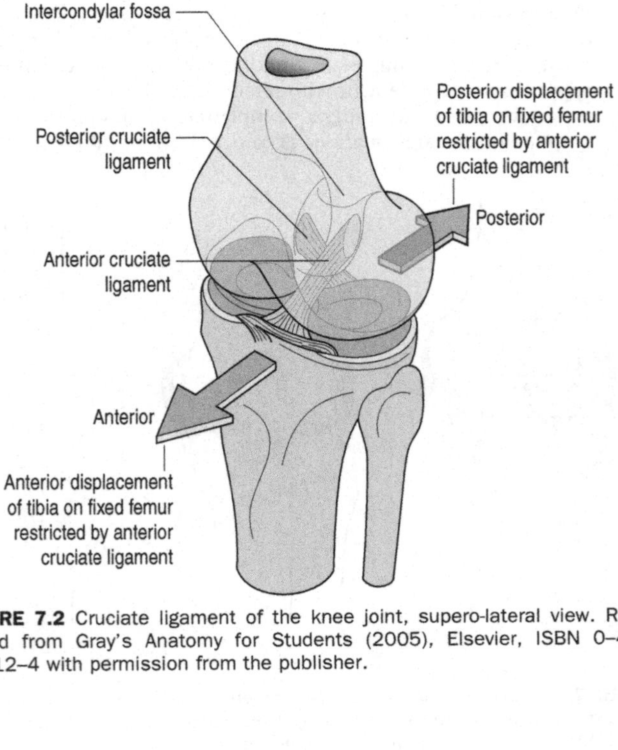


**FIGURE 7.2** Cruciate ligament of the knee joint, supero-lateral view. Reproduced from Gray's Anatomy for Students (2005), Elsevier, ISBN 0–443–06612–4 with permission from the publisher.

displacement, with ACL providing 30% of the restraint to medial displacement of the tibia (Palastanga et al 2002). Functionally the ACL should be considered having a restraining influence in all positions of the joint.

2. Isolated tears of the ACL are uncommon and are usually caused by a high-speed rotational injury over a forced hyperextended or flexed knee. Medial collateral ligament and medial meniscus tears are often associated with this type of injury (Dandy & Edwards 2003).

3. Effective repair of the ACL is impossible and very rarely used. The ligament crosses the synovial cavity of the knee and its torn ends are devitalised at the moment of injury and rapidly retract. Apposing two such structures with inert non-absorbable suture material does not produce a functioning ACL (Dandy & Edwards 2003). A full ACL reconstruction using a graft is the treatment of choice and there are different types of grafts that can be used.
   Types of graft:
   - Allografts – graft is donated from another individual
   - Xenografts – tissue donated from one species to another
   - Synthetic grafts
   - Collagen-based ligament grafts
   - Autografts – tissue is donated from one part of the body to another in the same individual.

   Reconstructive surgery using an autograft is the preferred choice for most surgeons. The most commonly used grafts for ACL reconstruction are patellar tendon and semitendinosus and gracilis (hamstring) tendon autografts (Bartlett et al 2001).

4. Harvesting a tendon graft from a previously healthy tendon has its disadvantages and rehabilitation risks. Patellar tendon autografts could lead to patella fracture, increase of patellofemoral pain and possible patellar tendon weakness and tear (Shaieb et al 2002). The patient is a carpenter and if one considers how much time he spends working on his knees, patellofemoral pain could delay his return to work.

5. Patients might see surgery as a 'quick fix' and expect to see an immediate improvement after surgery. Pain and swelling after an invasive procedure could be unexpected. To a lot of people joint pain and swelling can mean 'damage' and your patient might be anxious that 'something is wrong' and this could delay his return to work.

   The first step is to address his anxiety about his post-operative pain and swelling. You explain that this is common and does not predict surgical outcome. Managing swelling and pain is the first post-operative objective of an ACL rehabilitation programme and using the protocol as guidance you can reassure the patient that his presentation is expected rather than unexpected.

The second step is to address the patient's anxiety about work. His fear could make it difficult for him to problem solve that pain and swelling is not going to delay his rehabilitation. The majority of ACL reconstruction protocols are planned up to 12 months post surgery with specific targets at each rehabilitation stage. The therapist can explain the progression of each stage, emphasise the short-term goals and what the patient can do to achieve these goals. If the patient understands the post-operative progression and has realistic expectations, he will be empowered to take control of his rehabilitation and address his anxiety and fears.

6. Early research suggested that open kinetic chain (OKC) exercises can cause a greater anterior tibial displacement and put the graft at risk during the early rehabilitation period (Yack et al 1993). The opinion that OKC training of the knee extensors is more stressful for the ACL than close chain kinetic (CKC) exercises has dominated the management of early stage, post-operative rehabilitation programmes for ACLR (Morrisey et al 2000). Literature argues that anterior tibial displacement is just one consideration of many in ACL rehabilitation but the evidence to support the advantages of OKC exercises in early stage rehabilitation is not conclusive and CCK exercise for the first 12 weeks post ACL reconstruction are recommended by most surgeons protocols.



## Case Study 6

1. There are several classifications:

The Arbeitsgemeinschaft für Osteosynthesefragen (AO) uses a classification by position of fracture (McRae & Esser 2002):

a. Proximal
b. Central diaphyseal
c. Distal segments.

Another classification is based on many different factors (Coutts 2005a, Dandy & Edwards 2003):

a. Skin damage:
   - Open (compound): the skin is broken
   - Closed (simple); the skin remains intact
b. Shape or line of fracture:
   - Transverse or horizontal
   - Oblique/spiral
   - Comminuted: many bits
   - Crush
   - Greenstick (a bend in an immature bone, with a break in one of the cortices)

c. Displacement:
   - Un-displaced: although there is a clear break, the bone ends are in apposition
   - Displaced: bone ends do not meet
   - Impacted: bone ends have been firmly shunted together forming a firm though shortened bone
   - Stable: bone ends are held firmly by position or by surrounding tissues.

2. These are often abbreviated as 'ORIF' (open reduction internal fixation) (Coutts 2005). McRae and Esser (2002) describe the different types of ORIFs. These include screws, plates, intramedullary nails, locking nails, wires or nail-plates (Coutts 2005, McRae and Esser 2002). ORIF is often used when the patient has sustained multiple fractures. It provides the quickest form of stabilising a fracture resulting in stemming the blood loss which occurs when a bone is broken (Coutts 2005). This will not only reduce the pain and possible loss of function of a patient but also the shock that is experienced after multiple fractures.

3. Coutts (2005a) states that one of the problems with an ORIF is that it is invisible. One needs to look at it as a sort of scaffolding (Coutts 2005a, McRae & Esser 2002). This means that this patient will have to be non-weight bearing until initial callus formation has occurred which will be several weeks. He might think that he is more able to do things with his leg than he really is.

4. One needs to differentiate between union and consolidation.
   Table 7.2 gives an indication.
   Refer to Dandy & Edwards (2003) and McRae & Esser (2002) for more details.

5. - Delayed union (fracture takes longer than anticipated to heal)
   - Non-union (fracture does not heal in the anticipated time frame)



**TABLE 7.2 VARIATION IN HEALING TIMES OF FRACTURES IN DIFFERENT BONES**

| | Union | Consolidation |
|---|---|---|
| Proximal 1/3 humerus | 7–10 days | 3–4 weeks |
| Distal 1/3 radius | 4–6 weeks | 8–10 weeks |
| Proximal 1/3 femur | 4–6 weeks | 8–12 weeks |
| Distal 1/3 tibia | 6–8 weeks | 16–20 weeks |

- Mal-union (fracture heals in the appropriate time frame but there is an angulation/rotation)
- Myositis ossificans (often seen in patients with paraplegia, etc.; passive movements/stretching might predispose tissues to developing calcified masses but the evidence is inconclusive)
- Infection
- Muscle weakness (Coutts 2005a).

6. It is important to become aware that the patient and the team of health professionals looking after him might have very different views on the priorities of his rehabilitation. It is therefore absolutely vital that all goal and rehabilitation planning is collaborative. This might mean that the approach taken crosses disciplinary boundaries (inter-professional workings) in order to give the best go at recovery process (Steiner et al 2002). It is intended to avoid critical differences between the patient and the health care professionals dealing and working with him (Suarez et al 2001). All goals therefore have to be discussed early on in the rehabilitation process. There are some reports that state that collaborative goal setting is not just good practice but also a health status improving measure and able to increase efficiency of care (Stewart et al 2000).

The physiotherapist might wish to use the ICF (International Classification of Functioning, Disability and Health) model as a clinical problem-solving tool (Steiner et al 2002). This model implies that the ultimate goal of rehabilitation is to improve the patient's functional state and quality of life. Rehabilitation is a continuous process which starts on day 1 with the identification of the problems and needs of the patient (Steiner et al 2002) and the defining of the therapy goals.

The ICF classifies health and health-related components that describe body function and structures, activities and participation (ICIDH-2 1999). In Figure 7.3 you can see how these different components relate to each other. Each one of these can be expressed in both a positive and negative way, i.e. a component enhancing or ameliorating the overall outcome or adding to the burden of it. Steiner et al (2002) talk about the non-problematic aspects of health as those relating to the 'functioning' aspect whereas disability features are those that can be summarised under the headings of impairment, activity limitation and participation restriction.

This patient presents with quite a few relevant factors which will impact on this classic model. He will be out of action for a long time with his leg fracture (body functions and structures) but he is also the partial carer of his children (activity and participation) and he is self-employed (personal and environmental factors). All of these aspects are going to increase his anxiety which will need to be

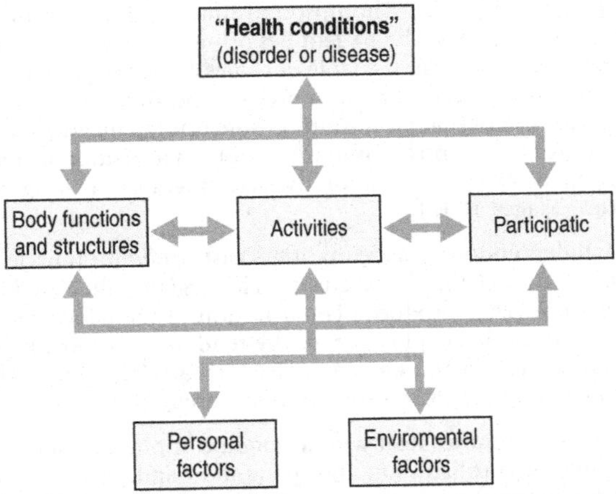


**FIGURE 7.3** How the components of the ICF relate to each other. Reproduced from ICDIH-2 (1999) with permission.



addressed by his physiotherapist. (Refer to fractured neck of femur and decompression case studies for more on this.)

Another model that might be useful in understanding the bio psychosocial challenges the patient faces is the Movement Continuum Model (Cott et al 1995). This idea incorporates all aspects of human life from cellular level to societal involvement in detailed and distinct parts – all of which could be assessed separately as well as globally. It might give you more ideas about integration of rehabilitation frameworks as well as patient-centred health care.

## Case Study 7

1. Achilles tendon injury (tendinopathy) is characterised by insidious onset of pain often noticed in a change in activity levels or training techniques and usually very stiff and painful in the morning. It can be resistant to treatment. Pathologically is non-inflammatory, with a degenerative or failed tendon healing response (Cook et al 2002). Although histopathologic studies have shown that ruptured Achilles tendons include clear degenerative changes before the rupture, many ruptures occur without any preceding signs or symptoms (Jarvinen et al 2001).

2. Diagnosis of tendon rupture is based on the history and physical findings. The patient will report the sensation of a blow to the tendon and a loss of function but may not be associated with considerable

pain (Cook et al 2002). Thompson's (Simmonds') test is performed to confirm diagnosis. The patient lies prone or kneels on a chair with the feet over the edge of the table or chair. While the patient is relaxed the examiner squeezes the calf muscles. A positive test is indicated by the absence of plantar flexion on squeezing. This indicates a third degree strain. It is important to note that plantar flexion may still be possible in this position by recruitment of the long flexor muscles (Magee 1997).

3. The Achilles tendon is made up of the gastrocnemius muscle (medial and lateral head) and the soleus muscle. Together they are known as triceps surae. They produce plantar flexion of the talocrural joint (ankle joint proper), and because the tendon passes just medial to the axes of the subtalar-talocalcaneonavicular (TCN) joints they also produce strong hindfoot supination (Levangie & Norkin 2001).

4. Acute tendon injuries heal with a standard triphasic response, i.e. inflammation, proliferation and maturation and a structure that resembles normal tendon organisation slowly reforms (Frank et al 1999) and are proceeded by a bleeding phase. An event in one phase will stimulate the following phase. Remodelling can go on for a very long time, i.e. up to 1 year (Watson 2007). For details of healing stages refer to www.electrotherapy.org

   For principles of tendon healing and repair as they apply to a ruptured TA refer to Hart et al (1988) – an old but authoritative source.



5. Changes in gait.

   First stage (NWB) with elbow crutches:

- Base of support becomes three point instead of two point
- Increased stance time on the unaffected leg
- Lower cadence (= steps/minute)
- Trunk muscles are stabilising to support weight on unaffected side and stabilising to hold leg up on affected side. The sustained loading may cause muscle fatigue.

Second stage (PWB):

- A four-point base of support
- More even swing/stance time when comparing affected with unaffected leg
- Cadence still lower but improves with time
- There is more control than when NWB
- Step length will start shorter.

Third stage (WB):

- Two-point base of support restored
- Unequal stance phase when comparing legs (shorter on the affected leg)

- Unequal swing phase when comparing legs (also shorter on the affected side)
- Resultant limp
- As remodelling continues and length/strength is restored then the stride length on the affected side will be restored.

6. Problems that may develop while using crutches:
   - Poor balance
   - Slipping, if rubber ferrules on bottom of crutches are worn
   - Backache if hand grips are too low and the patient is bending over while walking
   - Painful hands when taking too much weight through hands. Hand grips may need to be padded
   - Painful shoulders for same reason
   - Ulna neuritis due to compression of the ulna nerve with the hand in full dorsi flexion while weight bearing. Refer to Standring (2005) for nerve tract.

7. Exercises post plaster:
   - Physiological range of movement exercise will improve the circulation and positively influence the collagen alignment (Kannus et al 1997)
   - Stretching starts with the patient performing active physiologic dorsi flexion within limits of pain. Passive stretch starts with the tendon unloaded, i.e. NWB and the foot is pulled into dorsi-flexion using a band around the foot or something similar. This is gradually progressed to weight-bearing stretches
   - Isometric exercises progressing from small to large muscle contractions
   - Concentric exercises progressing from small to large muscle contractions.

   Eccentric contractions must be included in the rehabilitation (Alfredson et al 2004). It has been demonstrated that patients with painful TA treated conservatively have a better outcome than those treated only with concentric training (Mafi et al 2001).

## Case Study 8

1. Scoliosis is a 3-dimensional curvature of the spine occurring in the:
   - coronal plane – there is a lateral shift of the trunk on the pelvis
   - sagittal plane – there is a change in the lordosis/kyphosis balance
   - transverse (horizontal) plane – there is a rotation of the vertebra.

   Scoliosis can be congenital, neuromuscular or idiopathic. There is no known cause for idiopathic scoliosis. It most often develops in adolescents and progresses during the adolescent growth spurts. It can be detected by the Adam's forward bend test. As the patient bends over and a rotational deformity known as a rib hump can be seen while standing behind the patient (Reamy & Slakey 2001).

2. From regular X-rays the Cobb angle (Cobb 1948) can be taken, and the Risser value can be determined. Together these may indicate potential curve progression. The Cobb angle is the measurement of the curve. The Risser scale indicates the level of skeletal maturity. (Refer to Pashman 2006 for further details and pictures.)

3. Possible post-operative complications are:
   - respiratory – lung collapse, atelectasis, consolidation, effusion, pneumothorax, infection and fat embolism. Clinical evidence shows that deep breathing exercises and incentive spirometry both significantly reduce the incidence if post-operative pulmonary complications (Thomas & McIntosh 1994)
   - neurological – resulting from damage to spinal cord, haematoma compressing spinal cord or nerves in the critical period first 6–8 hours, causing paralysis (permanent/temporary) or altered sensation. Sympathetic changes. However, there is little risk of neurologic complications in idiopathic scoliosis whose neurologic status is normal preoperatively (Masatoshi et al 2004)
   - wound infection, poor healing and failure of metalwork
   - cast syndrome – normally occurs with good correction. Presents with continual projectile vomiting
   - post-operative haemorrhage, anaemia from blood loss
   - paralytic ileus, pancreatitis, superior mesenteric artery syndrome
   - pain.

4. It is generally felt that scoliotic patients 'hang into' their deformity thus increasing the inappropriate load bearing of growing bones (Stokes et al 2006). Following surgery this habitual posturing may strain the metalwork, and unnecessarily load the joints above and below the fusion. Education and correction using mirrors and positioning can increase the active correction of alignment obtained by the patient. This includes head centred over mid buttocks, shoulders level, scapulae level with equal prominence, hips level and symmetrical and equal distance between arms and body.

5. Precautions to be followed for 6–18 months to protect the fusion unless otherwise indicated are:
   - continuing with exercises and activities and returning to work or school by 6-week surgical review
   - log rolling to get in/out of bed
   - avoiding hip flexion beyond 90° and twisting of the spine
   - brace or corset worn 23.5 hours per day. This must only be removed for a seated wash. At 6/12 review with surgeon weaning out of the brace may begin and be complete after 2 weeks

- No sport for at least 6/12 or contact sport for 1 year
- Walking can be increased as tolerated.

Other limitations will depend on the degree of spinal stability and will be at the surgeon's discretion.

6. The MDT comprises:
   - consultant and surgical team
   - paediatrician
   - anaesthetist for pain management
   - nursing staff including health care assistants
   - physiotherapist for respiratory care and mobilising
   - occupational therapist, who will do a functional assessment prior to discharge
   - orthotist for casting of the brace
   - teacher, who will organise a home tuition referral. Home tuition will continue until the patient returns to school, usually between 4 and 6 weeks post operation
   - social worker, who will assess and contact local services to arrange discharge care package as required
   - dietician for provision of any food/nutrition supplements if deemed necessary
   - speech therapist for assessment.

7. Scoliosis may lead to multiple physical and psychosocial impairments depending on its severity. This includes function, body image, self image and quality of life (Freidel et al 2002).

   The patients who do well after surgery develop coping strategies to deal with:
   - wearing the brace for up to 6 months
   - restrictions on sport and exercise
   - fear of 'doing some wrong' or destabilising the surgery
   - large scars they may feel to be ugly.

   As with other disorders, any type of cosmetic surgery will affect patients in different ways depending on their underlying psychological makeup. Following surgery patients must be encouraged to resume a normal life within precautions as soon as possible.



## Case Study 9

1. Legg–Calvé–Perthes disease is a transient ischaemic necrosis of the capital femoral epiphysis which occurs in children between the age of 2 and 12 years (Chell & Dhar 2004). In 1910 it was described independently by the three authors after whom it is named. It is shortened to Perthes to acknowledge his recognition of its ischaemic nature. The exact cause is unknown. The incidence in the UK is 1 in 12 500; however, the geographical incidence varies nationally and

internationally. Boys are affected 3–5 times more than girls. Most cases are unilateral. The progress of the disease is divided into 2 phases: evolution and healing (for further details see Chell & Dhar 2004).

2. The classification system falls into two groups, those assessing the severity of the disease process and those predicting the long-term outcome. Disease severity is classified using the Salter–Thompson classification, Catterall classification and the lateral pillar classification A–C. In this case the patient has been classified as B which means that >50% height is maintained. The Stulberg classification on the other hand correlates with the long-term outcome of the hip and has five grades 1–5 (Coates et al 1990). (Refer also to Hefti & Clarke 2007.)
3. This is a sub-trochanteric surgical cutting of the femur and a realignment of the ends to allow healing in better alignment. The sub-trochanteric osteotomy is fixed with a plate pre-bent to 20° to ensure varus angulation (Joseph et al 1996, 2005).
4. The aim of conservative treatment is to minimise the deformity during the active phase of the disease and to reduce the incidence of osteoarthritis during adult life. It includes bed rest with or without traction and plaster casts (Petrie plasters) to maintain the abduction and internal rotation (Tidswell 1998). This patient's abduction orthosis allowed him to mobilise earlier without having to wear a plaster cast. It allowed him to walk with no restriction of activities unless pain or decreased range of movement occurred. However, adherence is often low with this (Herring et al 2004).
5. The patient will be in a double hip spica so activities must be devised around its obvious restrictions. The treatment activities should be appropriate for a child, i.e. through play (Department of Health 2003). The possible positions the patient will be able to maintain at this time will be semi-reclining, prone and supine.
   - Upper limbs: The aims will be for him to stay as strong as possible as he will need his upper limbs for crutch walking. The exercises need to maintain strength and endurance. Strength training involves lifting the maximum force with low repetitions to fatigue (Skinner 2005). This could be done in any of the starting positions above. He might have weights at home or improvise with tins of beans or bags of sugar. Every other day the weight could be increased. Endurance training involves many repetitions with a sub-maximal load. He could do press-ups and play skittles in prone or alternatively lie on a skateboard and propel himself along with his arms. Tom could keep a diary of his progress or utilise other means for maintaining his motivation such as a

graph to show progress. He could have a competition with his older brother. It is also important to involve his parents.

Additionally it is essential to include exercises for proprioception such as; lying prone with both hands on a ball and moving it from side to side as well as rolling it backwards and forwards with one hand.

## Case Study 10

1. Right-sided hemiplegia (now recognised as having a prenatal origin) means a typical hemiplegic gait with the weight on the left side only, retraction in the right hip and shoulder, curled toes of her right foot and a fisted hand on the same side. She will be 'toe' walking on the right side (Rodda & Graham 2001). The possible underlying factors for this are muscle weakness and imbalance, uncoordinated co-contraction, spasticity and disuse atrophy. She may also have a lack of recognition of her right side as well as a sensory deficit on that side (Neville & Goodman 2001).

2. Explain that it is very common for the umbilical cord to be found in this position due to the cramped quarters of the uterus. Furthermore, umbilical cords have mechanisms in place to help them keep functioning even when stretched. It is important, however, to remain sensitive to their concerns and possible mistrust of health care professionals (Nelson & Grether 1998).

3. Gait patterns can be identified and categorised by the use of instrumented motion analysis. Motion analysis provides a comprehensive gait evaluation. They quantify the nature and severity of neuromuscular and musculoskeletal abnormalities.

   The patient would be videoed while walking and an observational analysis produced. Reflective markers would have been placed on her limbs, pelvis and trunk to provide a 3-dimensional picture of joint motion (kinematics).

   Kinetic data are measures of the forces that cross the joints and the moments that cause the motion.

   An EMG analysis may be done which can provide a measure of muscles activity differentiating the action of each muscle which is correlated with the stance and swing phases of gait.

   Finally, joint kinematic and kinetic measurements can be analyzed with the EMG data to provide a comprehensive picture of the contributing factors to the patient's gait disorder (Coutts 2005b).

4. During this period the parents should be taught to encourage the patient to exercise the dorsiflexors (particularly tibialis anterior) and plantarflexors of her right leg in addition to her hip extensors. This will be carried out through the medium of play (Department of Health 2003 – refer to Perthes case study). This could be achieved

with ball play, all climbing activities (climbing frame, steps to a slide) walking on her toes, water play and swimming for example.

5. • Provide parents with clear messages regarding the goals of treatment and allow them to take part in the planning and decision making thus respecting their role as the patient's main carers (Litchfield & MacDougall 2002).
   • Don't overburden parents, fit exercises into their day-to-day activities.
   • Plan a weekly activity sheet with them and record any difficulties they have with the exercises.
6. • Sit out of the bed – suggestions: sit alongside patient to read a story. Get her to throw/catch a ball while sitting on the edge of the bed, 'post' a ball through the hoop in sitting.
   • Stand up with the plaster – suggestions: in standing play with a puzzle, tea set, thread beads, draw/paint.
   • Walk at least 10 m independently – prepare a fun course, kick/fetch a ball, push a pram along.
   • Go up and down stairs – a play slide or fetch a toy.
   • Be confident with the home exercise programme – prepare with her an exercise programme, draw pictures, paint it, etc. Prepare an exercise diary with smiley faces and stars. (For age-appropriate play refer to Chase 1994.)
7. A review of 11 studies looking at strengthening in cerebral palsy found evidence to suggest that, 'training can increase and may improve motor activity in people with cerebral palsy without adverse effects' (Dodd et al 2002).



## References

Adams M, Dolan P, Hutton W C 1986 The stages of disc degeneration as revealed by discogram. Journal of Bone and Joint Surgery 68B:36.

Alfredson H, Pietila T, Jonsson P et al 2004. Heavy load eccentric calf muscle training for the treatment of chronic Achilles tendinosis. American Journal of Sports Medicine 26(8):360–366.

Atkinson K 2005 Decision making and clinical reasoning in orthopaedics. In: Atkinson K, Coutts F, Hassenkamp A-M (eds) Physiotherapy in Orthopaedics: A Problem-Solving Approach, 2nd edn. Churchill Livingstone, Edinburgh.

Bartlett R J, Clatworthy M G, Nguyen T N V 2001 Graft selection in reconstruction of the anterior cruciate ligament. Journal of Bone and Joint Surgery 83B(5):625–634.

Borton D C, Walker K, Pirpiris M et al 2001 Isolated calf lengthening in cerebral palsy. Journal of Bone and Joint Surgery 83B:364–370.

Bunker T 2002 Rotator cuff disease. Current Orthopaedics 16:223–233.

Chase R A 1994 Toys, play and development. Journal of Perinatal Education 3(2):7–19.
Chell J, Dhar S 2004 Perthes Disease. Surgery 22(1):18–19.
Coates C J, Paterson J M H, Woods K R et al 1990 Femoral Osteotomy in Perthes Disease. Journal of Bone and Joint Surgery BR, 72:581–585.
Cobb J R 1948 Outline for the study of scoliosis. Instructional course lectures. American Academy of Orthopaedic Surgeons, Illinois 261–275.
Cook J L, Khan K M, Purdam C 2002 Achilles tendinopathy. Manual Therapy 7(3):121–130.
Cott C A, Finch E, Gasner D et al 1995 The movement continuum theory of physical therapy. Physiotherapy Canada 47:87–96.
Courtney P, Doherty M 2002 Key questions concerning paracetamol and NSAIDs for osteoarthritis. Annals of Rheumatic Diseases 61:767–773.
Coutts F 2005a Total joint replacements. In: Atkinson K, Coutts F, Hassenkamp A-M (eds) Physiotherapy in Orthopaedics: A Problem-Solving Approach, 2nd edn. Churchill Livingstone, Edinburgh.
Coutts F 2005b Gait analysis in the clinical situation. In: Atkinson K, Coutts F Hassenkamp A-M (eds) Physiotherapy in Orthopaedics, 2nd edn. Churchill Livingstone, Edinburgh.
Crawford H J, Jull G A 1993 The influence of thoracic posture and movement on range of arm elevation. Physiotherapy Theory and Practice 9:143–148.
Dandy D J, Edwards D J 2003 Essential Orthopedics and Trauma, 4th edn. Churchill Livingstone, Edinburgh.
De Palma A F 1973 Surgery of the Shoulder. J B Lipincott, Philadelphia.
Department for Health 2003 The National Service Framework for Children, Young People and Maternity Services Standard 3.7. HMSO, London.
Dodd K J, Taylor N F, Damiano D L 2002 A systematic review of the effectiveness of strength-training programmes for people with cerebral palsy. Archives of Physical Medicine and Rehabilitation 83:1157–1164.
Donatelli R A 1997 Physical Therapy of the Shoulder 3rd edn. Churchill Livingstone, Edinburgh.
Elstein A S, Shulman L S, Sprafka S A 1978 Medical Problem Solving. An Analysis of Clinical Reasoning. Harvard University Press, Cambridge.
Everett Y 2005 Muscle work, strength, power and endurance. In: Trew M & Everett T (eds) Human Movement: An introductory Text, 5th edn. Elsevier: Edinburgh.
Frank C, Shrive N, Hiraoka H et al 1999 Optimisation of the biology of soft tissue repair. Journal of Science and Medicine in Sport 2(3):190–210.
Freidel K, Petermann F, Reichel D et al 2002 Quality of life of women with idiopathic scoliosis. Spine 5:27(4).
Garden R S 1961 Low-angle fixation in the fractures of the femoral head. Journal of Bone and Joint Surgery 43B:647–663.
Gibson J 2007. Guide for Orthopaedic Surgeons and Therapists. Online. Available at http://www.theupperlimb.com 8 July 2007.

Gifford L 2006 Topical Issues in Pain 5. CNS Press, Falmouth.
Greenhalgh S, Selfe J 2006 Red Flags: A Guide to Identifying Serious Pathology of the Spine. Churchill Livingstone, Edinburgh.
Hart T J, Napoli R C, Wolfe J A et al 1988 Diagnosis and treatment of the ruptured Achilles Tendon. Journal of Foot Surgery 27(1): 30–39.
Hauer K, Specht N, Schuler M et al 2002 Intensive physical training in geriatric patients after severe falls and hip surgery. Age and Ageing 31:49–57.
Haq I, Murphy E, Darce J 2000 Osteoarthritis. Postgraduate Medical Journal 79:377–383.
Hefti F Clarke N M P 2007 The management of Legg–Calvé–Perthes disease: is there a consensus? Journal of Child Orthopedics 1:19–25.
Herring J A, Kim H T, Browne R 2004 Legg–Calvé–Perthes Disease Part II: Prospective Multicenter Study of the Effect of Treatment on Outcome. Journal of Bone and Joint Surgery 86:2121–2134.
Higgs J, Jones M 2000 Clinical reasoning in the health professions. In: Higgs J, Jones M (eds) Clinical Reasoning in the Health Professions, 2nd edn. Butterworth Heinemann, Oxford.
Higgs J, Titchen A 2000 Knowledge and reasoning. In: Higgs J, Jones M (eds) Clinical Reasoning in the Health Professions, 2nd edn. Butterworth Heinemann, Oxford.
ICDIH-2 1999 International Classification of Functioning and Disability. Beta-2 draft, full version. World Health Organization, Geneva, Switzerland.
Jarvinen T A, Kannus P, Paavola M et al 2001 Achilles tendon injuries. Current Opinion in Rheumatology 13(2):150–155.
Joseph B, Rao N, Mulpuri K et al 2005 How does a femoral varus osteotomy alter the natural evolution of Perthes' disease? Journal of Pediatric Orthopaedics 14:10–15.
Joseph B, Srinivas G, Thomas R 1996 Management of perthes disease of late onset in Southern India. Journal of Bone and Joint Surgery 78B(4):625–630.
Kannus P, Jozsa L, Natri A et al 1997 Effects of training, immobilization and remobilization on tendons. Scandinavian Journal of Medicine and Science in Sports 7:67–71.
Kibler W B 2000 Evaluation and diagnosis of scapulothoracic problems of the athelete. Sports Medicine and Arthroscopy Review 8:192–202.
Kibler W 1998 The role of the shoulder in athletic shoulder function. The American Journal of Sports Medicine 26(2):325–337.
Korpelainen R, Korpelainen J, Heikkinen J et al 2004 Lifestyle factors are associated with osteoporosis in lean women but not in normal and overweight women: a population-based cohort study of 1222 women. Osteoporosis International 14:34–43.
Levangie P K, Norkin C C 2001 Chapter 12 The ankle and foot complex. In: Levangie P, Norkin C Joint Structure and Function A Comprehensive Analysis, 3rd edn. FA Davis Company, Philadelphia.

Leone J M, Hansen A D 2005 Management of infection at the site of a total knee arthroplasty. Journal of Bone and Joint Surgery 87:2335–2348.
Litchfield R, MacDougall 2002 Professional issues for physiotherapists in family-centred and community-based settings. Australian Journal of Physiotherapy 48:105–111.
Mafi N, Lorentzon R, Alfredson H 2001 Superior short term results with eccentric calf muscle training in a randomized prospective multicentre study on patients with chronic Achilles tendinosis. Knee Surgery Sports Traumatology Arthroscopy 9:42–47.
Magee 1997 Chapter 13 Lower leg, ankle and foot. In: Magee D (ed) Orthopaedic Physical Assessment, 4th ed. Saunders, Philadelphia.
Marcus R, Wang O, Satterwhite J et al 2003 The skeletal response is largely independent of age, initial bone mineral density, and prevalent vertebral fractures in postmenopausal women with osteoporosis. Journal of Bone and Mineral Research 18:18–23.
Masatoshi Inoue, Shohei Minami, Yoshinori Nakata et al 2004. Preoperative MRI analysis of patients with idiopathic scoliosis. A prospective study. Spine 30(1):108–114.
McDevitt C A 1988 Proteoglycans of the intervertebral disc. In: Ghosh P (ed) The Biology of the Intervertebral Disc. CRC Press, Florida, p. 151.
McRae R, Esser M 2002 Practical Fracture Treatment, 4th edn. Churchill Livingstone, Edinburgh.
Messier S P, Loeser R F, Miller G D et al 2004 Exercise and dietary weight loss in overweight and obese older adults with knee osteoarthritis: the arthritis, diet, and activity promotion trial. Arthritis and Rheumatism 50(5):1501–1510.
Morrisey M C, Hudson Z L, Drechsler W I et al 2000 Effects of open versus closed kinetic chain training on knee laxity in the early period after anterior cruciate ligament reconstruction. Knee Surgery Sports Traumatology, Arthroscopy: Official Journal of the ESSKA 8:343–348.
Murray C J L, Lopez A D 1996 The Global Burden of Disease. World Health Organization, Geneva.
Nelson K B, Grether J K 1998 Potentially asphyxiating conditions and spastic cerebral palsy in infants of normal birth weight. American Journal of Obstetrics & Gynecology 179(2):507–513.
Neville B, Goodman R 2001 Congenital Hemiplegia. MacKeith Press, Cambridge.
Nicholas M, Molloy A, Tonkin L et al 2000 Manage Your Pain: Practical and Positive Ways of Adapting to Chronic Pain. ABC Books, Sydney.
Ostelo R W, de Vet H C, Waddell G et al 2003 Rehabilitation following first-time lumbar disc surgery: a systematic review within the framework of the Cochrane Collaboration. Spine 28(3):209–218.
Palastanga N, Field D, Soames R 2002 Anatomy and Human Movement, Structure and Function, 4th edn. Butterworth & Heinemann, Oxford.

Pashman R S 2006 eSpine: Adolescent Idiopathic Scoliosis. Online. Available http://www.espine.com/adolescent-scoliosis.htm 14 May 2007.
Peersman G, Laskin R, Davis J, Peterson M 2001 Infection in total knee replacement. A retrospective review of 6489 total knee replacements. Clinical Orthopaedics & Related Research 392:15–23.
Pincus T, Vlaeyen J, Kendall N et al 2002 Cognitive-behavioural therapy and psychosocial factors in low back pain. Spine 27:E133–E138.
Reamy B V, Slakey J B, 2001 Adolescent idiopathic scoliosis: review and current concepts. American Family Physician 64(1):324.
Ridgeway S, Wilson J, Charlet A et al 2005 Infection of the surgical site after arthroplasy of the hip. Journal of Bone and Joint Surgery 87B:844–850.
Rodda J, Graham H K 2001 Classification of gait patterns in spastic hemiplegia and spastic diplegia: a basis for a management algorithm. European Journal of Neurology 8(Suppl 5):96–108.
Rubin B D, Kibler W B 2002 Fundamental principles of shoulder rehabilitation: conservative to post-operative management. Arthroscopy: Journal of Arthroscopic and Related Surgery 18(9):29–39.
Shacklock M 2005 Clinical Neurodynamics: A New System of Musculo-Skeletal Treatment. Elsevier, Edinburgh.
Shaieb M D, Kan D M, Spencer K et al 2002 A prospective randomized comparison of patella tendon versus semitendinosus and gracilis tendon autografts for anterior cruciate ligament reconstruction. American Journal of Sports Medicine 30: 214–220.
Skinner J S P 2005 Exercise Testing and Exercise Prescription for Special Cases, 3rd edn. Lippincott, Williams and Wilkins, London.
Standring S 2005 Gray's Anatomy, 39th edn. The Anatomical Basis for Clinical Practice. Elsevier, Edinburgh.
Steiner W, Ryser L, Huber E et al 2002 Use of the ICF model as a clinical problem-solving tool in physical therapy and rehabilitation medicine. Physical Therapy 82:1098–1107.
Stewart M, Brown JB, Donner A et al 2000 The impact of patient-centered care on outcomes. Journal of Family Practice 49:769–804.
Stokes IA, Burwell RG, Dangerfield DH 2006 Biomechanical spinal growth modulation and progressive idiopathic scoliosis – a test of the vicious cycle pathenogenetic hypothesis. Summary of an electronic focus group debate. Scoliosis (Oct 18) 1:16.
Stulberg B N, Insall J N, Williams G W et al 1984 Deep vein thrombosis following total knee replacement. An analysis of six-hundred and thirty eight arthroplasties. American Journal of Bone and Joint Surgery 66:194–201.
Suarez A M E, Conner S B, Kendall C J, et al 2001 Lack of congruence in the ratings of patients' health status by patients and their physicians. Medical Decision Making 21:113–121.
Tidswell M 1998 Orthopaedic Physiotherapy. Mosby, London.
Thomas J A, McIntosh M 1994 Are incentive spirometry, intermittent positive pressure breathing, and deep breathing exercises effective in

the prevention of postoperative complications after abdominal surgery? A systematic overview and meta-analysis. Physical Therapy 74(1):3–10.
Vlaeyen J W, Linton S 2006 Are we fear-avoidant? Pain 124:240–242.
Watson T 2007 Electrotherapy. Tissue repair. Online. Available http://www.electrotherapy.org.
Yack H J, Collins C E, Whieldon T J 1993 Comparison of closed and open kinetic chain exercise in anterior cruciate ligament-deficient knee. American Journal of Sports Medicine 21:49–54.

# Case studies in a musculoskeletal out-patients setting

*Adrian Schoo, Nick Taylor, Ken Niere with a contribution from James Selfe*



## INTRODUCTION

Musculoskeletal problems are very common, and can be encountered in hospital emergency departments, orthopaedics, and out-patient physiotherapy (Carter & Rizzo 2007). It is not uncommon for in-patients who are admitted for another problem to be referred and treated in the ward or in the out-patient department for a musculoskeletal problem. The prevalence of specific conditions can vary between the different groups in the community. For example, sporting injuries are more likely to occur in the younger groups, whereas degenerative conditions such as osteoarthritis are more likely to occur as people progress in years.

Musculoskeletal problems can result in pain and functional limitations (disability), and represent a major burden to the society due to associated health care costs and loss of productivity (National Health Priority Action Council 2004). Musculoskeletal conditions, including arthritis, cause more disability than any other medical condition and affect one-third of all people with disability. Since part of the chronic disease burden is attributed to risk factors such as physical inactivity (Bauman 2004) people with musculoskeletal conditions are often referred to physiotherapy out-patients for management of their conditions.

As in other areas of physiotherapy practice, musculoskeletal assessment and treatment requires a systematic clinical reasoning approach (Edwards et al 2004). The clinical reasoning approach used in this chapter considers: (i) differential diagnoses based on assessment and clinical presentation; (ii) intervention based on the best evidence available; (iii) constant evaluation of therapy outcomes; (iv) adjustment of intervention programme in line with diagnosis and stage of progress; and (v) referring to or working together with other disciplines to exclude and or address confounding problems. In assessing and treating common musculoskeletal conditions and measuring progress it is important to use outcome measures that are valid and reliable, and that consideration must be given to impairments of body structure and function as well as activity limitation and participation restriction, such as ability to return to work. The World Health Organization's International Classification of Functioning, Disability and Health (ICF) provides a useful framework for physiotherapists in out-patients to assess patient functioning (Jette 2006). Referral to or working with other disciplines may involve tests such as X-rays or dynamic ultrasound scans, or the provision of orthotics to improve biomechanics. In addition to specific techniques, treatment may require education, ergonomic advice and the instruction of a home exercise programme to improve outcomes on function and pain.

There is an emerging and increasing body of research on the effectiveness of physiotherapy that provides the clinician in out-patients with an evidence base for their practice (Herbert et al 2001). For example, there is high level evidence that therapeutic exercise can benefit clients across broad areas of physiotherapy practice (Morris & Schoo 2004, Taylor et al 2007). In prescribing exercises it can be important to know whether the exercise programme is performed correctly and adhered to by the client. Conditions such as back problems or tendinopathies may be negatively affected by incorrect activity performance. Additional problems that can affect health outcomes are incorrect belief systems and mental health problems. For instance, people with osteoarthritis may think that movement harms the joint, but by not moving they put themselves at risk of developing problems associated with physical inactivity (e.g. increased morbidity and mortality due to cardiovascular problems or falls) (Philbin et al 1996). Also, people with chronic pain may be depressed and are, therefore, less likely to be interested in performing exercises, and may benefit from counselling (e.g. motivational interviewing). Screening patients for problems such as fear-avoidance behaviour and anxiety (Andrews & Slade 2001), asking about past and current exercise performance, motivating them if needed (Friedrich et al 1998) and demonstrating the prescribed exercises can assist in determining the likelihood of correct and consistent programme performance (Friedrich et al 1996b, Schneiders et al 1998).

We have selected common musculoskeletal conditions that are likely to be encountered in hospital out-patient departments. The different cases relate to younger and older people, females as well as males. A multitude of physical tests and outcome measures have been included together with clinical reasoning and evidence-based treatment options.

## CASE STUDY 1 JAW PAIN

### Subjective examination

| Subject | 34-year-old female office worker |
|---|---|
| HPC | Left sided headaches off and on for 3/12<br>Increasing pain of the left temporomandibular joint (TMJ) last 2/12<br>Pain at night, at rest, and when opening the mouth or chewing |
| PMH | Appendectomy<br>Stress at work |
| Aggravating factors | Biting a big apple<br>Chewing hard or tough food |
| Easing factors | Rest is better than chewing, although remains painful<br>Drinking fluid<br>Ice |
| Night | Wakes up because of pain<br>Grinds teeth when asleep (according to partner) |
| Daily pattern | Constant pain that worsens during and directly after opening the mouth or chewing |
| General health | Using prescribed sedatives due stress at work. No other problems reported |
| Attitude/ expectations | Given the symptoms she expects that it may take some time for them to settle |

| | |
|---|---|
| Pain and dysfunction scores | VAS current pain at rest = 3<br>VAS usual level of pain during chewing in the last week = 7<br>VAS worst level of pain during opening the mouth in the last week = 9 |

## Objective examination

| | |
|---|---|
| Palpation | Skin temperature (T*sk*) normal<br>Left TMJ painful on palpation<br>TMJ movement and clicking can be felt when placing the index finger in the auditory canal and opening the mouth<br>No signs of TMJ dislocation when comparing left with right |
| Muscle length | External pterygoid muscle feels tight and painful on opening of the mouth (palpation through the mouth) |
| Functional testing, including ROM and strength | Opening of the mouth is limited. It can accommodate two fingers only. Normally, the span is large enough to accommodate three fingers (Hoppenfield 1986)<br>Asymmetrical mandibular motion with severe swinging to the left when opening the mouth |

## Questions

1. What is your provisional diagnosis?
2. What signs and symptoms lead you to this diagnosis?
3. How will you address these in your treatment plan?
4. What kind of common and less common problems need to be excluded?
5. How likely is it that the patient's stress and teeth grinding contribute to the current complaint?
6. How will the expectations of the patient influence your treatment?
7. Is the patient likely to benefit from referral to other health professionals?

# CASE STUDY 2 HEADACHE

## Subjective examination

| | |
|---|---|
| Subject | 29-year-old male working on Help Desk in Information and Computer Technology |

| | |
|---|---|
| HPC | Gradual onset of headaches and cervical pain about 3/52 ago<br>Cannot recall precipitating incident<br>Headaches becoming more frequent (now daily) and lasting longer (up to 3 hours)<br>Has deep ache (non-throbbing) radiating from the back of the occiput to the right frontal region. Also complaining of stiffness like pain in the right side of the cervical spine. Neck pain and headache seem related (see Figure 8.1) |
| PMH | Car accident 10 years ago which led to cervical pain for about 3/52. No problems since apart from an occasional stiff neck |

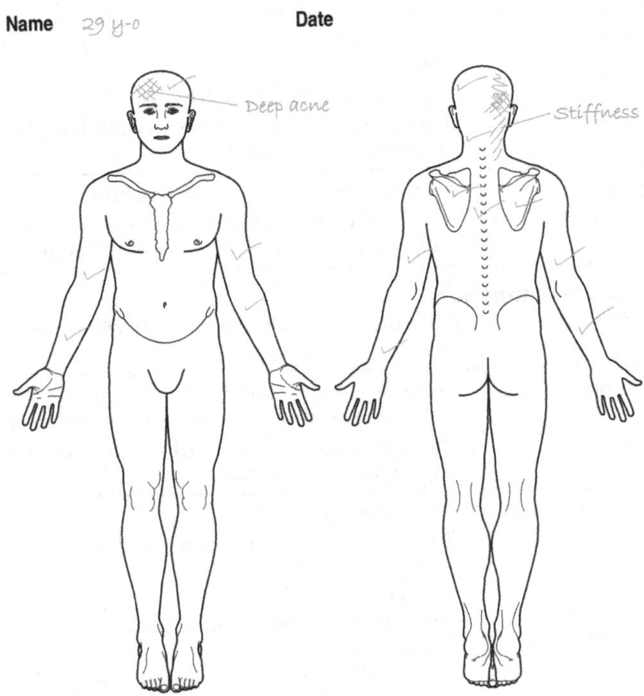


**FIGURE 8.1** Body chart – Case Study 2.

| | |
|---|---|
| **Aggravating factors** | Prolonged work at the computer (if more than 2 hours brings on headache)<br>Reversing the car reproduces slight cervical stiffness |
| **Easing factors** | Analgesia dulls the headache |
| **Night** | Sleep undisturbed |
| **Daily pattern** | Seems to depend on how long he has spent at the computer |
| **General health** | In good health, no weight loss<br>No complaints of dizziness, no nausea or vomiting<br>Assessed as being depressed, has been taking antidepressants over the last 3/12 |
| **Investigations** | No X-rays or other investigations at this stage |
| **Attitude/ expectations** | At the moment headache is not affecting him a lot but wanted to get it checked out in case it is something serious<br>Keen not to miss any work<br>Intends to continue normal recreation of sail boarding this weekend |
| **Pain and dysfunction scores** | Neck Disability Index: 14% Disability<br>VAS level of pain when headache is most severe (after working at the computer for 2 hours) = 6 |

## Physical examination

| | |
|---|---|
| **Observation** | Forward head posture with a slouched sitting posture |
| **Palpation** | Hypo-mobility of upper cervical joints on the right, with reproduction of local cervical pain<br>Increased muscle tone in right upper trapezius and right levator scapulae |
| **Movements** | *Active movements*<br>Right cervical rotation equals 60° with slight stiffness in neck<br>Left cervical rotation equals 75–80°<br>Limited cervical retraction, feels stiff<br>*Muscle function*<br>Decreased strength and endurance of the deep cervical neck flexors as determined by the cranio-cervical flexion test (Jull et al 1999) |

| | |
|---|---|
| **Neurodynamic testing** | Upper limb neurodynamic/tension test (base test): In 90° shoulder abduction and full external rotation, right elbow extension lacks 40° while left lacks 30°. Reproducing local neck pain, which is eased with cervical lateral flexion towards the right |
| **Neurological tests (tests of nerve conduction)** | Not assessed |

**Questions**

1. What is your provisional diagnosis?
2. What signs and symptoms led to your provisional diagnosis?
3. How will you address these in your treatment plan?
4. What kind of common and less common problems need to be excluded?
5. How relevant are work details for this patient?
6. How will the expectations of the patient influence your treatment?
7. Is the patient likely to benefit from referral to other health professionals?



## CASE STUDY 3 NECK PAIN – CASE ONE

### Subjective examination

| | |
|---|---|
| **Subject** | 32-year-old male accountant |
| **HPC** | Prolonged sitting (all day) at a conference 3/52 previously<br>Noticed onset of left lower cervical and interscapular pain at the end of the day<br>On waking the next morning pain had spread to the posterior aspect of the arm and forearm as far as the middle three fingers (see Figure 8.2)<br>Seen by doctor 1/52 ago. Doctor ordered plain X-rays including oblique views that did not show any abnormality<br>Has not improved at all since onset of symptoms |
| **Medical history** | High cholesterol, overweight, sedentary lifestyle<br>Minor neck complaints that usually settled within 2 or 3 days |

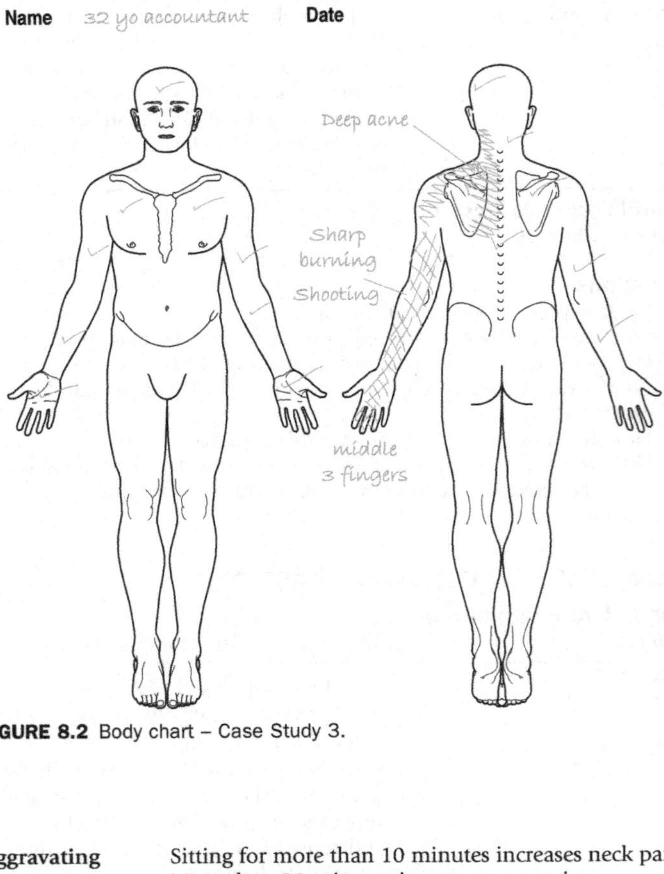


**FIGURE 8.2** Body chart – Case Study 3.

| | |
|---|---|
| **Aggravating factors** | Sitting for more than 10 minutes increases neck pain. More than 30 minutes increases arm pain<br>Looking up or to the left increases neck and arm pain<br>Lifting briefcase with left hand aggravates neck and interscapular pain |
| **Easing factors** | Neck pain relieved by lying supine<br>Arm pain relieved by lying supine with left arm above head |
| **Night** | Can sleep 2–3 hours at a time before being woken by increased neck and interscapular pain<br>Changing position helps to decrease the pain |

| | |
|---|---|
| **Daily pattern** | Increased symptoms with increased amounts of sitting, particularly if using computer |
| **Medication** | Was prescribed non-steroidal anti-inflammatory medication (Meloxicam) which helps take the edge off the neck pain |
| **Attitude/ expectations** | Wants to know what the problem is, particularly as the X-rays did not show any abnormality<br>Feels that something might be 'out' in his neck. If it could be 'put back in' the symptoms should resolve |

## Physical examination

| | |
|---|---|
| **Observation** | Sits with forward head posture |
| **Cervical active movements in sitting** | Extension reproduces pain in the neck and left arm at 30°. Movement occurs mainly in the upper and mid-cervical regions. Very little movement in the lower cervical or upper thoracic areas<br>Right rotation produces a stretching in the left cervical region at 75°<br>Left rotation reproduces left neck and interscapular pain at 40° |
| **Palpation** | Increased tone and tenderness noted in the left paraspinal muscles (cervical and upper thoracic) and left scalene muscles<br>Local pain and left arm pain reproduced by postero-anterior (PA) pressures over the spinous processes of C6 and C7 and over the C6 and C7 articular pillars on the left<br>Generalized stiffness noted with PA pressures in the mid and upper thoracic regions |
| **Segmental neurological examination** | Absent left triceps jerk<br>Weakness in left triceps (25% of right side)<br>Decreased sensation to light touch over the tip of the left middle finger |

## Questions

1. What is the most likely source of the patient's arm pain?
2. What is the most likely source of the patient's neck and interscapular pain?
3. What are other possible symptoms sources?

4. Are there reasons to be cautious in administering physiotherapy treatment?
5. What would an appropriate initial physiotherapy treatment involve?
6. What would a longer-term management programme include?
7. What is the likely prognosis?
8. Is referral to other health professionals warranted?

## CASE STUDY 4 NECK PAIN – CASE TWO

### Subjective examination

| Subject | 23-year-old female personal assistant |
|---|---|
| HPC | Rear end motor car accident 2/7 ago<br>Immediate onset of cervical pain and stiffness (left and right). Both pain and stiffness have been increasing. Pain is now constant<br>Vague headache started today (see Figure 8.3)<br>Seen by doctor yesterday who organised an X-ray (no abnormality detected) and referred patient to physiotherapy |
| PMH | Left knee reconstruction 3 years ago with good return of function since<br>No past history of neck complaints |
| Aggravating factors | Turning head to either side, especially if movement is quick<br>Travelling in car – took 20 minutes to settle after 30-minute car trip |
| Easing factors | Supine with head supported on one pillow<br>Felt a bit easier under hot shower |
| Night | Wakes often due to discomfort<br>Sleeps on 3 pillows<br>Difficulty turning in bed due to pain |
| Daily pattern | Constant pain that gradually worsens during the day |
| General health | Taking non-prescription analgesics every 4 hours on advice of doctor. No other medications<br>Not seeing the doctor for any other health problems |
| Attitude/ expectations | Anxious about prognosis<br>Worried about how much work she will have to miss as she only started in her current position 3/12 ago |

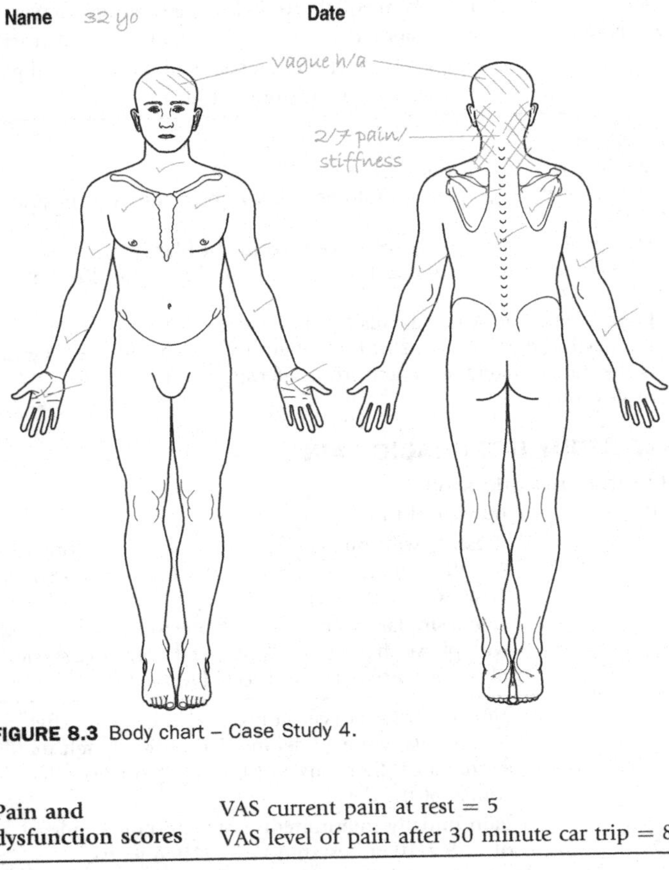


**FIGURE 8.3** Body chart – Case Study 4.

| | |
|---|---|
| Pain and dysfunction scores | VAS current pain at rest = 5<br>VAS level of pain after 30 minute car trip = 8.5 |

## Physical examination

| | |
|---|---|
| Observation | Walking slowly and all movements are guarded<br>Removes jacket slowly and with great care<br>Neck in slight protracted posture |
| Palpation | Generalized tenderness to light palpation of cervical spine (central, left and right)<br>Increased muscle spasm left and right paraspinal muscles<br>Further detailed palpation not possible because therapist wary of exacerbating symptoms |

| | |
|---|---|
| **Active movements** | Left rotation equals 30° before pain started increasing<br>Right rotation equals 35° before pain started increasing<br>Attempt to retract cervical spine caused increased pain<br>No other movements tested today |

## Questions

1. What is your provisional diagnosis?
2. Which of the signs and symptoms will you place on your priority list?
3. How will you address these in your treatment plan?
4. What kind of common and less common problems need to be excluded?
5. How relevant are work details for this patient?
6. How will the expectations of the patient influence your treatment?
7. Is the patient likely to benefit from referral to other health professionals?



## CASE STUDY 5 THORACIC PAIN

### Subjective examination

| | |
|---|---|
| Subject | 60-year-old male lawyer<br>Presents with bilateral lower thoracic pain with radiation of symptoms anteriorly to the lower sternal area (see Figure 8.4)<br>Had a similar problem 5 years previously that settled with physiotherapy which resolved after three sessions of passive mobilisation directed to the thoracic spine |
| HPC | Noticed onset of symptoms 4/52 previously after lifting pots while gardening. Pain initially felt in sternal area, then onset of thoracic pain over the course of the day<br>Pain initially intermittent, now constant at a level of VAS 2/10 at best and VAS 7/10 at worst |
| Medical history | Noticed 5 kg of weight loss in previous 4/52 that could not be explained by other factors<br>Had noticed intermittent, generalised, mild (VAS 1–2/10), aches and pains in trunk, arms and legs over the previous 3/12 that had worsened slightly over the previous 4/52 |
| Aggravating factors | Prolonged sitting for greater than 20 minutes at work would increase posterior and anterior chest pains to VAS 6/10 |

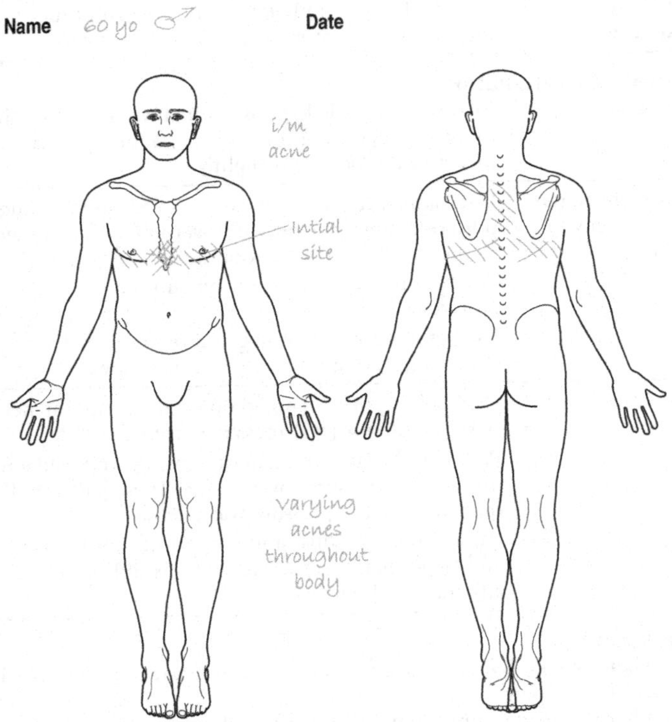


**FIGURE 8.4** Body chart – Case Study 5.



| | |
|---|---|
| **Easing factors** | Standing and walking for 10 minutes decreases all symptoms to VAS 2/10 |
| **Night** | Wakes 3–4 times each night with increased symptoms in thoracic and sternal areas. Has to get out of bed and walk around to ease pain. Tends to notice generalised aches and pains associated with increased sweating at night |
| **Daily pattern** | Dependent on amount of sitting during the day. More thoracic and sternal pain at end of day when sitting a lot |
| **Medication** | Nil |

| | |
|---|---|
| **Attitude/ expectations** | Expects that physiotherapy will ease symptoms as they did for a past episode of similar pain |

## Physical examination

| | |
|---|---|
| **Observation** | Increased thoracic kyphosis noted while sitting. Able to actively correct sitting posture, although this increases thoracic pain slightly |
| **Thoracic active movements in sitting** | Extension is restricted by about 50% and reproduces posterior thoracic pain with overpressures localised to the mid/lower thoracic spine<br>Thoracic rotation feels stiff but no pain reproduced<br>Flexion is normal in range and reproduces a stretching feeling in the mid thoracic area |
| **Palpation** | Generalised stiffness noted on midline and unilateral postero-anterior (PA) pressures from T2–T10<br>Posterior thoracic and anterior pain reproduced with midline PA pressures over T7–T8. These pains settled quickly once the pressure was released<br>Palpation of the ribs, inferior part of the sternum and upper part of rectus abdominis did not reveal any increased tenderness |

## Questions

1. What are your hypotheses regarding the likely source of the thoracic and sternal pains?
2. What would an appropriate initial physiotherapy treatment involve?
3. Are there examination findings that would make you suspect a non-musculoskeletal source of the symptoms?
4. What are red flags?
5. Is referral to other health professionals warranted?

# CASE STUDY 6 LOW BACK PAIN – CASE ONE

## Subjective examination

| | |
|---|---|
| Subject | 44-year-old male bank manager |
| HPC | 4/7 ago bent to reach into boot of car and felt slight backache. Thought it would settle so played golf anyway.<br>Next morning severe low back pain with aching pain radiating down the back of the right leg to just below |

**Name** 40 yo **Date**

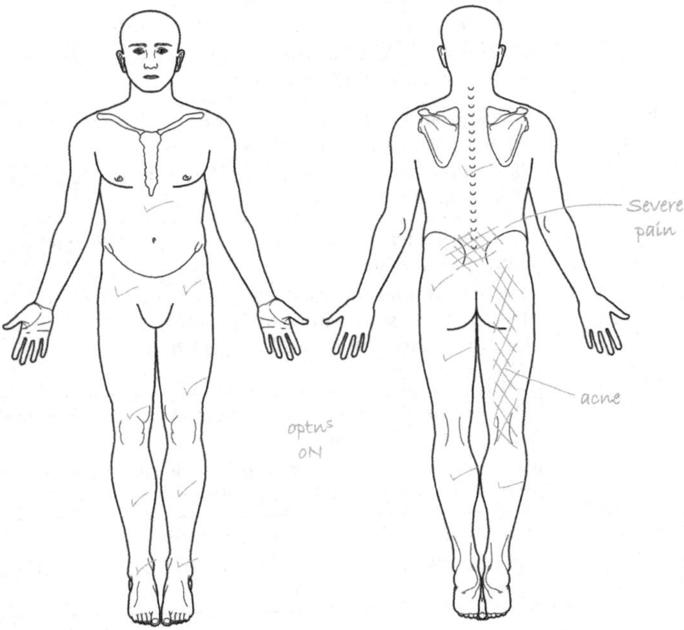


**FIGURE 8.5** Body chart – Case Study 6.

| | |
|---|---|
| | the knee. Has no pins and needles or numbness (see Figure 8.5) |
| **PMH** | Has had four or five episodes of low back pain over the last 8 years, usually settles quickly in 2 or 3 days<br>Has not required treatment with previous episodes |
| **Aggravating factors** | Finds it difficult to put shoes and socks on in the morning<br>After driving to work (about 40 minutes) found leg pain had worsened<br>Can only sit for about 15 to 20 minutes at a time at work<br>Has noticed that sneezing increased back and leg pain |

| | |
|---|---|
| **Easing factors** | Lying on back eventually relieves the leg pain<br>Standing and walking seem to help a little |
| **Night** | Pain gradually eases after initial discomfort<br>Is waking at night but finds can get back to sleep quite quickly when changes position |
| **Daily pattern** | Back stiff and aches getting out of bed first thing in the morning but eases after shower<br>Back pain is worse by the end of the day, and leg pain is more constant by the end of the day |
| **General health** | Taking non-steroidal anti-inflammatories (NSAIDs) with slight improvement<br>At recent annual review doctor advised to increase physical activity to reduce weight (BMI 26.4) and adjust diet (cholesterol 6.4). Otherwise fit and well |
| **Attitude/ expectations** | Very keen not to miss club Stableford golf competition this weekend (in 3/7)<br>Intending to cope with work as best he can. Very busy at work so reluctant to take time off |
| **Pain and dysfunction scores** | Oswestry Disability Score: 36% Disability<br>VAS level of pain after 40 minute car trip: back = 8, leg = 6 |



## Physical examination

| | |
|---|---|
| **Observation** | Slight left-sided contralateral list (when observed from behind in standing shoulders are to the left relative to the hips)<br>Changes position regularly when in sitting position |
| **Palpation** | Increased tone, right erector spinae in the lumbar region<br>Central postero-anterior pressures over the lumbar spine reproduced back pain (but not leg pain) at L4 and L5<br>Unilateral pressures were painful on the right at L4 and L5 |
| **Movements** | *Active movements*<br>■ Lumbar flexion in standing limited (2 cm below the knee)<br>■ Lumbar extension in standing markedly limited<br>■ Left and right rotation (assessed in sitting) both more than 60° |

- Attempt to correct contralateral list led to increased back pain

*Repeated active movements*

- Flexion in standing repeated 10 times led to increased back pain and increase of leg pain
- Extension in standing repeated 15 times abolished leg pain, and increased range – back pain remained
- Repeated correction of contralateral list (side gliding to the right) led to reduced central back pain and slightly increased range

*Neurodynamic tests*

- Straight leg raise: right = 70° left = 70°
- Slump test not evaluated

*Neurological tests (tests of nerve conduction)*

- Muscle strength in myotomes L3 to S1, left = right
- Sensation in dermatomes L2 to S1, left = right
- Reflexes (patella tendon and Achilles), brisk left = right

## Questions

1. What is your provisional diagnosis?
2. What is the likely source of the right leg pain?
3. Which of the signs and symptoms will you place on your priority list?
4. How will you address these in your treatment plan?
5. What kind of common and less common problems need to be excluded?
6. How relevant are work details for this patient?
7. How will the expectations of the patient influence your treatment?
8. Is the patient likely to benefit from referral to other health professionals?



## CASE STUDY 7 LOW BACK PAIN – CASE TWO

### Subjective examination

| | |
|---|---|
| Subject | 49-year-female assembly worker at automotive manufacturer |
| HPC | Complaining of increasing back pain over the last 14/12. Back pain is in the central low back region and radiates into both gluteal regions – no leg pain (see Figure 8.6). Has been off work for the last 6/12 with no improvement in pain<br>Injured back when installing car upholstery 14/12 ago. Initially had 3/7 off work and experienced some slow improvement over the first 3/12 |

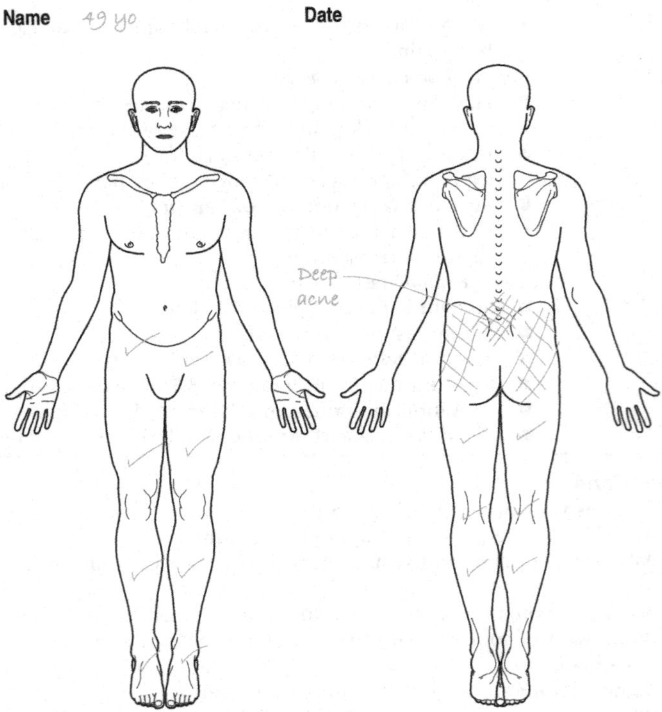


FIGURE 8.6 Body chart – Case Study 7.



| | |
|---|---|
| | Has had manipulative physiotherapy involving manipulation, mobilisation and traction with no benefit. Also tried chiropractic without benefit |
| PMH | 15-year history of intermittent low back pain usually no more than a few days off work<br>Cholecystectomy 6 years ago |
| Aggravating factors | Prolonged walking or standing (more than 15 minutes) increases ache<br>Prolonged sitting (more than 15 minutes) increases ache<br>Unable to do weekly shopping or housework as these activities aggravate the ache |

| | |
|---|---|
| **Easing factors** | Lying down but only for about 30 minutes, as gets stiff when lying in one position for too long |
| **Night** | Finds it difficult to get comfortable, wakes when turning<br>Not getting good-quality sleep any more |
| **Daily pattern** | Gradually worse by the end of the day |
| **General health** | Has gained weight over the last 14/12 (about 6 kg)<br>Assessed as being depressed, has been taking antidepressants over the last 3/12 |
| **Investigations** | X-ray shows mild bilateral degeneration of the L4–5 facets<br>CT scan shows a minor disc bulge at L4–5 and L5–S1 with no nerve root involvement |
| **Attitude/ expectations** | Has reduced activity level to avoid aggravating back<br>Believes that if she can find the right practitioner then they will fix her<br>Very concerned with the CT scan report and the diagnosis of disc pathology<br>Has been more short-tempered with family and friends since her back problem began<br>Her spouse has been very supportive and has willingly taken over tasks such as housework and shopping |
| **Pain and dysfunction scores** | Oswestry Disability Score: 72% Disability<br>VAS level of pain after 15 minutes of standing or sitting = 7.5 |

## Physical examination

| | |
|---|---|
| **Observation** | Exhibits pain behaviours including grimacing, and placing hand on back<br>Changes position regularly when sitting and standing<br>Walking pattern is slow and guarded |
| **Palpation** | Central palpation of the lumbar spine at L1, L2, L3, L4 and L5 painful<br>Unilateral pressures are painful left and right at L1, L2, L3, L4 and L5 |

| | |
|---|---|
| Movements | *Active movements*<br>■ Lumbar flexion in standing limited (2 cm above the knee)<br>■ Lumbar extension in standing moderately limited (estimated half of expected range)<br>■ Left and right rotation (assessed in sitting) both about 40°<br>*Neural mobility tests*<br>■ Straight leg raise on right = 50° left = 50°<br>■ Able to fully extend knee in upright sitting<br>■ Slump test not evaluated<br>*Neurological tests (tests of nerve conduction)*<br>■ Normal no abnormality detected |

## Questions

1. What is your provisional diagnosis?
2. How do you interpret the X-ray and CT scan reports?
3. Which of the signs and symptoms will you place on your priority list?
4. How will you address these in your treatment plan?
5. What kind of common and less common problems need to be excluded?
6. How relevant are work details for this patient?
7. What are yellow flags and how are they relevant for this patient?
8. Is the patient likely to benefit from referral to other health professionals?



# CASE STUDY 8 SHOULDER PAIN

## Subjective examination

| | |
|---|---|
| Subject | 47-year-old female factory worker<br>Right arm dominant |
| HPC | Right shoulder pain which started 1/52 ago when dragging a heavy item onto the conveyor belt. Routinely she has to pull, lift, and reach overhead |
| PMH | Low back pain episodes since work-related lifting injury<br>Asthma and frequent coughing |
| Aggravating factors | ■ At work: Overhead work, lifting and carrying boxes<br>■ In transit: Driving car, riding a bike with wide handlebars.<br>■ At home: Preparing meals, working at the computer, knitting |

| | |
|---|---|
| **Easing factors** | Rest<br>Avoiding overhead work or holding elbows out when lifting or carrying items |
| **Night** | Wakes frequently because of pain, particularly when sleeping on the painful shoulder |
| **Daily pattern** | Constant nagging pain that worsens during activities as mentioned above (see aggravating factors) |
| **General health** | Asthma attacks. Smokes. Using bronchodilatators as needed |
| **Attitude/ expectations** | Is afraid that she may need to look for another job due to experiencing increasing shoulder problems at work<br>Wants better duties within the factory as some of her colleagues have managed to do |
| **Pain and dysfunction scores** | VAS current pain at rest = 3<br>VAS usual level of pain during aggravating activity in the last week = 7<br>VAS worst level of pain in the last week = 9<br>Shoulder Pain and Disability Index (SPADI): Pain score = 60%, Disability score = 45%, Total score = 50.8% (Roach et al 1991) |

## Objective examination

| | |
|---|---|
| **Standing with arms relaxed** | Shoulders protracted and depressed (right > left)<br>Right shoulder abducted and elbow flexed<br>Hyper kyphosis<br>Shortness of breath with upper chest breathing |
| **Palpation** | Skin temperature (T*sk*) normal<br>Tenderness of subscapularis, supraspinatus and serratus posterior superior with palpable trigger points<br>Painful insertion of subscapularis and supraspinatus on the humerus<br>Palpable click on shoulder abduction |
| **Muscle length and strength** | Tightness of the subscapularis, pectoralis minor<br>Weakness of rhomboids, supraspinatus |

| | |
|---|---|
| **Functional and other testing, including ROM** | Painful arc when abducting arm (90–115° abduction) with audible click (VAS rises to 6 during this impingement)<br>Hawkins and Kennedy impingement test (compressing the subacromial tissues by internal rotation in 90° shoulder flexion) was positive (Ginn 2003) and VAS rises to 8<br>Apprehension test for shoulder stability and SLAP lesion tests were negative, indicating integrity of joint capsule, labrum and ligaments (Brukner et al 2001e, Ginn 2003, Hoppenfield 1986)<br>Shoulder elevation reduced by 10° with early scapular movement when comparing with left shoulder (VAS rises to 5)<br>Pain on resistance against external rotation and abduction (VAS rises to 8)<br>Reduced internal rotation and adduction strength when pushing palm of the hand on the table when sitting at the table (VAS rises to 7)<br>Difficulty placing right hand behind back. Positive Gerbers' test (resisting against hand when patient is pushing hand away from the spine (VAS rises to 8) |

## Questions

1. What is your provisional diagnosis?
2. What signs and symptoms lead you to this diagnosis?
3. Describe the mechanism that can leads to this condition.
4. How will you address these signs and symptoms in your treatment plan?
5. What kind of common and less common problems need to be excluded?
6. Can patient's asthma and hyper kyphosis contribute to the shoulder complaint?
7. How will the expectation of the patient influence your treatment?
8. Is it possible that outcome measures do not reflect the severity of pain and disability experienced by the patient?
9. Is the patient likely to benefit from referral to other health professionals?

## CASE STUDY 9 ELBOW PAIN

### Subjective examination

| | |
|---|---|
| Subject | 39-year-old male carpenter<br>Right hand dominant |
| HPC | Right lateral elbow pain off and on for at least 5/12. Insidious onset<br>Worsened 4/52 ago when his nail gun broke down and he was forced to use a hammer all day<br>Severe pain and reduced strength, particularly when using his arm during activities such as gripping, holding and lifting. Pain radiates into forearm<br>No history of locking |
| PMH | Fractured ribs 3 years ago due to fall at work. Landed on his right side, and elbow was pushed into the ribs. No elbow symptoms until 5/12 ago<br>Never experienced any symptoms of the cervical or thoracic spine<br>Minor injuries such as an ankle sprain, mainly due to sport |
| Aggravating factors | Firm gripping (e.g. pliers)<br>Hammering<br>Screw driving<br>Using a jackhammer<br>Driving (car has no power steering)<br>Closing a tap<br>Knocking the elbow |
| Easing factors | Rest<br>Ice |
| Night | Constant ache. Lying on elbow or pulling up the blanket makes it worse |
| Daily pattern | Constant pain that worsens during and directly after activity |
| General health | No other health problems reported. Not using any medication or receiving any other medical care |

| | |
|---|---|
| **Attitude/ expectations** | Is disappointed that his elbow problem hasn't improved over time as his other injuries did<br>Experiencing increasing problems at work. Is afraid that he will lose his job<br>One of his colleagues experienced major improvement after physiotherapy treatment and he hopes that it will help him too<br>Expects that it may take some time since he wants to stay at work |
| **Pain and dysfunction scores** | VAS current pain at rest = 4<br>VAS usual level of pain during activity in the last week = 8<br>VAS worst level of pain in the last week = 9–10<br>Upper Extremity Functional Index (UEFI) 35/80 (Stanford et al 2001) |

## Objective examination

| | |
|---|---|
| **Arm at rest while standing** | Elbow flexed (right > left)<br>Wrist flexed (right > left)<br>Forearm supinated (right > left) |
| **Palpation** | Skin temperature (T*sk*) normal<br>Lateral epicondyle extremely painful with some palpable swelling<br>Tenderness extensor carpi radialis brevis and longus<br>Thickening in extensor carpi radialis brevis (ECRB)<br>Difficult to palpate for tenderness of capitellum radii due to surrounding tissue swelling and pain |
| **Muscle length** | ECRB – tight (flexion and ulnar deviation of the wrist, pronation of the forearm, and slight extension of elbow)<br>Extensor carpi radialis longus – tight (flexion and ulnar deviation of the wrist, pronation of the forearm, and complete extension of elbow) |
| **Functional testing, including ROM and strength** | Elbow extension showed pain in at end of ROM (VAS rises to 6)<br>Forearm pronation/supination showed full ROM (VAS rises to 5) |

CHAPTER EIGHT

| | |
|---|---|
| | Reduced grip strength (VAS rises from 4 to 9 during firm gripping)<br>Difficulty opening pushing door handle and opening door (VAS rises to 7)<br>Difficulty lifting an object with palm of hand facing down (VAS rises to 8)<br>Resistance against dorsiflexion in a dorsiflexed position of the wrist, with fist closed, caused severe pain on the lateral side of the elbow |

**Questions**

1. What is your provisional diagnosis?
2. What signs and symptoms lead you to this diagnosis?
3. Describe the mechanism that can lead to the condition
4. What will you include in your treatment plan?
5. What kind of common and less common problems need to be excluded?
6. How likely does the patient's previous fall contribute to the current complaint?
7. How will the expectations of the patient influence your treatment?
8. Is the patient likely to benefit from referral to other health professionals?



## CASE STUDY 10 HAND WEAKNESS AND PAIN

### Subjective examination

| | |
|---|---|
| Subject | 56-year-old woman who works part-time as a kindergarten assistant<br>Right hand dominant |
| HPC | Pain, numbness and tingling noticed in right hand (particularly in the thumb, index and middle fingers) over the last 6/52, especially at night. Insidious onset<br>Has started to have difficulty using right hand for gripping and it is starting to affect work as a kindergarten assistant and tennis<br>Feels it is getting worse, because pain is now extending up the forearm. Is now waking her during the night |
| PMH | Diagnosed with non-insulin-dependent diabetes 5 years ago, currently well controlled with diet and exercise (walks for 45 minutes three times a week and plays social tennis twice a week) |

| | |
|---|---|
| | Knee arthroscopy with partial left medial menisectomy 12 years ago after tennis injury, recovered well |
| **Aggravating factors** | Gripping (tennis racquet after 1 set, a feeling of weakness)<br>Opening jars<br>Packing up play equipment at kindergarten<br>Sleeping |
| **Easing factors** | Gets a little relief from changing position and shaking out wrist<br>Aspirin (started aspirin 2/52 ago on advice of GP), may have helped a little |
| **Night** | Now waking every night (once only) with right wrist pain and numbness |
| **Daily pattern** | Symptoms are dependent on activity. Finds it is painful at end of shift at the kindergarten and after tennis. Otherwise not troubling too much during the day |
| **Attitude/ expectations** | Enjoys her regular exercise (especially tennis) so is keen to get the problem fixed<br>She has friends who had surgery for something that sounded similar so is not sure why she was referred to physiotherapy or how it might help |
| **Pain and dysfunction scores** | VAS current pain at rest = 1.5<br>VAS worst level of pain in the last week = 7<br>Levine symptom severity scale = 1.9/5.0<br>Levine functional status scale = 1.4/5.0 |

## Physical examination

| | |
|---|---|
| **Observation** | No abnormality detected<br>No wasting of right thenar eminence |
| **Palpation** | Slight reduction to light touch on the palmar surface of the right thumb and 1st and 2nd finger |
| **Movement (right side)** | Wrist flexion = 60°, no pain<br>Wrist extension = 55°, no pain<br>Wrist supination = 90° from mid-prone, no pain |

| | |
|---|---|
| | Wrist pronation = 90° from mid-prone, no pain<br>Finger IP flexion OK, no pain<br>Finger MCP flexion OK, no pain<br>Thumb flexion, abduction and opposition OK, no pain |
| **Functional testing, including ROM and strength** | Grip strength assessed on Jamar dynamometer (right = 27 kg with VAS = 3, left = 35 kg)<br>Phalen's test (sustained bilateral wrist flexion) reproduced numbness on palmar surface of index and middle after 45 seconds<br>Upper limb tension test with a median nerve bias: reproduced right hand symptoms which eased on release of shoulder depression (Butler 2000) |

## Questions

1. What is your provisional diagnosis?
2. What are the anatomical relationships that explain your provisional diagnosis and the patient's symptoms and signs?
3. Explain the significance of the night symptoms and the positive Phalen's sign.
4. Are there other assessment techniques that could be used to confirm the provisional diagnosis?
5. Find out what items the Levine symptom severity and functional status scales assesses (Levine et al 1993) and then discuss how this patient rates.
6. Which of the symptoms and signs will you place on your priority list?
7. How will you address these in your physiotherapy treatment plan?
8. Are there other problems that could be contributing to the symptoms?
9. The patient has some friends who had surgery for something similar. What is the role of surgery for this condition?

# CASE STUDY 11 GROIN PAIN

## Subjective examination

| | |
|---|---|
| **Subject** | 17-year-old male student<br>Playing in high-level senior soccer team with training three times a week in addition to a match on the weekend |

| | |
|---|---|
| | Plays as midfielder<br>Right foot dominant |
| **HPC** | About 4/12 ago noticed slight stiffness in groin the morning after a strenuous match. Insidious onset<br>Gradually got worse until about 2/12 ago could not train or play without right-sided groin pain. Performance was also waning with a loss of power and acceleration<br>On advice of team trainer rested from all training and playing for 6/52, but on resumption of training 2/52 ago groin pain returned immediately. Seen by GP who ordered X-rays and a bone scan, and referred him to physiotherapy |
| **PMH** | Well-controlled asthma. Uses one puff of a preventer daily (Flixitide). Rarely needs to use reliever (Ventolin)<br>Episode of Osgood–Schlatters syndrome when 14 years old after joining soccer development squad. Resolved after 1 year through modification of activity<br>Otherwise well and not seeing the doctor for any other condition |
| **Aggravating factors** | Running, especially when sprinting and when cutting (changing direction)<br>Kicking, especially when taking a corner<br>No pain on sneezing or coughing |
| **Easing factors** | Avoidance of aggravating activities |
| **Night** | Sleep unaffected |
| **Daily pattern** | Symptoms are dependent on activity. Now affecting whenever tries to run or kick a ball<br>Notices in morning, takes 10 to 15 minutes to ease |
| **Attitude/ expectations** | Concerned that the problem appears to be getting worse. Had thought it would just go away<br>Receives payment for playing in soccer team which he had planned to continue to help support his studies at university |

| | |
|---|---|
| **Pain and dysfunction scores** | VAS current pain at rest = 0<br>VAS worst level of pain in the last week = 9 (kicking across from a corner)<br>VAS worst level of pain in the last week = 8 (when attempting to sprint) |

**Physical examination**

| | |
|---|---|
| **Observation** | In standing, no obvious wasting or pelvic asymmetry<br>With walking, observed excessive pelvic tilting (obliquity) in the frontal plane |
| **Palpation** | Tender to palpation at tendon attaching to right medial inferior pubic ramus<br>Trigger point tenderness to muscle belly distal to medial inferior pubic ramus<br>Tender at right side of pubic symphysis |
| **Movement** | Right hip flexion = 130°, no pain = left<br>Right hip extension = 25°, no pain = left<br>Right hip abduction = 45°, pain (VAS = 3), left = 55°<br>Right hip internal/external rotation = left |
| **Functional testing** | ■ Squeeze test (patient supine with hip flexed 45°, examiner places fist between patient knees, and asks patient to bilaterally adduct) reproduced right groin pain (VAS = 4)<br>■ Resisted straight-leg right hip adduction reproduced right groin pain (VAS = 4)<br>■ Right hip quadrant (passive hip flexion, adduction and internal rotation) only very slight pain, similar to discomfort when tested on the left side<br>■ Thomas test (slight restriction on right compared to left with only slight reproduction of pain (VAS = 0.5) when hip flexion resisted)<br>■ Abdominal muscle testing:<br>1. global muscles, only slight pain (VAS = 1) on resisted abdominal flexion<br>2. stabilising muscles, assessed in supine with a pressure cuff biofeedback unit placed in the small of the back. He could increase the pressure in the cuff |

| | |
|---|---|
| | from 40 to 43 mmHg for 3 seconds 4 times before unwanted activity from global muscles was observed<br>■ Standing on one leg (Trendelenburg test), only slight drop of pelvis observed, within normal limits (<10°) |
| **Investigations (completed 1/52 ago)** | X-ray: no abnormality detected<br>Bone scan: indicated some increased uptake in the right inferior pubic region |

## Questions

1. What is your provisional diagnosis?
2. What are the key findings from your examination that led to your provisional diagnosis?
3. What other common causes of groin pain did you consider in making your diagnosis?
4. What are some less common causes of groin pain that you need to consider when examining this patient? Briefly explain why these are considered unlikely at this stage.
5. What is Osgood–Schlatter's disease and what is its relevance to the current condition?
6. What are the significance of the bone scan findings and the assessment of the abdominal stabilising muscles, and do these findings tie in with the other assessment findings?
7. Which of the symptoms and signs will you place on your priority list?
8. How will you address these in your physiotherapy treatment plan?

## CASE STUDY 12 HIP AND THIGH PAIN

### Subjective examination

| | |
|---|---|
| Subject | 38-year-old female<br>Right leg dominant |
| HPC | Right lateral hip and thigh pain that can radiate to knee<br>Started approximately 1/12 ago<br>Woke up with pain after a long shopping day |
| PMH | Overweight (BMI ≥27)<br>Neck pain and headaches |
| Aggravating factors | Walking<br>Sleeping on right side<br>Sleeping on a hard mattress |

| | |
|---|---|
| **Easing factors** | Rest and ice |
| **Night** | Wakes up frequently, particularly when lying on right side, or on left side with right hip in adduction and knee resting on the mattress |
| **Daily pattern** | Pain during and after prolonged standing and walking |
| **General health** | Overweight. No other problems reported. Not using any medication |
| **Attitude/ expectations** | Is not sure whether treatment will provide immediate relief, but hopes that at least she will be able to sleep better. Between pain experienced at night and her youngest child waking up and demanding attention she does not get much sleep and feels fatigued |
| **Pain and dysfunction scores** | VAS current pain at rest before activity = 2<br>VAS usual level of pain when waking up at night = 8<br>VAS usual level of pain during and after activity in the last week = 7<br>VAS worst level of pain in the last week = 9<br>Lower Extremity Functional Scale 48/80 (Binkley et al 1999) |

## Objective examination

| | |
|---|---|
| **Standing** | Visibly overweight<br>Wide hips, but knees are touching each other<br>Valgus position of knees and ankles<br>Pronated feet with reasonable longitudinal arches |
| **Palpation** | Although skin temperature (T*sk*) around hip and along the thigh appeared normal, that of the posterior aspect of the trochanter may have been a little elevated<br>Tenderness of the iliotibial tract and the bony posterior aspect of the greater trochanter, with a boggy feeling around the location of the bursa (Hoppenfield 1986) |

| | |
|---|---|
| **Muscle length** | Tensor fasciae latae – tight<br>Gluteus medius – tight<br>Gluteus minimus – tight |
| **Functional testing, including ROM and strength** | Walking with a positive Trendelenburg and with pronated feet<br>Difficulty lifting opposite hip in standing and when walking (VAS rises to 4)<br>Flexing and adducting the hip during the swinging phase of the right leg when walking slowly is associated with an audible and palpable click on the lateral side of the hip, whereas the standing phase of the right leg is associated with pain and difficulty holding the pelvis horizontal<br>Resisting abduction in supine showed reduced strength on right side<br>Joint mobility appeared normal, although combined hip flexion, adduction and internal rotation of the hip (in supine) felt tight and was associated with lateral hip pain and pain along the lateral side of the thigh<br>True leg length discrepancy (Hoppenfield 1986). Left leg almost 3 cm shorter than right leg |

## Questions

1. Based on the information presented, what is your provisional diagnosis?
2. What signs and symptoms lead you to this diagnosis, and what is the likely mechanism that contributes to the problem?
3. How will you address these in your treatment plan?
4. What kind of common and less common problems need to be excluded?
5. What are the biomechanical factors that could contribute to the current complaint?
6. How will the expectations of the patient influence your treatment?
7. Is the patient likely to benefit from referral to other health professionals?

## CASE STUDY 13 MEDIAL KNEE PAIN

### Subjective examination

| | |
|---|---|
| Subject | 32-year-old female<br>Right leg dominant |
| HPC | Injured right knee during skiing 5/7 ago. Did the splits and twisted right knee. Right knee showed some swelling |
| PMH | Concussion 3 years ago<br>Minor injuries such as an ankle sprain |
| Aggravating factors | Moving objects on the floor by pushing with medial side of the right foot<br>Getting into the driver's side of a car (steering wheel on right)<br>Turning sharply to the left when walking<br>Lying on left side with right knee unsupported |
| Easing factors | Walking in a straight line<br>Rest |
| Night | Wakes up with pain when knee is unsupported or in complete extension |
| Daily pattern | Pain and swelling worsen with prolonged standing and as the day goes on<br>No locking of the knee, although occasionally it clicks and seems to give way |
| General health | No other health problems reported. Not using any medication or receiving any other medical care |
| Attitude/ expectations | Very positive. Is convinced that the injury will heal with good management and is prepared to do the work that is required<br>Misses regular running and court sport and wants to return to these activities as early as possible |
| Pain and dysfunction scores | VAS current pain at rest = 1<br>VAS when getting into a car = 5<br>VAS when pushing with foot against an object = 9<br>The knee injury and osteoarthritis outcome score (KOOS): Pain = 56% (Roos et al 1998) |

## Objective examination

| | |
|---|---|
| **Standing** | Weight bearing on left leg, right knee flexed<br>Right patella not completely visible due to some swelling<br>Knee valgus when extending knee (right = left) |
| **Gait** | Shorter right stand phase<br>Limited right knee extension when pushing off |
| **Palpation** | Skin temperature (T*sk*) normal<br>Medial collateral ligament painful on palpation<br>Patella not ballotable (the patella is ballotable when underlying synovia lifts it off the femur. Tapping on the patella causes it to bounce on the femur) with knee in extension<br>When joint fluid is manually forced from the suprapatellar pouch and from the lateral side of the knee to the medial side of the knee (sweep test), gentle tapping on this swelling causes the fluid to travel to the lateral side of the knee with visible swelling that pulses with the tapping (Hoppenfield 1986)<br>Tenderness at the level of the posterior attachment of the medial meniscus |
| **Muscle length** | NAD |
| **Functional testing, including ROM and strength** | Full knee flexion and extension, although medial knee pain at end of ROM (VAS rises to 3 on full flexion and 5 on full extension)<br>External knee rotation with knee in 90° flexion proved painful (VAS rises to 6)<br>Applying valgus stress to the right knee with knee in 30° flexion caused medial knee pain and some joint line opening on the medial side compared with left knee (VAS rises to 5). Although there was laxity compared with left knee, there |

| | |
|---|---|
| | was a noticeable end point during this valgus testing<br>Apleys' distraction test caused medial knee pain (VAS rises to 4)<br>Anterior drawer sign was negative<br>Apley's compression test caused no pain, clicking or locking<br>McMurray test for medial meniscus was negative (testing lateral meniscus was not appropriate and would have caused unnecessary stress on the medial collateral ligament) |

## Questions

1. What is your provisional diagnosis?
2. What signs and symptoms lead you to this diagnosis?
3. How will you address these in your treatment plan?
4. What kind of common and less common problems need to be excluded?
5. Given patient's history, what needs to pointed out to assist the healing process?
6. How will the expectation of the patient influence your treatment?
7. Is the patient likely to benefit from referral to other health professionals?



## CASE STUDY 14 ANTERIOR KNEE PAIN

### Subjective examination

| | |
|---|---|
| Subject | 26-year-old female physical education teacher<br>Right side dominant |
| HPC | Bilateral knee pain right > left insidious onset started approximately 1 year ago has gradually got worse<br>Diffuse pain 'unable to put finger on it' lateral and inferior to patella (see Figure 8.7)<br>No history of giving way or locking<br>No report of visible swelling but patient states 'it sometimes feels swollen even though it doesn't look swollen'<br>No history of altered temperature sensations, knee feeling cold or hot |
| PMH | 18/12 ago had RTA and suffered whiplash injury. Received physiotherapy and this does not bother |

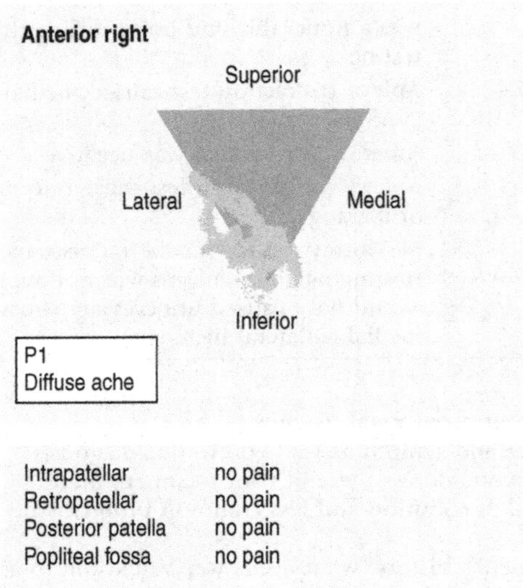


**FIGURE 8.7** Knee body chart – Case Study 14.



| | |
|---|---|
| | her now. Was off work for a couple of months and put weight on (2 kg) which she has found hard to lose<br>No history of patella dislocation or subluxation |
| **Aggravating factors** | Stairs<br>Squatting<br>Running<br>Driving |
| **Easing factors** | Nothing in particular |
| **Night** | No problems |
| **Daily pattern** | None – depends on what activities she does on that particular day |
| **General Health** | No other health problems reported, not taking any medications or under any other medical care |
| **Attitude/ expectations** | Expresses frustration at not being able to do job properly<br>Also frustrated by inability to loose weight |

| | |
|---|---|
| | Very high level of expectation that physiotherapy will 'cure' her problem quickly |
| **Pain & dysfunction scores** | VAS current pain = 4<br>VAS usual level of pain in the last week = 4<br>VAS worst level of pain in the last week = 8<br>Modified Functional Index Questionnaire (MFIQ) 33 points |

## Objective examination

All of the following are approximately symmetrical bilaterally

| | |
|---|---|
| **Palpation** | Skin temperature (T*sk*) normal<br>Patellar size normal<br>Slight posterior tilt of pole of patella into fat pad which is slightly puffy<br>Patellar tendon length normal<br>Tibial tubercle normal size |
| **Muscle length** | Rectus femoris – tight (in prone passive heel to buttock 30 cm)<br>Hamstrings – tight (in supine with hip flexion at 90° active knee extension 35°)<br>Gastrocnemius – tight (in supine knee full extension with full passive dorsi-flexion – active plantar flexion reduced <10°) |
| **Standing posture** | *Feet*<br>■ Great toes – mild hallux valgus (great toes deviated laterally)<br>■ Medial longitudinal arches flattened<br>*Knees*<br>■ Slight genu recurvatum (knee hyperextension)<br>■ Slight genu valgus (knock knees)<br>■ Reduced quadriceps bulk |
| **Functional testing** | *Walking*<br>■ No pain<br>■ Knee flexion at heel strike bilaterally<br>*Stairs*<br>■ Ascent VAS rises to 5<br>■ Descent VAS rises to 6<br>■ During descent quadriceps demonstrate inability to control the movement effectively |

## Questions

1. What is your provisional diagnosis?
2. Which items will you include on your priority problem list?
3. How will you manage your problem list?
4. How do you interpret the patient's report of no actual swelling visible but a sensation of swelling being present?
5. Does the patient's previous road traffic accident have any relevance to her current complaint?
6. How will the patient's expectation of physiotherapy influence your management?
7. Would you consider it relevant to refer this patient to any other health professionals?

## CASE STUDY 15 CALF PAIN

### Subjective examination

| | |
|---|---|
| **Subject** | 55-year-old male tennis player<br>Right leg dominant |
| **HPC** | Left calf pain. Sudden onset 1/52 ago when playing tennis<br>Did not warm up before the game<br>Five minutes in the game it felt like someone hit him in the calf with a tennis ball. Had problems walking, although this has improved day by day. Is now able to walk and jog on the flat without discomfort |
| **PMH** | Coronary bypass surgery 6 years ago<br>Low back pain off and on |
| **Aggravating factors** | Running<br>Fast walking uphill, particularly when pushing off with foot |
| **Easing factors** | Rest |
| **Night** | No problems |
| **Daily pattern** | No pain except when running or going for long or fast uphill walk<br>No cramps |
| **General health** | Overweight (BMI = 27)<br>Fitness has improved after coronary bypass |
| **Attitude/ expectations** | Wants to keep up fitness because of his weight and past heart condition |

| | |
|---|---|
| | Finds it frustrating that calf pain limits his needed level of activity<br>Pain and dysfunction scores<br>VAS during demanding physical activity = 6 |
| **Objective examination**<br>Standing | NAD. No swelling or differences in skin colour, or varicose veins |
| Palpation | Skin temperature (T*sk*) normal<br>Some tenderness in the medial head of the gastrocnemius, and a slight palpable gap in the muscle belly |
| Muscle length | Some tightness and pain on maximum calf stretch with knee straight (gastrocnemius), but not with knee bent (soleus) |
| Functional testing, including ROM, strength and specific tests | Repeated unilateral heel raises caused pain at maximum lift (VAS rises to 6)<br>Unilateral hopping caused pain when pushing off (VAS raises to 5), but not on landing<br>Slump test as well as SLR were negative, even SLR with added dorsiflexion and eversion or inversion (Butler 2000)<br>Homan's sign was negative (Hoppenfield 1986)<br>Arteries palpable (a. poplitea, a. dorsalis pedis, a. tibialis posterior) |

## Questions

1. What is your provisional diagnosis?
2. What signs and symptoms lead you to this diagnosis?
3. How will you address these in your treatment plan?
4. What kind of common and less common problems need to be excluded?
5. Can the patient's coronary condition or occasional low back pain explain current symptoms?
6. How will the expectations of the patient influence your treatment?
7. Is the patient likely to benefit from referral to other health professionals?

# CASE STUDY 16 ACHILLES PAIN

## Subjective examination

| | |
|---|---|
| Subject | 43-year-old male<br>Right leg dominant |
| HPC | Right Achilles pain<br>Insidious onset, started approximately 3/12 ago |
| PMH | Overweight (BMI $\geq$27)<br>Diet-controlled diabetes |
| Aggravating factors | Jogging or brisk walking<br>Compression bandage |
| Easing factors | Rest and ice |
| Night | No problems |
| Daily pattern | Achilles pain, particularly during and after prolonged activities such as walking and jogging. Pain and stiffness seem to ease at the start of activity but worsens as the activity prolongs. Pain is worst after these physical activities |
| General health | Type 2 diabetes which is controlled by diet and exercise. Not using any medication or receiving any other medical care apart from regular health checks that include blood glucose and weight |
| Attitude/ expectations | Wants to remain physically active to control type 2 diabetes, but is frustrated that the Achilles tendon problem limits his ability to perform the more intensive forms of physical activity he likes doing<br>Given the time for the problem to develop, he expects that it will take some time for the symptoms to settle. He is prepared to do whatever it takes to assist the healing process and his return to jogging |
| Pain and dysfunction scores | VAS current pain at rest before activity = 3<br>VAS usual level of pain at the start of activity in the last week = 2<br>VAS usual level of pain after activity in the last week = 7<br>VAS worst level of pain in the last week = 8 |

## Objective examination

| | |
|---|---|
| Standing | Pronated feet with fallen longitudinal arches<br>Valgus of ankles with Achilles tendon deviation (right > left)<br>Visibly overweight |
| Palpation | Skin temperature (T*sk*) normal<br>Local thickening of midway the Achilles tendon with tenderness over a length of approximately 1 cm<br>Slight crepitus palpable during plantar/dorsiflexion |
| Muscle length | Soleus – tight (is not able to squat down while maintaining heel pressure on the floor)<br>Hamstrings – tight |
| Functional testing, including ROM and strength | Walking with pronated feet. Valgus of heel noticeable (VAS lowers to 2)<br>Jogging on spot shows increased knee and hip action when pushing off rather than ankle action (VAS rises to 4)<br>Difficulty with slow heel raises, does not seem to have enough calf strength to lift (VAS increases to 5) |

## Questions

1. What is your provisional diagnosis?
2. What signs and symptoms lead you to this diagnosis?
3. Describe the mechanism that can lead to the condition.
4. How will you address these signs and symptoms in your treatment plan?
5. What kind of common and less common problems need to be excluded?
6. How likely does BMI of 27 or over contribute to the current complaint?
7. How will the expectation of the patient influence your treatment?
8. Is the patient likely to benefit from referral to other health professionals?

# CASE STUDY 17 ANKLE SPRAIN

## Subjective examination

| | |
|---|---|
| Subject | 26-year-old female basketball player<br>Right leg dominant |
| HPC | Injured right ankle during basketball training the previous night by landing on someone's foot and rolling ankle<br>Excruciating pain at the time of the injury and inability to weight bear<br>Initially there was an egg-shape swelling visible on the anterolateral side of the right ankle. Within a couple of hours the whole ankle was swollen<br>The trainer applied RICE (rest, ice, compression bandage, elevation of leg) immediately after injury which helped at the time. Pain and swelling worsened when joining other players for drinks after the training and travelling home |
| PMH | Multiple mild ankle sprains of both ankles over the last 10 years<br>Episode of pain behind the ankle when running cross country 3 years ago. Pain ceased when she stopped running<br>Was prescribed foot orthotics due to flat feet |
| Aggravating factors | Sitting or standing with foot down on floor, even without weight bearing<br>Weight bearing (WB)<br>Moving ankle, particularly inversion and plantar flexion<br>Knocking or bumping into objects |
| Easing factors | RICE<br>Partial weight bearing (PWB), or non-weight bearing (NWB) |
| Night | Constant discomfort and mild pain, particularly when left leg rests on right ankle |
| Daily pattern | Swelling and discomfort is worse as the day goes on |
| General health | No other health problems reported. Not using any medication or receiving any other medical care |

| | |
|---|---|
| **Attitude/ expectations** | Although worse than previously experienced she is confident that the ankle will heal with proper care and wants to prevent another injury if possible<br>Wants to continue her favourite sport as soon as possible for reasons of health and wellbeing. Also, she developed many contacts through basketball and enjoys company of others |
| **Pain and dysfunction scores** | VAS level of pain when foot down, but NWB = 3–4<br>VAS level of pain during WB = 8<br>Lower Extremity Functional Scale 46/80 (Binkley et al 1999) |

## Objective examination

| | |
|---|---|
| **Standing with right foot on floor, although PWB** | Swelling right ankle, but no bruising visible<br>Pes plani valgi (left > right due to WB on left foot and PWB on right foot)<br>Achilles tendon deviation due to valgus position of ankle |
| **Palpation** | Skin temperature (T*sk*) felt warmer, although this may be attributed to the compression bandage that was removed prior to the examination<br>Although there was tenderness around the ankle, lateral as well medial, the anterior talofibular ligament was most painful on palpation<br>The lateral malleolus as well as the medial malleolus felt intact<br>In applying the Ottawa ankle rules (Stiell et al 1994), there was no excessive bony tenderness of the posterior aspects of both malleoli peripherally over at least the last 6 cm. No tenderness over the base of the fifth metatarsal or navicular bone<br>Achilles tendon proved slightly tender on medial side, although there was no palpable swelling |

| | |
|---|---|
| **Joint stability and ROM** | Anterior drawer test proved painful on anterolateral side of right ankle and was associated with more anterior movement when compared with left ankle<br>Talar tilt was negative<br>Passive inversion and plantar flexion were painful and slightly limited |
| **Muscle length** | Right soleus seemed tight (dorsal flexion of ankle with knee bent), although it was not possible to test muscle length well. Left soleus was tight with slight medial tenderness at end of the stretch<br>Hamstrings were both tight (right = left) |
| **Functional testing, including ROM and strength** | Inversion and plantar flexion ROM was limited (VAS rises to 6)<br>Dorsiflexion of the ankle during lunging was limited<br>Balance and proprioception could only be tested by standing on left leg with eyes closed. Maintaining balance proved difficult for her and was associated with excessive ankle movement and arm compensation |



## Questions

1. What is your provisional diagnosis?
2. What signs and symptoms lead you to this diagnosis?
3. How will you address these in your treatment plan?
4. What kind of common and less common problems need to be excluded?
5. How likely do patient's pes plani valgi contribute to the current complaint?
6. How will the expectations of the patient influence your treatment?
7. Is the patient likely to benefit from referral to other health professionals?

## CASE STUDY 18 FIBROMYALGIA

### Subjective examination

| | |
|---|---|
| Subject | 23-year-old female nurse |
| HPC | Chronic and general musculoskeletal pain and stiffness with no specific cause. |

| | |
|---|---|
| | Pain started 3 years ago when she was studying nursing. Although she finished her study, she experienced problems with concentrating, and comprehending and memorising information<br>Constant fatigue. Can sleep for many hours, but does not wake up refreshed<br>Experienced fewer problems 2 years ago when she went hiking with friends after finishing her study, but problems slowly returned after starting her new job as a nurse |
| **PMH** | Headaches off and on |
| **Aggravating factors** | Working at night<br>Does not want to rely on taking prescribed analgesic medication |
| **Easing factors** | Rest |
| **Night** | Wakes up frequently |
| **Daily pattern** | Pain is constant. Although the pain can shift to different regions and vary in intensity, it mostly is a vague and general pain |
| **General health** | Feels tired constantly, and down at times<br>Using tricyclic and reuptake inhibitor medication to increase serotonin and norepinephrine levels in the central nervous system |
| **Attitude/ expectations** | Feels down. Is disappointed that pain has not improved. Experiencing increasing problems at work due to bodily pain, headaches and constant fatigue, particularly when starting a new work shift. Has been told by her physician that exercise may help to improve her condition |
| **Pain and dysfunction scores** | VAS current pain at rest = 3<br>VAS worst level of pain in the last week = 7<br>The Kessler 10 (K-10), a measure of anxiety and depressive symptoms, showed a score of 24 (22–50 = high) (Andrews & Slade 2001)<br>The Hospital Anxiety and Depression Scale (HADS) consists of items for anxiety and for depression. The aggregated score was 15 (11–21 = moderate to severe anxiety and depression) (Zigond & Snaith 1983) |

### Objective examination

| | |
|---|---|
| General posture in standing | Poor posture (round shouldered, increased cervical lordosis)<br>Poorly developed muscles |
| Palpation | Skin temperature (T*sk*) normal<br>Tenderness of many muscles with palpable trigger points, particularly the suboccipital muscles, descending part of the trapezius, serratus posterior superior and quadratus lumborum |
| Functional testing, including ROM and strength | General joint mobility and muscle length were acceptable; accept suboccipital muscles, descending part of the trapezius, serratus posterior superior, quadratus lumborum and hamstrings were tight<br>Abdominals were weak |



### Questions

1. What is your provisional diagnosis?
2. What signs and symptoms lead to this diagnosis?
3. How will you address these in your treatment plan?
4. What kind of common and less common problems need to be excluded?
5. Can patient's headaches be related to her current musculoskeletal condition?
6. How will the expectation of the patient influence your treatment?
7. Is the patient likely to benefit from referral to other health professionals?

## ANSWERS TO CHAPTER 8: CASE STUDIES IN MUSCULOSKELETAL OUT-PATIENTS

### Case Study 1

1. TMJ disorder.

2. Masticatory muscle pain at rest and during chewing, localised tenderness or pain of the TMJ joint, and reduced oral opening (depression of the jaw). Treatment of these symptoms may be effective. Unfortunately, many interventional studies that have been conducted so far are of poor methodological quality and results should be interpreted with caution. Some of the limitations are lack of consensus on defining the disorder, inclusion and exclusion criteria, and using sound (valid and reliable) outcome measures.

3. Improvements in oral opening have been found with:
   a. muscular awareness relaxation therapy
   b. biofeedback training; and
   c. low-level laser therapy treatment (McNeely et al 2006, Medlicott & Harris 2006).

   In addition:
   i. Active exercises and manual mobilisations may be effective, and proprioceptive re-education may be more effective than placebo treatment or occlusal splints (Medlicott & Harris 2006).
   ii. Compared with no treatment a stabilisation splint may assist in decreasing the severity of pain at rest, on palpation and when depressing the jaw (Al-Ani et al 2005). In fact, the type of splint (stabilisation splint, soft splint or non-occluding palatal splint) does not seem to make a difference in clinical outcome (Turp et al 2004).
   iii. Acupuncture may be effective (Turp et al 2004).
   iv. The use of ultrasound therapy in the treatment of TMJ joint disorder is not justified (van der Windt et al 1999).

4. Problems that can cause TMJ disorders include asymmetrical dentition, TMJ dislocation due to hyper extension of the neck, muscle cramps due to low blood calcium levels, tension of the external pterygoid muscles and TMJ osteoarthritis. The Chvostek test (tapping the area of the parotid gland) can be an indicator for low blood calcium levels when the masseter muscle twitches.

5. Given that muscular awareness relaxation therapy and biofeedback training has shown some effectiveness in the treatment of TMJ disorder, it seems relevant to reduce muscle tension that can be caused by stress. Also, a soft splint may reduce the impact of teeth grinding on teeth as well as TMJ symptoms.

6. The expectation that it will take time is justified. Given the symptoms and level of evidence it will be important for the patient to understand that this condition is likely to improve when all factors are being addressed (including stress reduction), and that programme adherence is needed (including wearing a splint at night).

7. The patient may benefit from referral to a dentist or an advanced dental technician for assessment of occlusion problems due to asymmetrical dentition and/or the provision of a splint.



### Case Study 2

1. Cervicogenic headache. The headache is unilateral and there are symptoms and signs of neck involvement with restriction of range

(right rotation), ipsilateral pain and hypo-mobility on cervical palpation, and headache brought on by sustained postures (sitting at the computer for 2 hours with a forward head posture) (Sjaastad et al 1998).

2. The main findings that led to the provisional diagnosis are:
   a. the restricted range of right rotation and the right-sided palpatory findings in the upper cervical spine
   b. the second main group of findings placed on the priority list are factors that could be considered as contributing factors, such as the decreased strength and endurance of the deep cervical flexors and the poor posture of the cervical spine. It is possible the past history of the car accident 10 years ago might be related to the poor muscle function now observed.

3. The initial focus of management is to address the musculoskeletal impairment (Jull & Niere 2004). Education is important to explain to the patient that your assessment indicates that his headache appears to be related to some stiffness and dysfunction in his neck and that treatment aimed at easing that dysfunction should help his headaches.

   Manual therapy directed at the upper cervical spine on the right can be an effective technique in restoring range of right rotation and relieving symptoms of cervicogenic headache (Bronfort et al 2004a). As well as mobilising the cervical spine directly, the therapist could trial mobilising the cervical spine indirectly via neurodynamic techniques (note that the upper limb tension test was positive on the right side) (Refshauge & Gass 2004).

   Specific low-load exercises to improve function of the deep cervical flexor muscles could also be taught (Jull et al 2002). Initially, exercises focus on the patient being able to isolate the deep cervical flexors; in supine the patient should 'drop their chin towards their chest' and aim to maintain for 10 seconds (repeat 10 times, twice daily), without any superficial muscle activity. There is evidence that physiotherapy combining manual therapy and muscle training exercises can result in improvements in headache frequency and duration with benefits lasting up to 12 months (Jull et al 2002).

   There is a lack of evidence to support the use of electrotherapy modalities in the treatment of cervicogenic headache (Kroeling et al 2005).

4. The patient has expressed some concern that his headaches may be serious:
   a. Red flags that might be indicative of serious pathologies such as cancer, infection or vascular disorders like sub-arachnoid haemorrhage, include sudden onset of severe headache not related

to activity, constant unremitting pain, headaches progressively worsening, significant night pain, the first or worst headache in the patient's life, headache associated with fever, nausea or vomiting, or headaches related to a change in cognition, neurological signs or neck rigidity (Jull & Niere 2004).

b. It is also important for the physiotherapist to be able to distinguish between cervicogenic headache, tension type headache and migraine. Migraines can have a pulsating or throbbing quality and are likely to be severe with nausea, vomiting and/or photophobia as accompanying features (IHS 2004). They are often triggered by stress or by certain foods, such as chocolate. Migraines in the acute phase also respond to serotonergic medication. Tension type headaches are typically bilateral in nature, less likely to be severe and rarely associated with nausea, vomiting, photophobia or phonophobia (IHS 2004).

5. Prolonged sitting at the computer is a significant precipitating factor. Regular interruption of sitting with standing and stretching should be encouraged and correction of the forward head posture with cervical retraction exercises should be performed frequently while sitting. Correction of lumbar and thoracic posture and/or changes in workstation set up may be necessary to help achieve this.

6. The patient has a positive expectation and is keen to continue with work and recreational activities. This should help with compliance relating to exercises and postural correction. The concern he had that he might have something serious should be addressed by careful education regarding the diagnosis and proposed treatment and by monitoring his condition.

7. The patient is likely to respond well to physiotherapy directed principally to his upper cervical spine. If he does not get better or if his symptoms worsen he should be referred to a medical practitioner for further investigation to rule out serious pathology or other causes of headache such as migraine.



## Case Study 3

1. The most likely source of the patient's arm pain is irritation of the 7th cervical nerve root. The reason we think that the C7 nerve root is irritated is because:
   - the quality of the pain (sharp, shooting, well localised) is consistent with that of nerve root irritation (also known as radicular pain or radiculopathy)
   - the symptoms are associated with examination findings of decreased triceps strength and absence of triceps deep tendon reflex, suggestive of impaired conduction in the C7 nerve root.

2. The most likely cause of his neck and interscapular pain is pathology affecting a lower cervical intervertebral disc, probably between C6 and C7:
   - Referred pain from deep somatic structures such as the intervertebral disc is commonly described as deep, dull and aching. Cloward (1959) showed that stimulation of cervical intervertebral discs could produce pain in the interscapular area, although a more recent study by Tanaka et al (2006) suggested that the cervical nerve roots themselves could also refer pain into this area.
   - There is likely to be a high inflammatory component as the pain is constant and tends to be worse in the mornings. Reproduction of arm pain with cervical extension and left rotation is consistent with nerve root compromise as these movements have been shown to decrease the diameter of the cervical intervertebral foraminae (Ordway et al 1999). Similarly, postero-anterior vertebral pressures are also likely to create an extension type movement of the cervical spine, also leading to foraminal narrowing and nerve impingement.



3. Other possible sources of pain include the lower cervical zygapophysial joints (Dwyer et al 1990). The cervical paraspinal muscles and scalenes on the left could also contribute to the symptoms.

4. In this case the physiotherapist should take care not to perform any procedure that might lead to an exacerbation of the condition, particularly with respect to the arm pain which is likely to be neural in origin. Careful monitoring of symptoms within the initial treatment session and in follow-up sessions as well as re-evaluation of the neurological findings in follow-up sessions should alert the physiotherapist to changes in the likely pathology and its effect on nerve function.

5. An appropriate initial treatment would involve:
   - education as to the likely causes and mechanisms of the symptoms and reassurance that even radicular pain usually settles. The patient should be advised to continue with normal activities of daily living while avoiding movements and postures that exacerbate his arm pain
   - manual techniques may be appropriate to decrease load on the affected segments by improving mobility in adjacent areas (e.g. mobilisation or manipulation to improve thoracic mobility). Manual techniques may help to decrease pain by stimulation of non-nociceptive afferent neural pathways (e.g. large amplitude passive mobilisation). Relief of neural compromise may be achieved by techniques that increase intervertebral foramen

diameter (e.g. manual traction or contralateral rotation mobilisation)
- Gentle soft-tissue massage or local heat may be used to decrease tone and tenderness in the paraspinal and scalene muscles.

6. Longer-term management should aim to address the likely contributing factors. Workstation set up, sitting posture, thoracic mobility, general health and fitness levels may need to be improved to attain an optimal outcome.

7. The prognosis is likely to be good as patients with radicular pain have been shown to have good recovery rates, usually within months (Heckmann et al 1999).

8. Referral back to doctor would be helpful for investigations that confirm pathology or rule out other soft tissue lesions. Oral prednisolone is sometimes recommended for cervical disc prolapses. Although this appears to be useful clinically for some patients, studies have not shown this to be the case on a population level. Progressing neurological deficit or signs of spinal cord compression (e.g. gait disturbances or bilateral upper or lower limb sensory deficits) would be grounds for urgent referral to a medical practitioner:

   *What happened to this patient?*

   This patient was referred back to the doctor as the symptoms were not settling after three treatment sessions, spanning 2/52. He was subsequently referred to a neurosurgeon who ordered an MRI that showed a large C6–7 prolapse (see Figure 8.8). The neurosurgeon prescribed oral prednisolone at a dose of 50 mg daily for 7 days during which time the arm eased, increased strength was noted in the left triceps muscle and a triceps reflex was elicited, although significantly diminished in relation to the right side. In this case surgical intervention was not required. Surgery may have been indicated if there had been progressive, functionally important motor deficit or if the pain had persisted for more than 6–12 weeks (Carette & Fehlings 2005).

## Case Study 4

1. Whiplash associated disorder. This case would be classified as grade 1 or grade 2. It is not grade 3 as there are no neurological signs (WAD guidelines 2001). This is a soft tissue sprain of the cervical spine that may or may not include bone and joint involvement. Structures that could be affected include the cervical muscles, ligaments, zygapophyseal joints, discs, and spinal and sympathetic nerves.

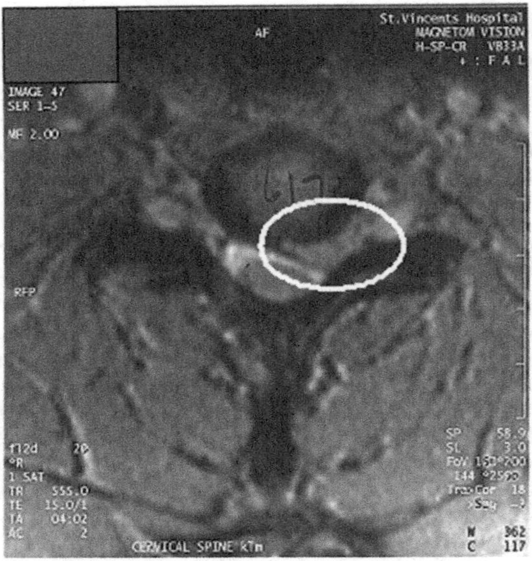


**FIGURE 8.8** MRI showing left sided C6–7 disc prolapsed.



2. Pain increasing to high levels (8.5 on VAS) during car trip that takes 20 minutes to settle. This indicates that there is an inflammatory component to the condition, possibly associated with peripheral and central nervous system sensitisation, and tells the clinician that they need to be careful of doing too much assessment or treatment.

   The other sign that that will be placed high on the priority list is the markedly reduced range of neck rotation movement to the left and right.

3. The main priority at this stage is to reduce pain levels and promote optimal soft tissue healing in conjunction with facilitating pain-free active range of motion:
   - Explanation and education play an important role at this stage with positive messages of reassurance and advice to remain relatively active (Borchgrevink 1998, Rosenfeld 2000). For example, instruct the patient that walking puts less strain on her neck than sitting. Also she should be advised to only sleep with one pillow as extra pillows can push the neck away from a neutral position into flexion or lateral flexion. A short period off work may need to be arranged if work is exacerbating her symptoms

and alternative duties cannot be arranged. The patient may need to return to the doctor to receive adequate medication for pain relief; non-opioid analgesics and NSAIDS can be used in the short term to relieve pain (WAD guidelines 2001). We could advise that at this early stage ice could give more relief to symptoms than heat. There is a lot of debate among clinicians about whether a soft collar could be useful to give relative rest to the neck, but clinical guidelines recommend that soft collars not be prescribed for grade 1 and 2 sprains (WAD guidelines 2001).

- There is limited evidence that active treatment such as exercise is more beneficial than passive modalities (Verhagen et al 2004). To help promote pain-free movement, gentle range of motion exercises in a non-stressful position such as rotation in supine should be prescribed (McKinney et al 1989).

4. The most common problem that needs to be excluded is the possibility of spinal fracture. The decision rules of Hoffman et al (2000) can be applied to help rule out when X-rays are not required. The five criteria are:
   - no midline cervical tenderness
   - no neurological deficit
   - normal alertness
   - no intoxication
   - no painful distracting injury.

   Applying these criteria would allow 12% of trauma victims to avoid X-ray without risk. Our patient has had an X-ray that has cleared the neck of any significant fracture.

   The other factors that the clinician needs to be alert to are the persistence or development of signs that are associated with poor outcome. These may include generalised hyperalgesia, indicative of maladaptive central sensitisation and evidence of psychological impairments such as excessive fear avoidance behaviour and post-traumatic stress reactions (Sterling et al 2005).

5. Work details are very relevant for this patient. This would require further questioning but a large amount of the time sitting and working on a key board would place a high level of stress through the cervical spine. Also, the patient has only been in her current position for a relatively short time so it might make it more difficult to arrange time off work or modified hours and duties.

6. The patient appears anxious about her prognosis and about how the injury will affect her employment. Although a level of anxiety is understandable, it is thought too much anxiety may contribute to symptoms becoming chronic. It is still too early to predict prognosis but at this stage the physiotherapist should allay anxiety with

reassurance and clear explanations, and treat the injury as a simple sprain.

7. The patient may benefit from referral back to their doctor to make sure that pain cover is adequate. Psychological distress may be helped by psychological referral while symptoms associated with persistent central sensitisation may be helped by appropriate medication or a treatment programme incorporating cognitive behavioural principles.

## Case Study 5

1. The thoracic and sternal symptoms are consistent with a predominantly mechanical disorder affecting the thoracic spine:
   - The patient reported that lifting pots brought on his symptoms.
   - The resulting pains were predictably aggravated and eased by mechanical factors (prolonged sitting and standing/walking respectively). Kellgren (1939) demonstrated that deep somatic structures such as ligaments and muscles in the thoracic spine could refer pain to the lateral and anterior chest walls. The thoracic intervertebral discs could also be a source of local and referred pain.

2. An appropriate initial physiotherapy treatment could include passive mobilisation and postural advice:
   - The patient reported that he had experienced a favourable result with passive mobilisation for a similar problem 5 years earlier. Given the relationship between decreased thoracic mobility and production of symptoms on active and passive motion testing, gentle passive mobilising would be an appropriate starting point for treatment. Specific PA pressures at the T7–8 level would be reasonably expected to decrease pain and increase range of movement.
   - It could be hypothesised that sitting with the thoracic spine in flexion for long periods and the generalised restriction of thoracic extension are contributing factors. The factors could be addressed by improving postural awareness, regular postural correction when sitting and by exercises and/or manual therapy to improve range of thoracic extension.

3. Although the behaviour of the thoracic and sternal pain indicates a mechanical disorder the physiotherapist should always be alert to the possibility of serious pathology as a source of spinal pain. This may include primary or metastatic tumours, inflammatory conditions, infective disorders or referral from visceral disorders. Increased pain at night may be associated with non-mechanical disorders, although

it may also be associated with awkward sleeping postures or lack of support provided by the sleeping surface (mattress and/or pillow). For this case the presence of widespread, albeit mild, aches and pains that are worse at night, associated night sweats and unexplained weight loss should alert the physiotherapist to the possible presence of non-mechanical pathology. This non-mechanical pathology could be mimicking the musculoskeletal signs and symptoms, could be causing the musculoskeletal signs and symptoms via viscero-somatic connections or may be incidental to the musculoskeletal signs and symptoms (Grieve 1994).

4. The term 'red flags' has been used to describe examination findings that might be suggestive of serious pathology:
   - Features of cauda equina syndrome (especially urinary retention, bilateral neurological symptoms and signs, saddle anaesthesia)
   - Significant trauma
   - Weight loss
   - History of cancer
   - Fever
   - Intravenous drug use or steroid use
   - Patient aged over 50 years
   - Severe, unremitting night-time pain
   - Pain that gets worse when patient is lying down.

5. The presence of a number of 'red flags' (night pain, unexplained weight loss, night sweats and generalised aches and pains) makes referral to a medical practitioner a priority to investigate the possibility of serious pathology:

   *What happened in this case?*

   The treating physiotherapist in this case did treat the patient with gentle passive mobilising over T7–8 that improved thoracic extension on reassessment. Postural advice and exercises were also provided along with a letter to the GP outlining concerns about the possibility of serious pathology. The patient was referred for further investigations including bone scans and magnetic resonance imaging (MRI) which revealed a large mediastinal tumour, later diagnosed as non-Hodgkin's lymphoma (see Figures 8.9 and 8.10). The patient later reported that the physical treatment had been of great benefit in relieving his thoracic and sternal pain (even at night), but that the generalised aches and pains had not changed. This would indicate that the musculoskeletal dysfunction probably caused symptoms, largely independent of those associated with the lymphoma. The patient made a full recovery with appropriate medical management based mainly around chemotherapy.

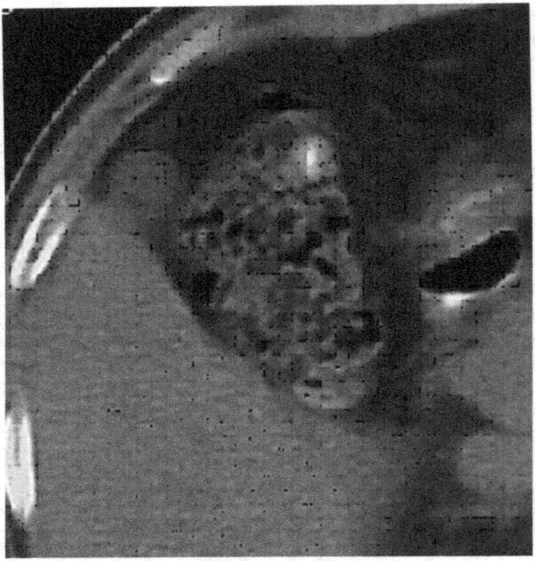

FIGURE 8.9 MRI showing large mediastinal lymphoma.

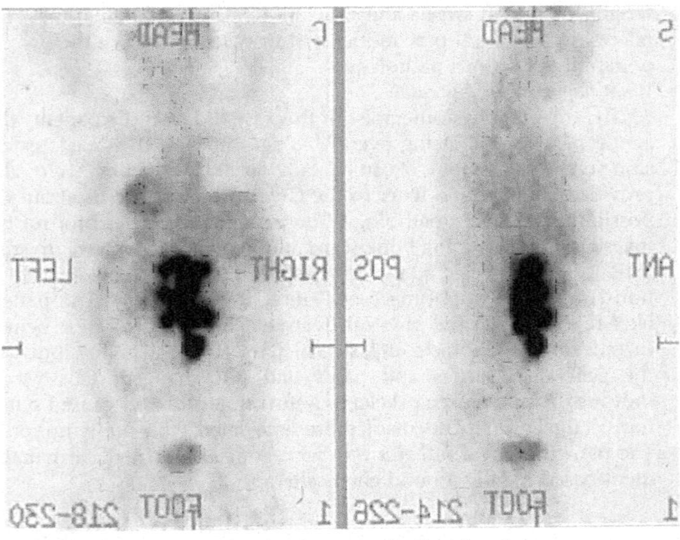

FIGURE 8.10 Bone scan showing large mediastinal lymphoma.

## Case Study 6

1. Discogenic low back pain due to injury to one of the lower lumbar discs. Flexion when repeated and or sustained is an aggravating activity; and unloading (lying supine) and relative extension are easing activities.
2. The right leg pain is likely to be referred pain caused by nociceptive input from pain sensitive structures in the lumbar spine. The leg pain is unlikely to be due to nerve root irritation (radicular pain). This is because segmental neurological testing and neurodynamic tests did not reveal any abnormality. Also, the quality of pain was described as an ache which is commonly attributed to somatic referred pain. Radicular or peripheral neurogenic pain is commonly described as lancinating, sickening, boring or burning. Also, there was no report of pins and needles or numbness which commonly accompany pain associated with compromise of peripheral nerves.
3. The main symptom placed on the priority list is the increased back and leg pain after the 40-minute car journey.

   The main signs on the priority list are the pain responses to repeated movement. Examination suggests that repeated flexion makes things worse (it peripheralises the pain) and repeated extension and side-gliding to the right can make things better (centralise the pain).
4. The presentation is consistent with McKenzie's description of the posterior derangement syndrome (McKenzie and May 2003). When there is a clear pattern that movement in one direction can help and movement in the opposite direction can make the pain worse then the physiotherapist has clear guidelines for treatment:
   a. First, the patient needs to minimise sustained and repeated lumbar flexion. This could include trying to reduce time in sitting, using a support to help maintain the lumbar lordosis during sitting, and possibly taping to remind him not to bend too much.
   b. Second, the patient needs to practice the movements that help to ease or centralise his pain. Based on clinical experience, McKenzie recommends that the side gliding exercise should be done before the repeated extension exercise. These exercises may be done 10 to 15 times and may need to be done hourly throughout the day. Systematic reviews of trials of the McKenzie approach for treating acute low back pain have reported some evidence of short-term benefits in pain and disability (Clare et al 2004, Machado et al 2006).
   c. Spinal manual therapy could also be another effective therapy in the acute phase (Bronfort et al 2004b). This could involve rotation mobilisation, unilateral PA pressures or central PA pressures

(effectively repeated localised extension mobilisation) as described by Maitland et al (2006).

5. A not uncommon problem that must be considered at this stage is if the patient has an irreducible herniated lumbar disc. The absence of neurological signs and the positive responses to movement testing suggest that the disc is still intact.

   A less common problem could be if the pain is due to a secondary tumour in the spine. On this presentation this is unlikely, as he presents with mechanical back pain affected by movement, there is no unexplained weight loss, there is only a relatively small inflammatory component to the pain (able to sleep at night), and the patient had a recent medical check-up when overall he was evaluated as being fit and well. Another rare problem that could be excluded is cauda equina syndrome, compression on the distal bundle of nerve roots. Although this patient has no other signs of nerve root compression cauda equina should be excluded by asking if he has had any bladder and bowel dysfunction.

6. Work details are relevant for this patient. It may be difficult for him to avoid prolonged sitting at work. However, his managerial position means that he may be able to arrange his day and working environment to minimise the stress on his back.

7. The patient has a positive attitude to his back pain. His attitude of coping while his back gets better is likely to be helpful. There is evidence that advice to stay active is effective for short-term pain relief and long-term improvement in function in acute low back pain (van Tulder et al 2006).

8. At this stage the patient should not require referral to another practitioner. The prognosis is reasonable, especially as his pain centralises on repeated movement and his past history indicates that there may be a quick resolution of symptoms. If he doesn't respond to treatment in the first 4 weeks then he should be referred back to his doctor for further investigations. For simple mechanical backache X-rays are not recommended in the first 6 weeks (Waddell et al 1999).



### Case Study 7

1. Chronic low back pain with cognitive and affective components, exacerbated by physical deconditioning due to long-term inactivity. Original injury 14/12 ago may have involved injury to low back structure but symptoms and disability have become chronic and are out of proportion with the original tissue damage.

2. The radiological reports are minor and could almost be regarded as normal age-related changes. The correlation between radiological

changes and patient symptoms is very poor (Schwarzer et al 1995). In other words there are many people who would have reports as bad as this but who have never reported any back pain or any absence of work from back pain.

The other problem with the reports is that the patient believes that they legitimise her condition and reinforce her belief that she has a serious back condition.

3. The main findings placed on the priority list are:
   a. that the patient has not worked for 6/12. Once someone has been off work for more than 6/12 the chances of them successfully returning to work are very low (Waddell 2004)
   b. the number of positive yellow flags exhibited by this patient (New Zealand Acute Low Back Pain Guide 2004) (see below)
   c. the likelihood of physical deconditioning (although not formally assessed) evidenced by the patient's stated avoidance of activity, her increase in weight and her slow walking speed.

4. The management of chronic low back pain is based on the biopsychosocial model of health care with recognition of the psychological and social factors contributing to pain and disability. This patient will need physical treatment to address her musculoskeletal dysfunction but she will also need support and help to cope with pain and to restore normal attitudes and behaviours (Waddell 2004):
   a. Physical rehabilitation aims to improve physical functioning with an active incremental exercise programme, setting achievable goals. There is strong evidence that exercise can reduce pain levels, improve functioning and reduce sick leave in people with chronic low back pain (Hayden et al 2005, Kool et al 2004). Passive modalities are discouraged in the management of people with chronic low back pain as they reinforce patient dependence on therapist.
   b. Psychological support involves helping patients to overcome barriers to progress by encouraging well behaviour and using self-management techniques such as promoting self-efficacy (the belief that you can do something). The physiotherapist has an important role in explaining pain mechanisms to the patient. Professional referral for psychological support may be necessary.
   c. Vocational management is very important and should include workplace assessment, a return to work programme with incremental graduated return to full duties.

   This biopsychosocial model of care can be difficult for a physiotherapist to implement in isolation and in the hospital out-patient setting. Multidisciplinary functional restoration programmes with a coordinated approach to assessment and management have proven effective in improving return to work and reducing sick leave for people with chronic low back pain (Guzman et al 2001). When effective these functional restoration programmes are intensive and can run for up to 40 hours a week for at least 3 weeks. Some hospitals might run programmes like these but as a physiotherapist in an out-patient setting you may need to organise referral to a functional restoration programme if your hospital does not offer this type of programme.

An important component of managing chronic low back pain is relapse management, as exacerbations are almost inevitable. Relapse management includes discussing triggers, coping strategies and an agreed plan for resumption of normal activity and return to self-management.

5. The patient has already been thoroughly screened and investigated medically. We can be confident that there is no serious pathology. The patient will be concerned about the significance of the minor disc bulge. However, there is no evidence of nerve root irritation (no referred pain, normal neurological testing).

6. Work details are relevant. A successful return to work programme will involve a workplace assessment and a plan for graduated return to work. This will involve liaison between the automotive manufacturer, the patient's insurer and the clinician.

   Also, people with back pain doing manual work who have low levels of job satisfaction are more likely to develop chronic symptoms (New Zealand Acute Low Back Pain Guide 2004).

7. The patient exhibits many yellow flags (New Zealand Acute Low Back Pain Guide 2004). Yellow flags are psycho-social risk factors that increase the risk of developing or perpetuating chronic low back pain. Yellow flags relate to: (a) attitudes and beliefs about back pain such as believing that pain and damage and is harmful; (b) behaviours such as fear avoidance behaviour; (c) compensation issues; (d) diagnostic and treatment issues such as catastrophizing from the results of diagnostic tests; (e) emotions, such as a tendency to a low mood or depression; (f) family, such as withdrawal from social interaction or having a partner who is a willing accomplice in the perpetuation of disability; and (g) work, such as being involved in manual work and being unhappy at work. This patient has many positive yellow flags. These yellow flags must be addressed if we are to help with her condition and highlight the importance of the psychosocial component of management.

8. Because of the importance of the multidisciplinary approach this patient is likely to require referral to other health professionals such as psychologists, exercise physiologists and specialists who can help coordinate return to the work place.

## Case Study 8

1. Rotator cuff condition with symptoms of supraspinatus tendon impingement and subscapularis involvement.
2. Painful arc on abduction with audible click, pain and weakness on resisting subscapularis as well as supraspinatus activity.
3. Within the domain of shoulder pain, rotator cuff conditions can be caused by an inter-relationship between soft tissue laxity (i.e. ligament) resulting in glenohumeral laxity, impingement (e.g. due to bursitis or osteophytes) resulting in tendon compression and cuff lesions (Allingham & McConnell 2003). Therefore, treatment is likely to be more effective when all possible factors that can cause laxity, impingement or lesion of the cuff are considered. These include:
   a. Poor mobility of the thoracic spine
   b. Muscle imbalance (tightness and or weakness)
   c. Poor posture (e.g. hyperkyphosis, protracted or depressed shoulders) that result in abnormal scapular movement and sub-acromial impingement
   or
   d. Degenerative changes of the acromioclavicular joint due to trauma and or osteoarthritis.
4. As with back pain each of the possible contributing factors need to be examined and included in the treatment plan as appropriate (Kent et al 2005). This means that instead of lumping groups of symptoms together (e.g. rotator cuff symptoms) it has been suggested to split and recognise factors that cause laxity, impingement and/or lesion and provide treatment as the clinician sees fit. So far:
   a. an exercise programme that includes stabilisation exercises of the scapula, functional shoulder exercises and thoracic mobilisation is likely to be effective in short-term recovery and longer-term functioning of rotator cuff disease
   b. the combination of exercise and mobilisation has shown to enhance outcomes
   c. ultrasound and pulsed electromagnetic field therapy has shown to only improve pain in case of calcific tendinitis, and laser therapy only symptoms associated with adhesive capsulitis (Green et al 2003).

Allingham and McConnell (2003) described the various components of a rehabilitation programme that can be individualised to address the multiplicity factors that can be involved in the aetiology of shoulder pain.

5. *Common* shoulder problems that can cause pain are strain or tendinopathy of the rotator cuff (supraspinatus, subscapularis, infraspinatus and teres minor), glenoid labral tear, glenohumeral instability or dislocation, acromioclavicular sprain and/or fractured distal end of the clavicle, and muscle strain or tear of the pectoralis major or long head of the biceps. Other common causes of shoulder pain can be based on referred pain from the cervical or thoracic spine, or pathology of the brachial plexus.

   *Less common* causes of shoulder pain are suprascapular or long thoracic nerve entrapment. Problems not to be missed include thoracic outlet syndrome (e.g. cervical rib), circulation problems (e.g. axillary vein thrombosis), bone tumour, or referred pain from diaphragm or organs (e.g. heart, gallbladder, spleen, apex of the lungs, or duodenum) (Brukner et al 2001e).

   Although adhesive capsulitis of the glenohumeral joint, calcification tendinopathy or tear in one of the muscles of the rotator cuff, or a fracture of the neck of humerus, coracoid process or scapula are less common in sports medicine (Brukner et al 2001e), they can be more common in middle-aged and older people.



6. As explained in the third answer, thoracic mobility (or rather lack of) and poor scapular stability can cause tissue impingement and cause rotator cuff problems. Since poor respiration in asthma can be associated with thoracic dysfunction, it is important to include breathing and thoracic mobilisation exercises if needed.

7. Although modified duties at work can reduce impingement until scapular movement and stability have improved, it is not always accepted by the employer. Educating the patient, careful monitoring, and liaison with employer can enhance the outcome of the rehabilitation process.

8. Using outcome measures such as the Upper Extremity Functional Index (Stratford et al 2001) or the Croft Disability Questionnaire (Croft et al 1994) do not measure pain and disability associated with overhead activities as the SPADI does. Although cross-sectional comparison of different shoulder questionnaires can show comparable overall validity and patient acceptability, it is important to include overhead activities since overhead work is an important aspect of her daily work. An additional benefit of the SPADI is that it is responsive to change, quick to complete, and scores are not likely to change in stable subjects (Paul et al 2004).

9. Corticosteroid injections can be beneficial in reducing symptoms (Green et al 2003). Also, an ultrasound scan can assist with assessing the degree of tendon degeneration as well as showing the presence of bursitis, whereas an X-ray can exclude calcific tendinitis or degenerative joint changes of the acromioclavicular joint. MRI can exclude problems in the glenohumeral joint (e.g. labral tears).

## Case Study 9

1. Lateral epicondylitis or tennis elbow (i.e. extensor tendinopathy of ECRB).
2. Pain when gripping, hammering, screw driving, pushing doorhandle, closing a tap and knocking the elbow. Positive tennis elbow test (resistance against dorsiflexion in dorsiflexed position of the wrist with closed fist), palpable swelling in ECRB. Localised tenderness/pain.
3. The process leading to the development of ECRB tendinopathy may involve poorly designed equipment, incorrect technique, overuse and excessive tissue loading, inadequate blood supply, degenerative tendon changes and microscopic tears and scarring with continued use (Brukner et al 2001b). This can result in pain reduced strength during gripping and lifting.
4. Local friction or gentle massage, and gentle stretching can help to improve local blood supply and tightness. In addition, ultrasound treatment has been found to have some benefit (van der Windt et al 1999). Along with local treatment of swelling and pain, addressing the cause of the problem requires:
   a. adherence to alternative or modified duties at work
   b. the use of properly designed equipment
   c. adequate manual handling techniques
   d. counterforce bracing to minimise the risk of overloading
   e. avoiding tight gripping
   f. avoiding high load repetitive activities, such as hammering
   g. using ergonomically designed tools, non-slip grip, and the use of power tools and longer levers.
5. Common problems that can cause elbow and forearm pain are extensor tendinopathy of ECRB, referred pain from cervical or thoracic spine, shoulder joint or increased neural tension. Neurodynamic testing can be very helpful to exclude neural tissue involvement (Butler 2000).

   Less common causes are articular injuries, primary degenerative arthritis (which is not uncommon in men aged 30–50), inflammatory arthropathy (with synovitis and effusion of the radiohumeral joint), radiohumeral bursitis, entrapment neuropathy of the radial nerve or posterior interosseous nerve.

A cause that is not to be missed is osteochondritis dissecans of the capitellum radii (Brukner et al 2001b, Perko & Prosser 2003), or other joint problems associated with occupational use of vibrational tools in the industry (Bovenzi et al 1987).

6. The fall is unlikely to be related to the current condition. Although there is a possibility that the articular cartilage may have been damaged as a result of the fall, the patient never experienced locking of the joint and did not report pain until 5/12 ago. Given the serious flare up of pain at the time of sudden, strenuous and prolonged muscle activity of the elbow/forearm, the positive tennis elbow test, and absence of cervical or thoracic spine symptoms or shoulder pain, the preferred provisional diagnosis is lateral epicondylitis, and probably ECRB tendinopathy.

7. The expectation that it will take time is justified. It will be important for the patient to understand that this degenerative condition is different from other conditions he has had over the years. Understanding that local treatment is likely not to be sufficient to slow down or halt to process that led to the development of ECRB tendinopathy, and that programme adherence is needed, and is likely to enhance outcomes of the interventional programme.

8. An ultrasound scan can assist with assessing the degree of tendon degeneration as well as showing the presence of a bursa, whereas an X-ray can exclude osteochondritis dissecans, degenerative joint changes, or heterotopic calcification (Brukner et al 2001b). There are not great benefits to be expected from corticosteroid and or local anaesthetics injection (Hay et al 1999).



## Case Study 10

1. Carpal tunnel syndrome.

2. Carpal tunnel syndrome is caused by compression of the median nerve as it courses through the carpal tunnel. Compression can be caused by anything that reduces the space in the tunnel such as extra fluid, and inflammation and thickening of the lining of the tendons. The median nerve is responsible for sensation to the palmar surface of the thumb, index, middle and half the ring finger which is consistent with the area of sensory deficits. The median nerve also has a motor supply to the muscles of the thenar eminence (flexor pollicis brevis, abductor pollicis brevis and opponens pollicis) as well as the first two lumbricals. Alterations in motor supply for this patient are seen in the reduced grip strength measured on the right side. The fact that there is no observable wasting of the thenar muscles is probably because it has only been a problem for a relatively short time and the symptoms are not severe.

3. Phalen's sign is positive in this patient because sustained flexion of the wrist for 45 seconds started to reproduce her symptoms. Sustained flexion can reproduce symptoms because full flexion reduces the space available in the carpal tunnel, thereby increasing compression on a vulnerable median nerve. Night symptoms are characteristic of carpal tunnel syndrome. It is thought that night symptoms are due to sustained flexion of the wrist, which occurs with relaxation of the wrist during sleep.

4. Other assessment techniques that could be performed to confirm the diagnosis of carpal tunnel syndrome include:
   - Nerve conduction tests: expect slowing of conduction of the median nerve as it passes through the carpal tunnel. Can also observe absence of the sensory nerve action potential and prolonged terminal motor latency (Oh 1993).
   - Sensory deficits in the lateral three and a half fingers could be quantified, for example by measuring two-point discrimination or by using von Frey filaments to quantify reductions in light touch.
   - Any changes in motor conduction could be more fully examined by using a device to measure pinch grip, as well as overall grip strength.

5. The Levine symptom severity scale was designed specifically to assess the severity of symptoms and functional status of people with carpal tunnel syndrome. The scales are highly reliable ($r = -\cdot 91 - \cdot 93$), internally consistent, and highly responsive to clinical change (Levine et al 1993):
   a. The symptom severity scale measures 11 items on a 5-point scale. Items assess the severity and frequency of pain, numbness, tingling and weakness during the day and at night.
   b. The functional status scale measures the average score of 8 items on a 5-point scale from no difficulty (score = 1) to cannot do at all due to my hand or wrist symptoms (score = 5): writing, buttoning of clothes, holding a book while reading, gripping of a telephone, opening of jars, household chores, carrying of grocery bags, and bathing and dressing.

   The patient scored 1.9 on the symptom severity scale which means for most items she only had mild symptoms, and no symptoms on a few of the items. The patient scored 1.4 on the functional status scale. This score was obtained because she reported mild-to-moderate difficulty on a few of the items (e.g. moderate difficulty with opening jars score for item = 3), but no difficulty (score = 1) on items such as writing, buttoning of clothes, and bathing and dressing. Overall the Levine scales indicate that the patient has mild symptoms at this stage, with a mild functional deficit.

6. Symptoms and signs placed on the priority list are:
   - waking once each night
   - Phalen's sign reproduces numbness after 45 seconds
   - grip strength reduced on right side to 27 kg
   - Levine's symptom severity scale = 1.9
   - Levine's functional status scale = 1.4
   - positive upper limb tension test with median nerve bias.

   These items will be used as outcome measures to monitor patient's progress during her course of physiotherapy.

7. The physiotherapy treatment plan is:
   - explanation/education: a clear explanation of the diagnosis and how increased pressure in the carpal tunnel compressing the median nerve can account for her symptoms and signs. At this stage the patient can be instructed to maintain her levels of physical activity including playing tennis. The role of physiotherapy and how it fits in with medical and surgical management should be clearly explained to this patient
   - prescription and fitting of an off-the-shelf nocturnal resting splint for the right wrist. The purpose of the splint is to prevent the right wrist falling into flexion during the night. There is evidence from randomised controlled trials that splints worn during the night for a period of 6/52 can reduce symptoms and improve function in people with carpal tunnel syndrome (O'Connor et al 2003, Werner et al 2005)
   - prescription of nerve and tendon gliding exercises. The clinical findings of altered neurodynamics in the upper limb tension test with a median nerve bias suggests this might be a useful approach. Also there is evidence from a randomised controlled trial that nerve and tension gliding exercises could be a useful adjunct in the management of carpal tunnel syndrome (Akalin et al 2002).

     Starting position neck and shoulder neutral and elbow supinated and flexed 90°. Each exercise repeated 10 times 5 times each day with each position maintained for 5 seconds:

     i. Tendon gliding positions: Fingers placed in five positions – straight, hook, fist, tabletop and straight fist.
     ii. Median nerve gliding positions: fist, wrist neutral fingers and thumb extended, wrist and fingers extended thumb neutral, wrist fingers and thumb extended, opposite hand applies gentle stretch to thumb extension
   - ultrasound, but not at this stage. Although there is evidence that intensive ultrasound therapy (20 sessions at 1 MHz, 1.0 W/cm, pulsed mode 1:4, 15 minutes per session) can lead to improvements in carpal tunnel syndrome (Ebenbichler et al 1998,

CHAPTER EIGHT

Bakhtiary & Rashidy-Pur 2004), in many busy departments it is not feasible to apply this intervention when there are other treatment options available.

8. The positive upper limb tension test, with a median nerve bias and reproduction of symptom with movement of a body part a long way from the wrist (shoulder depression) should make the physiotherapist consider whether any dysfunction in the cervical spine could be contributing to her symptoms. Next appointment will include a brief examination of the cervical spine (including active movements with overpressures, combined movements and palpation) to confirm that it is not contributing to her symptoms.

   The patient's type 2 diabetes may have made her more susceptible to developing carpal tunnel syndrome. Carpal tunnel syndrome is more common in people with diabetes (Gulliford et al 2006). However, since her diabetes is currently well controlled by diet and exercise the management of her carpal tunnel syndrome will not change.

9. Surgery for carpal tunnel syndrome involves releasing the carpal ligament to relieve pressure on the median nerve. It is usually done with local anaesthetic and performed as a day procedure. It is a successful procedure with success rates of 90% reported 18/12 after surgery (compared with a 75% success rate after splinting) (Gerritsen et al 2002). If this patient doesn't respond to physiotherapy within 6/52 or her symptoms worsen then surgery will be likely to be recommended by her doctor.



## Case Study 11

1. Adductor-related groin pain.
2. The key assessment findings that led to the diagnosis of adductor related groin pain were:
   a. pain reproduced in squeeze test and resisted adduction
   b. pain reproduced on adductor length test
   c. pain reproduced on palpation near the origin of adductor longus muscle at its attachment to the inferior pubic ramus
   d. pain reproduced by dynamic activities involving hip flexion and adduction (running especially when cutting, and kicking across the body as when crossing a ball from a corner)
3. Other common causes of groin pain considered included:
   a. Iliospoas-related groin pain
   b. Abdominal-wall-related groin pain (e.g. posterior inguinal wall weakness)
   c. Pubic bone stress-related groin pain (e.g. osteitis pubis)

4. Some less common causes of groin pain considered included:
   - Hip osteoarthritis. The negative finding from the X-ray and the quadrant test (right = left, with slight discomfort) makes this unlikely.
   - Referred pain from the lumbar spine or sacroiliac joint. No reports of lumbar pain or buttock pain on the right side. Also, strong findings from tests of the adductor longus make the lumbar spine unlikely to be the key source of pain.
   - Obturator nerve entrapment as it enters the adductor compartment. Key assessment findings are weakness of resisted adduction and reduced sensation over the distal part of the medial thigh, especially after the patient has been exercised to reproduce his symptoms (Bradshaw et al 1997). This has not been assessed in this patient so must be retained as a possible alternative hypothesis.
   - Stress fracture of the neck of femur or pubic ramus or a slipped upper femoral epiphysis. X-rays are negative and these might be expected to show the fracture as the condition has been present for a couple of months. The bone scan is negative for the neck of femur and indicated only slightly increased uptake in the inferior pubic bone, so this diagnosis is unlikely.
   - Serious pathology including intra-abdominal abnormalities or tumours. The patient was examined and screened by the doctor 2/52 ago, the patient reports that otherwise he is well, there is a clear mechanical pattern to the reproduction of his symptoms, and only indications of slight inflammation, making serious pathology unlikely.

5. Osgood–Schlatter's disease is an osteochondritis that occurs at the growth plate of the tibial tuberosity. Repeated pull of the patellar tendon can cause inflammation and partial avulsion of the tibial tuberosity, leading to a painful and prominent bump. It is a relatively common condition in adolescents who play a large amount of sport. As in this patient it usually resolves with modification of activity. It is not directly relevant for this patient, except that it tells us that he has a history of overuse sports-related injury.

6. The patient appears to have primary pathology that is adductor related but patients with relatively longstanding groin pain often present with evidence of a number of pathologies, all related to an overuse syndrome affecting the pelvic region (Bradshaw & Holmich 2007):
   - The patient is showing some signs of pubic bone stress, as evidenced by the tenderness to palpation about the pubic symphysis and the light radionuclide uptake in the region seen on the bone

scan. The interpretation is that this indicates that he has had the adductor-related problem for some time and that it is now overloading into some stress on the pubic bone.

- The patient demonstrates poor control of his abdominal stabilising muscles. In the testing procedure described we expect someone with good control to be able to complete 10 × 10 second holds increasing the pressure of a cuff placed in the small of the back from 40 to 50 mmHg (Richardson et al 2004). Our observation of his walking indicated increased lateral tilting of the pelvis, which may also be related to poor stabilisation of the pelvis. This lack of pelvic control could be a contributing factor that has put greater stress on the adductor muscles and pelvis and is consistent with research demonstrated impaired transversus abdominis activity in patients with longstanding groin pain (Cowan et al 2004).
- The other entities that are believed to be associated with the sequelae of longstanding groin pain are related to iliopsoas and abdominal wall related pathologies. Iliopsoas related pathology would be suspected if resisted hip flexion on the right from the Thomas test position reproduced pain. Indicators of abdominal wall related pathology include reproduction of pain in resisted trunk flexion and reproduction of pain on coughing and sneezing (both factors negative in this patient) as well as a tender dilated superficial inguinal ring (not assessed in this patient) (Swan & Wolcott 2006).

7. Symptoms and signs placed on the priority list are:
   - pain on resisted adduction (including squeeze test)
   - pain on length test
   - pain on palpation of origin of adductor longus
   - pain on running
   - pain on kicking
   - lack of pelvic control (poor control of abdominal stabilising muscles).

   These items will be used for reassessment to monitor patient progress during her course of physiotherapy.

8. The physiotherapy treatment plan is based on active treatment. A high-quality randomised controlled trial compared a graduated active physiotherapy regime to increase muscle strength with a control group receiving passive modalities such as stretching, massage and electrotherapy modalities. Treatment was 3 times a week for a minimum of 8/52. It was shown that people with groin pain in the active group were more than 12 times more likely to return to their usual sporting activity after 4/12 than were people in

the passive treatment group (Holmich et al 1999). The principles of the active treatment programme are (Bradshaw & Holmich 2007):

- pain-free exercise
- reduce sources of load on the pelvis. For example adductor muscle tone could be reduced with soft-tissue treatment
- improve lumboplevic stability. A core stability programme as described by Richardson et al (2004) will be an important component of this patient's treatment
- strengthen the adductor muscles using a progression of static exercises (e.g. isometric adduction with a ball placed between feet) and dynamic exercises (e.g. standing abduction and adduction using pulleys (Holmich et al 1999). Training is completed 6 days a week with dynamic exercises typically completed in 5 sets of 10 repetitions on 3 days and static exercises emphasising control completed on the alternate 3 days
- progression to return to soccer based on pain-free progression of load and activity, such as a progression from brisk walking to straight-line running, to lateral running.



## Case Study 12

1. Trochanteric bursitis.

2. A snapping hip is not uncommon during activities such as stair climbing, and does not have to cause major symptoms. However, weakness of the gluteus medius, tightness of the tensor fasciae latae and leg-length discrepancy can cause added soft-tissue pressure on the bursa and friction during movement. This mechanism can lead to an aching sensation in mild cases and more severe pain in cases of an inflammation and swelling of the trochanteric bursa. Although the palpable swelling and boggy feeling around the bursa may suggest an inflammation of the bursa, current evidence indicates gluteus medius or minimus muscle involvement in the development of trochanteric symptoms rather then the bursa (Alvarez-Nemegyei & Canoso 2004).

3. Minimising local pressure on the trochanteric area by placing a pillow between the legs and maintaining hip abduction while lying on either side in bed can prevent waking up at night. Also, a softer mattress and a folded blanket placed above the pelvis can reduce pressure on the trochanteric area when lying on the affected side. Treatment may include:
   a. Icing, local friction or gentle massage to reduce swelling and pain, and to improve blood supply at the trochanteric muscle insertion
   b. Stretching the tensor fasciae latae and iliotibial tract, and strengthening the glutei medius and minimus, which addresses the

muscle imbalance. Minimising tissue compression and friction is likely to reduce irritation and inflammation

c. Activity modification, proper footwear and weight loss can assist in minimising the risk of tissue overloading.

4. Iliotibial band friction syndrome is a common cause of lateral knee pain and can be associated with pain along the iliotibial tract, although the disorder is more common in endurance sports (Ellis et al 2007). Factors such as weakness of the hip abductors and tightness of the iliotibial tract can cause compression and friction of the tissues against the lateral epicondyle of the femur, particularly during 30° flexion and internal rotation of the tibia (Fairclough et al 2006). Although different from trochanteric bursitis (or muscle insertion inflammation), treatment of iliotibial band syndrome is fairly similar.

   Less common causes of lateral hip thigh and knee pain are referred pain from neural tissues or the lumbar spine, or biceps femoris tendinopathy. Causes that need not be missed are common peroneal nerve injury or, in younger people, a slipped capital femoral epiphysis or Perthes' disease (Brukner & Khan 2001b).

5. Together with biomechanical factors such as difference in leg length, muscle imbalance, and valgus and pronation problems, obesity is likely to increase compression when walking and climbing.

6. Performing the home exercise programme on a regular basis, icing before going to bed, and reducing compression by maintaining hip abduction when asleep is likely to assist in reducing irritation. Improved sleep and being less fatigued may help with maintaining correct pelvic position when walking.

7. NSAIDs or a corticosteroid injection in addition to physiotherapy treatment can assist in decreasing the symptoms. Proper footwear and foot orthotics can assist in minimising internal rotation of the tibia during ambulation.

   Ultrasound scans can assist with assessing the soft tissues in the trochanteric area to refine the diagnosis. Radiography can exclude slipped capital femoral epiphysis or Perthes' disease.

## Case Study 13

1. Medial collateral ligament sprain (grade 2).

2. Gapping of the medial joint line (laxity of medial collateral ligament) together with local pain on applying a force in valgus direction, although there was a marked end point. Painful distraction test and pain on full knee extension and external rotation. Some knee effusion (in cases of grade 1 sprain there is no swelling or ligament laxity).

3. Avoiding forces on the knee in the direction of valgus. Supportive taping or wearing a knee orthosis can help to achieve knee alignment and avoid stress on the medial collateral ligament when resuming sporting activities. Application of ice to soft tissue injuries may have some benefit in the very acute stage (Bleakley et al 2004). Closed chain exercises are well tolerated when strengthening the quadriceps, particularly when avoiding end of ROM. Open chain quadriceps exercises such as lifting a weight with knee in extension can cause medial knee pain due to stress on the medial collateral ligament. Over time knee stability needs to be actively maintained during activities such as bouncing on a trampoline, skipping, and changing direction while walking or running.
4. Common problems that can cause medial knee pain include medial collateral ligament sprain, medial meniscus tear, patellar dislocation and articular cartilage injury.

   Less common causes of medial knee pain and swelling are bursitis (e.g. pes anserine) and haematoma of the bursa or the lower part of the quadriceps. Medial knee pain causes that are not to be missed include avulsion fracture or tibia plateau fracture. Patients in their adolescence can have knee pain due to osteochondritis dissecans, whereas in chronic conditions reflex sympathetic dystrophy can be the cause of ongoing knee pain after injury (Brukner et al 2001d).
5. Given the active lifestyle of the patient and that she is likely to want to return to sporting activities early, it is important to point out the time it takes for ligaments to heal after a sprain and for the patient to be cautious. Use of external support by either taping or wearing an orthotic device, as well as her own ability to actively stabilise during function, are important to minimise the chance of re-injury.
6. The positive attitude of the patient and adherence to the exercise programme is likely to assist treatment outcome.
7. An ultrasound scan can assist with assessing the extent of the ligament tear. An X-ray can exclude an avulsion fracture or osteochondral fracture. MRI can be helpful to exclude a lesion of the medial meniscus.



## Case Study 14

1. This patient had a diagnosis of patellofemoral pain syndrome (PFPS). The age and gender of this patient are very typical of PFPS patients who present to the NHS for physiotherapy (Clark et al 2000, Selfe et al 2001, 2006). PFPS patients commonly describe diffuse bilateral pain of insidious onset of their condition. Published data for the NHS show that bilateral pain occurs in over 50% of patients (Selfe et al 2001). It is common to find that one leg is worse than the

other. The aggravating factors listed are typical and occur when the patellofemoral joint is being loaded.

2. • Muscle tightness
   • Posterior patella tilt
   • Fat pad swelling
   • Poor eccentric quadriceps control.

3. • *Muscle tightness.* The three muscles tested can influence the mechanics of the patellofemoral joint if they are tight and a home stretching programme should be instigated. These muscles have one thing in common: they are bi-articular. They are predisposed to tightness due to the complexity of their mechanism of action in closed kinetic chain activities as there is simultaneous concentric and eccentric contraction occurring at the opposite end of the same muscle.
   • *Posterior patella tilt and fat pad swelling.* Taping may help to provide pain relief by having an unloading effect on the fat pad and it may help to improve quadriceps control. The mechanism of the effect of taping is a very controversial subject and is currently poorly understood. However, there is agreement in the literature that taping does provide pain relief (Selfe 2004).
   • *Poor eccentric quadriceps control.* The quadriceps eccentrically act like a large shock absorber. Addressing the poor control will decrease the stress loading on the patellofemoral joint. However, it is important that the patient is pain free when carrying out rehabilitation exercises (Dye et al 1999, McConnell 1986).



4. This is quite a common report. Spencer et al (1984) found that 20 ml of saline will inhibit the vastus medialis and 50/60 ml will inhibit both rectus femoris and vastus lateralis. Iles et al (1990) suggest that any degree of joint effusion will have an inhibitory effect. The knee joint is the largest joint in the body and it is possible that there is enough space inside the joint capsule to contain 20 ml of swelling, which the patient will be able to feel, without it appearing visible to a therapist.

5. In an indirect way, yes. Due to the whiplash injury the patient's activity levels were reduced and she put weight on. This increased the loading on her knees, when she resumed her activities her knees were loaded above her 'envelope of function' which caused 'supraphysiological overload' (Dye et al 1999). This caused the homeostatic balance of her knees to be compromised and pain and dysfunction gradually developed.

   Another reason that weight may increase is due to 'comfort eating' which occurs due to depressed mood because of being unable to carry out her job properly. This is a very sensitive issue and problems associated with weight control can be associated with other underlying emotional problems, so clinicians have to proceed carefully in this area.

There often emerges a 'Catch 22' situation as one of the keys to weight loss is exercise. However, this may aggravate the patellofemoral symptoms. Clinicians need to be sensitive to this issue and plan rehabilitation activities carefully in order not to provoke the very problem that the patient is seeking help for.

6. Having very high expectations of what physiotherapy will be able to do is very common and this needs to be managed carefully if frustration and disappointment are to be avoided.

   It is important from the outset to work in partnership with the patient in order to establish realistic and achievable aims. Patient explanation is really important especially surrounding timescales. It is obvious to therapists that a condition which has taken 1 year to develop is not going to be resolved in one 30-minute session, patients often have a different perspective. It is important that the patient is treated holistically and that a biopsychosocial approach is adopted.

7. As some alterations to the normal shape of the foot and great toe have been identified, which could potentially contribute to PFPS, a referral to a podiatrist may be considered appropriate. However, the research evidence supporting the use of orthotics is not strong (Selfe 2004).



## Case Study 15

1. Symptoms agree with a grade one calf strain and generally take less then 2 weeks to subside (Brukner et al 2001c).

2. The sudden onset 1/52 ago when he felt like someone hit him in the calf with a tennis ball is a classic example of a muscle tear. A palpable gap in the muscle belly, localised pain and pain at end of the lift during unilateral heel raises the diagnosis.

3. In very acute and more severe cases RICE (rest, ice, compression and elevation) is indicated, and crutches are needed to reduce muscle loading. Subsequent treatment may include:
   a. Taping or a non-elastic bandage to provide external support to the muscle membrane during contraction and to enable patients to return to activity as early as possible. An additional benefit of this external support is the massage effect and the rhythmic increases of internal pressure caused by muscle contraction during physical activity which is likely to assist in removing

swelling. It is advisable to continue the use of external support for another couple of weeks, particularly during sporting activities

b. Gentle massage (avoiding pointy techniques at the location of the tear) and stretching can also be beneficial at this point of time

c. Finally, the value of warming up before intensive forms of physical activity needs to be reinforced.

4. Common muscle problems that can cause calf pain are gastrocnemius or soleus strain, contusion or cramp, or a delayed onset of muscle soreness after intensive physical activity. Another common cause of calf pain can be the result of referred pain that originates from the lumbar spine.

   Less common causes can relate to muscle compartment syndromes (superficial or deep posterior compartment), stress fracture of tibia or fibula) or the circulatory system (varicose veins, or entrapment or endofibrosis of the popliteal or external iliac arteries).

   Other less common causes include referred joint (superior tibiofibular) or soft tissue pain (posterior capsule, posterior cruciate ligament, or Baker's cyst) (Brukner et al 2001c).

   Causes that are not to be missed are circulation problems such as arterial insufficiency or deep venous thrombosis (Brukner et al 2001c).

5. Given his medical history and his age, it is important to recognise circulatory problems or back pathology. Current symptoms are not likely to be related to coronary or other circulatory problems, pathology of the lower back, or a stress fracture. There were no signs of thrombosis, arteries were palpable, nerve stretches were negative and landing during hopping did not cause any discomfort.

6. Given his medical history the patient is keen to maintain his level of physical activity. Although the injury is not severe and symptoms are likely to cease within 1 week, it is important for the patient to understand how he can avoid re-injury. In addition, there is value in explaining that calf pain can be related to other problems and that he should be in contact if the problem persists.

7. An ultrasound scan can assist with assessing the extent of the muscle tear, whereas a Doppler scan or venography can be employed when suspecting venous thrombosis. Elevated pressure testing during and after exercise is indicated when there is suspicion of superficial compartment syndrome. A MRI or nuclear scan can be useful when problems persist to exclude stress fractures or other problems.

## Case Study 16

1. Achilles tendinopathy.

2. Achilles pain, particularly during and after prolonged activities such as walking and jogging. Pain and stiffness seem to ease at the start of activity but worsens as the activity prolongs. Thickening of the Achilles tendon with associated tenderness. Crepitus during plantar/dorsiflexion.

3. The process leading to the development of Achilles tendinopathy may involve inappropriate increases in frequency, intensity and or duration of physical activity. Problems can be compounded by poor running technique and or footwear, resulting in overuse and excessive tissue loading, inadequate blood supply, degenerative tendon changes and microscopic tears and scarring with continued use (Brukner et al 2001a).

4. A treatment programme may include different modalities:
   a. Advice on footwear, weight loss (if needed) and training to minimise the risk of overloading
   b. An eccentric strengthening exercise programme of the calf muscles has shown dramatic decreases in pain (Alfredson et al 1998)
   c. Icing, local friction or gentle massage, and gentle stretching can help to decrease inflammation and improve local blood supply and tightness
   d. Ultrasound treatment has been found to have some benefit in tendinopathy of the extensor carpi radialis brevis (van der Windt et al 1999).



5. Retrocalcaneal bursitis and Achilles tendinopathies such as partial tears, tendinosis or paratendonitis are common problems that can cause pain in the Achilles region. Achilles bursitis, Sever's disease, posterior impingement syndrome or referred pain from the lower back or neural tissues are less common. Achilles problems that need not to be missed include a complete rupture of the tendon or symptoms related to an inflammatory arthropathy (Brukner et al 2001a).

6. Both, diabetes and having a BMI of 27 or over are factors that have been associated with the onset of Achilles tendinopathy. The biomechanical forces caused by extra weight and the Achilles tendon deviation due to the patient's pronated feet with fallen longitudinal arches are compounding factors.

7. It will be important for him to realise that minimising the impact of biomechanical factors is likely to be of great benefit, and that obtaining foot orthotics and dietary advice will enhance the

outcome. Although it will take time to lose weight, pain can decrease dramatically after 12 weeks of heavy-load eccentric calf muscle training. In addition to the eccentric exercise programme he could swim or use a rowing machine to expand energy.

8. A podiatrist can provide appropriate orthotics and correct alignment of the Achilles tendon by correcting foot and ankle position. It is important to prevent any whipping action from the Achilles tendon as a result of over pronation during brisk walking and jogging (Clement 1984). In addition, the patient may benefit from dietetic support and aim for a BMI of 25.

   The amount of local fluid (degree of hypoechogenity) can be assessed by sonography. Ultrasound scans can assist with assessing discontinuity of the Achilles tendon fibres. Finally, MRI scanning can complement assessing appearance of the tendon (Brukner et al 2001a).

## Case Study 17

1. Sprained anterior talofibular ligament with a Grade 1+ to 2– tear.
2. The following symptoms are important indicators:
   a. Egg-shaped swelling over the anterior talofibular ligament immediately after the injury
   b. Localised tenderness/pain
   c. Positive anterior drawer test
   d. Pain on weight bearing
   e. Painful and slightly reduced inversion and plantar flexion of the ankle.
3. Instability of the ankle, over pronation during loading and poor proprioception are factors that need to be addressed. At the same time, symptoms such as pain and swelling need to subside. The evidence so far is:
   a. ultrasound treatment appears to be of little value. Van der Windt et al (2002) found that only one study reported positive effects on pain and swelling, whereas the results of four placebo-controlled trials demonstrated no significant improvements in the treatment of ankle sprains
   b. although ice may not be better than compression, there is limited evidence that ice in addition to exercise is effective after ankle sprain (Bleakley et al 2004)
   c. compared with immobilisation, intervention that requires functional forms of physical activity appears to produce better results (Kerkhoffs et al 2002). This may include ambulation in the pool during the acute stage, and proprioceptive exercises as progress is made and weight tolerated

d. supervised exercises such as stabilisation exercises as part of an individualised treatment regimen may result in greater reduction in swelling and faster return to work (van Os et al 2005)
e. exercise therapy such as stabilisation exercises has been found to improve functional instability and decrease the risk of re-injury after an acute ankle sprain, although no effects were found on postural sway in those with functional instability (van der Wees et al 2006)
f. according to van der Wees and colleagues (2006) the use of a wobble board is likely to be effective in the prevention of recurrent ankle sprains
g. manual mobilisation of dorsiflexion in view of increasing range of motion may have some effect at the start, although clinical relevance is limited (van der Wees et al 2006). Functional activity is likely to produce similar results.

4. Common problems as a result of ankle injury are sprained ligaments, particularly the lateral ones. Whereas a less severe sprain may only involve the anterior talofibular ligament, a severe one can even affect the posterior talofibular ligament. When the calcaneofibular ligament is torn the talar tilt test will be positive. In patients with mild symptoms single leg standing and hopping can be appropriate for use during assessment.

   Less common problems include medial ligament sprain (i.e. deltoid ligament) or fractures (e.g. malleoli, base of fifth metatarsal, tibial plafond, lateral or posterior process of the talus, trigonum or anterior process of calcaneus, or dislocation and or tendon rupture). Ankle conditions not to be missed include a torn syndesmosis (Brukner & Khan 2001a). Achilles tendinopathy can occur with loading and excessive movement of the tendon due to overpronation (Clement et al 1984).

5. Pes plani valgi (flat feet) are associated with hyper mobility of the foot and poor Achilles tendon alignment. The multiple sprains and past episode of pain in the Achilles region indicate that this has been a longstanding problem.

6. The positive outlook and determination to return to her sport can assist motivation to perform and maintain the required exercise regimen. At the same time she needs to realise that by addressing biomechanical factors she is less likely to sustain injuries or develop problems that jeopardise long-term performance of this leisure activity.

7. An X-ray can exclude avulsion fractures of the distal end of the fibula and the base of the fifth metatarsal, or confirm the intactness of the

tibiofibular syndesmosis. A podiatrist can provide the patient with foot orthotics that correct ankle position and Achilles tendon alignment, and that are suitable for sport. Proper orthotics together with footwear that provide maximum support (i.e. sewn on heel cup, pronation bar, side reinforcement that links with shoe laces) assist in stabilising the ankle.

## Case Study 18

1. Fibromyalgia (FM) and depression.

2. Slow information-processing, experienced problems with concentrating, and comprehending and memorising information has been associated with fibromyalgia (Glass 2006). Fibromyalgia is a painful and disabling chronic musculoskeletal condition that commonly affects women (Arnold 2006).

3. Exercise in combination with education and psychologically based intervention such as CBT has shown more consistent and positive results than other modalities in the treatment of patients with FM (Adams & Sim 2005). So far, there is little or no support for most types of electrotherapy (Sim & Adams 1999). Mind–body therapy together with exercise and antidepressants if needed are likely to have a synergistic effect, although this needs further research (Hadhazy et al 2000).

   Trigger point therapy over a limited period of time may be useful to reduce muscle symptoms. She may be able to continue progress by adding muscle stretches to her exercise programme and maintaining correct posture.

4. Although FM is a common cause of diffuse chronic musculoskeletal pain, it is important to be aware of rheumatic diseases that can mimic FM and that can cause joint destruction, organ damage, or threaten life if undetected and untreated. Diseases to exclude are systematic lupus erythematosus, polymyalgia rheumatica, rheumatoid arthritis, ankylosing spondylitis and osteoarthritis (Hwang & Barkhuizen 2006).

   Increasing levels of physical activity can be beneficial for both FM and mental health. The health and quality of life benefits of physical activity and exercise in people with depression or anxiety have been well established (Babyak et al 2000, Biddle et al 2000, Byrne & Byrne 1993, Scully et al 1998).

5. FM can be associated with headache symptoms. Although there are profound differences between FM and tension-type headache, pathogenic mechanisms partly overlap and they can share clinical features (Lenaerts & Gill 2006).

6. Although exercise adherence is likely to be enhanced by being referred by the physician, depression can negatively impact on consistent performance. Also, it will be important to employ a stepwise approach and to avoid disappointment due to increased fatigue, stiffness and or pain. Education, an exercise diary, regular follow-up (e.g. by telephone) can assist in maintaining performance over time.

7. Radiographic imaging, laboratory testing, and specific questioning around the key features of rheumatic diseases such as systematic lupus erythematosus, polymyalgia rheumatica, rheumatoid arthritis, ankylosing spondylitis and osteoarthritis can assist in considering these as an alternative diagnosis (Hwang & Barkhuizen 2006). Involvement of a psychologist or counsellor is important.



## References

Adams N, Sim J 2005 Rehabilitation approaches in fibromyalgia. Disability & Rehabilitation 27(12):711–723.
Akalin E, El O, Peker O et al 2002 Treatment of carpal tunnel syndrome with nerve and tendon gliding exercises. American Journal Physical Medicine Rehabilitation 81(2):108–113.
Al-Ani Z, Gray R J, Davies S J et al 2005 Stabilization splint therapy for the treatment of temporomandibular myofascial pain: a systematic review. Journal of Dental Education 69(11):1242–1250.
Alfredson H, Pietila T, Jonsson P et al 1998 Heavy-load eccentric calf muscle training for the treatment of chronic Achilles tendinosis. American Journal of Sports Medicine 26:360–366.
Allingham C, McConnell J 2003 Conservative management of rotator cuff, capsulitis and frozen shoulder. In: Prosser R, Conolly W B (eds), Rehabilitation of the Hand and Upper Limb. Butterworth Heinemann, Edinburgh, p. 241–250.
Alvarez-Nemegyei J, Canoso J 2004 Evidence-based soft tissue rheumatology: III: trochanteric bursitis. Journal of Clinical Rheumatology 10 (3):123–124.
Andrews G, Slade T 2001 Interpreting scores on the Kessler Psychological Distress Scale (K10). Australian and New Zealand Journal of Public Health 25(6):494–497.
Arnold L M 2006 Biology and therapy of fibromyalgia. New therapies in fibromyalgia. Arthritis Research & Therapy 8(4):212.
Babyak M, Blumenthal J, Herman S et al 2000 Exercise treatment for major depression: maintenance of therapeutic benefit at 10 months. Psychosomatic Medicine 62(5):633–638.
Bakhtiary A H, Rashidy-Pur A 2004 Ultrasound and laser therapy in the treatment of carpal tunnel syndrome. Australian Journal of Physiotherapy 50(3):147–151.
Bauman A 2004 Health benefits of physical activity for older adults – epidemiological approachs to the evidence. In: Morris M E, Schoo A M M

(eds) Optimizing Exercise and Physical Activity in Older People. Butterworth Heinemann, Edinburgh, p. 1–25.
Biddle S, Fox K, Boutcher S 2000 Physical activity and psychological well-being. Routledge, London.
Binkley J M, Stratford P W, Lott S A et al 1999 The Lower Extremity Functional Scale (LEFS): scale development, measurement properties, and clinical application. Physical Therapy 79(4):371–383.
Binkley Jill M, Stratford Paul W, Lott Sue Ann et al 1999 The North American Orthopaedic Rehabilitation Research Network. Physical Therapy 79:371–383.
Bleakley C, McDonough S, MacAuley D 2004 The use of ice in the treatment of acute soft-tissue injury: a systematic review of randomized controlled trials. American Journal of Sports Medicine 32(1):251–261.
Borchgrevink G E 1998 Acute treatment of whiplash neck sprain injuries. A randomized trial of treatment during the first 14 days after a car accident. Spine 23(1):25–31.
Bovenzi M, Fiorito A, Volpe C 1987 Bone and joint disorders in the upper extremities of chipping and grinding operators. Int Arch Occup Environ Health 59(2):189–198.
Bradshaw C, Holmich P 2007 Chapter 24 Longstanding groin pain. In: Brunker P, Khan K (eds) Clinical Sports Medicine, 3rd edn. McGraw-Hill, Sydney.
Bradshaw C, McCrory P, Bell S et al 1997 Obturator nerve entrapment: a cause of groin pain in athletes. American Journal of Sports Medicine 25 (3):402–408.
Bronfort G, Nillson N, Haas M et al 2004a Non-invasive physical treatments for chronic/recurrent headache. Cochrane Database Syst Rev 3: CD001878.
Bronfort G, Haas M, Evans RL et al 2004b Efficacy of spinal manipulation and mobilization for low back pain and neck pain: a systematic review and best evidence synthesis. Spine 4(3):335–356.
Brukner P, Khan K 2001a Acute ankle injuries. In: Brukner P, Khan K (eds) Clinical Sports Medicine, 2nd edn. McGraw-Hill, Sydney, p. 553–573.
Brukner P, Khan K 2001b Lateral, medial and posterior knee pain. In: Brukner P, Khan K (eds) Clinical Sports Medicine, 2nd edn. McGraw-Hill, Sydney, p. 495–507.
Brukner P, Khan K, Alfredson H 2001a Pain in the Achilles region. In: Brukner P, Khan K (eds) Clinical Sports Medicine, 2nd edn. McGraw-Hill, Sydney, p. 535–552.
Brukner P, Khan K, Bell S 2001b Elbow and forearm pain. In: Brukner P, Khan K (eds) Clinical Sports Medicine, 2nd edn. McGraw-Hill, Sydney, p. 274–291.
Brukner P, Khan K, Bradshaw C 2001c Calf pain. In: Brukner P, Khan K (eds) Clinical Sports Medicine, 2nd edn. McGraw-Hill, Sydney, p. 524–534.
Brukner P, Khan K, Cooper R et al 2001d Acute knee injuries. In: Brukner P, Khan K (eds) Clinical Sports Medicine, 2nd edn. McGraw-Hill, Sydney, p. 426–463.

Brukner P, Khan K, Kibler W B 2001e Shoulder pain. In: Brukner P, Khan K (eds) Clinical Sports Medicine, 2nd edn. McGraw-Hill, Sydney, p. 229–273.
Butler D S 2000 The sensitive nervous system. Unley: Noigroup Publications.
Byrne A, Byrne D 1993 The effect of exercise on depression, anxiety and other mood states. Journal of Psychosomatic Research 37(6):565–574.
Carette S, Fehlings M G 2005 Clinical practice. Cervical radiculopathy. N Engl J Med 353(4):392–399.
Carter S K, Rizzo J A 2007 Use of outpatient physical therapy services by people with musculoskeletal conditions. Physical Therapy 87 (Mar 20 [Epub ahead of print]).
Clare H A, Adams R, Maher C G 2004 A systematic review of efficacy of McKenzie therapy for spinal pain. Australian Journal of Physiotherapy 50(4):209–216.
Clark D I, Downing N, Mitchell J et al 2000 Physiotherapy for anterior knee pain: a randomised controlled trial. Annals of the Rheumatic Diseases 59(9):700–704.
Clement D B, Taunton J E, Smart G W 1984 Achilles tendinitis and peritendinitis. Etiology and treatment. American Journal of Sports Medicine 12:179–184.
Cloward R B 1959 Cervical discography. A contribution to the etiology and mechanism of neck, shoulder and arm pain. Annals of Surgery 150:1052–1064.
Cowan S M, Scache A G, Brukner P et al 2004 Delayed onset of transversus abdominis in longstanding groin pain. Med Sci Sports Exerc 36 (12):2040–2045.
Croft P, Pope D, Zonca M et al 1994 Measurement of shoulder related disability: results of a validation study. Annals of the Rheumatic Diseases 53(8):525–528.
Dwyer A, Aprill C, Bogduk N 1990 Cervical zygapophyseal joint pain patterns. I: A study in normal volunteers. Spine 15(6):453–457.
Dye S F, Staubli H U, Biedert R M et al 1999 The mosaic of pathophysiology causing patellofemoral pain: therapeutic implications. Operative Techniques in Sports Medicine 7:46–54.
Ebinbichler G R, Resch K L, Nicolakis P et al 1998 Ultrasound treatment for treating carpal tunnel syndrome: a randomised sham controlled trial. BMJ 316(7133):731–735.
Edwards I, Jones M, Carr J et al 2004 Clinical reasoning strategies in physical therapy. Physical Therapy 84(4):331–335.
Ellis R, Hing W, Reid D 2007 Iliotibial band friction syndrome – a systematic review. Manual Therapy, [Epub ahead of print](Jan 5).
Fairclough J, Hayashi K, Toumi H et al 2006 The functional anatomy of the iliotibial band during flexion and extension of the knee: implications for understanding iliotibial band syndrome. Journal of Anatomy 208 (3):309–316.

CHAPTER EIGHT

Ginn K 2003 Functional anatomy and assessment. In: Prosser R, Conolly W B (eds) Rehabilitation of the Upper Limb. Butterworth Heinemann, Edinburgh, p. 236–241.

Glass J M 2006 Cognitive dysfunction in fibromyalgia and chronic fatigue syndrome: new trends and future directions. Current Rheumatology Reports 8(6):425–429.

Green S, Buchbinder R, Hetrick S 2003 Physiotherapy interventions for shoulder pain. Cochrane Database of Systematic Reviews(2):CD004258.

Grieve G P 1994 The Masqueraders. In: Boyling J D, Palastanga N (eds) Grieve's Modern Manual Therapy of the Vertebral Column, 2nd edn. Churchill Livingstone, Edinburgh, p. 841–856.

Gulliford M C, Latinovic R, Charlton J et al 2006 Increased incidence of carpal tunnel syndrome up to 10 years before diagnosis of diabetes. Diabetes Care 29(8):1929–1930.

Guzman J, Esmail R, Karjalainen K et al 2001 Multi-disciplinary rehabilitation for chronic low back pain: systematic review BMJ 322:1511–1516.

Hadhazy V A, Ezzo J, Creamer P et al 2000 Mind-body therapies for the treatment of fibromyalgia. A systematic review. Journal of Rheumatology 27(12):2911–2918.

Hay E M, Paterson S M, Lewis M et al 1999 Pragmatic randomised controlled trial of local corticosteroid injection and naproxon for treatment of lateral epicondylitis of elbow in primary care. British Medical Journal 319:964–968.

Hayden J A, van Tulder M W, Tomlinson G 2005 Systematic review: strategies for using exercise therapy to improve outcomes in chronic low back pain. Annals of Internal Medicine 142:776–785.

Heckmann J G, Lang C J, Zobelein I et al 1999 Herniated cervical intervertebral discs with radiculaopathy: an outcome study of conservatively or surgiczally treated patients. Journal of Spinal Disorders 12(5):396–401.

Herbert R D, Maher C G, Moselely A M et al 2001 Effective physiotherapy. BMJ 323:788–790.

Hoffman J R, Mower W R, Wolfson A B et al 2000 Validity of a set of clinical criteria to rule out injury to the cervical spine in patients with blunt trauma. National Emergency X-Radiography Utilization Study Group. New England Journal of Medicine 343(2):94–99.

Holmich P, Uhrskhou P, Ulnits L et al 1999 Effectiveness of active physical training as treatment for long-standing adductor-related groin pain in athletes: randomised trial. Lancet 353(9151):439–443.

Hoppenfield S 1986 Physical Examination of the Spine and Extremities. Appleton-Century-Crofts, New York.

Hwang E, Barkhuizen A 2006 Update on rheumatologic mimics of fibromyalgia. Current Pain & Headache Reports 10(5):327–332.

Iles J F, Stokes M, Young A 1990 Reflex actions of knee joint afferents during contraction of the human quadriceps. Clinical Physiology 10:489–500.

International Headache Society (IHS) Classification Subcommittee. The International Classification of Headache Disorders, 2nd edn. Cephalalgia 2004;24 (Suppl 1).
Jette A M 2006 Toward a common language for function, disability, and health. Physical Therapy 86(5):726–734.
Jull G, Barrett C, Magee R et al 1999 Further clinical clarification of the muscle dysfunction in cervical headache. Cephalalgia 19:179–185.
Jull G, Trott P, Potter H et al 2002 A randomized controlled trial of exercise and manipulative therapy for cervicogenic headache. Spine 27: 1835–1843.
Jull G A, Niere K R 2004 The cervical spine and headache. In: Boyling J D, Jull G A (eds) Grieve's Modern Manaul therapy, 3rd edn. Churchill Livingstone, Edinburgh, p. 291–309.
Kellgren J H 1939 On the distribution of pain arising from deep somatic structures with charts of segmental pain areas. Clinical Science 4:35–45.
Kent P, Marks D, Pearson W et al 2005 Does clinician treatment choice improve the outcomes of manual therapy for nonspecific low back pain? A meta-analysis. Journal of Manipulative & Physiological Therapeutics 28(5):312–322.
Kerkhoffs G M M J, Rowe B H, Assendelft W J J et al 2002 Immobilization and functional treatment for acute lateral ankle ligament injuries in adults. Cochrane Database of Systematic Reviews(3):CD003762.
Kool J, de Bie R, Oesch P et al 2004 Exercise reduces sick leave in patients with non-acute non-specific low back pain: a meta-analysis. Journal of Rehabilitation Medicine 36:49–62.
Kroeling P, Gross A, Houghton P E 2005 Electrotherapy for neck disorders. Cochrane Database Syst Rev 2:CD004251.
Lenaerts M E, Gill P S 2006 At the crossroads between tension-type headache and fibromyalgia. Current Pain & Headache Reports 10(6):463–466.
Levine D W, Simmons B P, Koris M J et al 1993 A self-administered questionnaire for the assessment of severity of symptoms and functional status in carpal tunnel syndrome. JBJS 75A:1585–1592.
Machado L A, de Souza M S, Ferreira P H et al 2006 The McKenzie method for low back pain: a systematic review of the literature with a meta-analysis approach. Spine 31(9):254–262.
Maitland G D, Hengeveld E, Banks K et al 2006 Maitland's Verterbal Manipulation, 7th edn. Butterworth Heinemann, Edinburgh.
McConnell J 1986 The management of chondromalacia patellae: a long term solution. Australian Journal of Physiotherapy 32(14):215–223.
McKenzie R A, May S 2003 The Lumbar Spine: Mechanical Diagnosis and Therapy Vols 1 and 2, 2nd edn. Spinal Publications New Zealand Ltd, Waikanae.
McKinney L A, Dornan J O, Ryan M 1989 The role of physiotherapy in the management of acute neck sprains following road-traffic accidents. Archives of Emergency Medicine 6(1):27–33.

McNeely M L, Armijo Olivo S, Magee D J 2006 A systematic review of the effectiveness of physical therapy interventions for temporomandibular disorders. Physical Therapy 86(5):710–725.
Medlicott M S, Harris S R 2006 A systematic review of the effectiveness of exercise, manual therapy, electrotherapy, relaxation training, and biofeedback in the management of temporomandibular disorder. Physical Therapy 86(7):955–973.
Morris M E, Schoo A M M 2004 Optimizing Physical Activity and Exercise in Older People. Butterworth Heinemann, Edinburgh.
National Health Priority Action Council 2004 National Action Plan 2004-2005 for Arthritis and Musculoskeletal Conditions. Canberra: Australian Government Department of Health and Ageing.
New Zealand Acute Low Back Pain Guide 2004 ACC, Wellington.
O'Connor D, Marshall S, Massy-Westropp N 2003 Non-surgical treatment (other than steroid injection) for carpal tunnel syndrome. Cochrane Database Syst Rev 1:CD003219.
Oh S J 1993 Clinical Electromyography: Nerve Conduction Studies, 2nd edn. Williams & Wilkins, Baltimore .
Ordway N R, Seymour R J, Donelson R G et al 1999 Cervical flexion, extension, protrusion, retraction: a radiographic segmental analysis. Spine 24(3):240–247.
Paul A, Lewis M, Shadforth M F et al 2004 A comparison of four shoulder-specific questionnaires in primary care. Annals of the Rheumatic Diseases 63(10):1293–1299.
Perko M, Prosser R 2003 Soft tissue injuries – epicondylitis biceps tendon repair. In: Prosser R, Conolly W B (eds) Rehabilitation of the Hand and Upper Limb. Butterworth Heinemann, Edinburgh, p. 228–233.
Philbin E F, Ries M D, Groff G D et al 1996 Osteoarthritis as a determinant of an adverse coronary heart disease risk profile. Journal of Cardiovascular Risk 3(6):529–533.
Refshauge K, Gass E 2004 Musculoskeletal Physiotherapy: Clinical Science and Evidence-Based Practice, 2nd edn. Butterworth Heinemann, Oxford.
Richardson C, Hodges P, Hides J 2004 Therapeutic Exercise for Lumbopelvic Stabilization: A Motor Control Approach for the Treatment and Prevention of Low Back Pain, 2nd edn. Churchill Livingstone, Edinburgh.
Roach K E, Budiman-Mak E, Songsiridej N et al 1991 Development of a shoulder pain and disability index. Arthritis Care Res 4(4):143–149.
Roos E M, Roos H P, Lohmander L S et al 1998 Knee Injury and Osteoarthritis Outcome Score (KOOS) – Development of a self-administered outcome measure. The Journal of Orthopaedic and Sports Physical Therapy 28(2):88–96.
Rosenfeld M, Gunnarsson R, Borenstein P 2000 Early intervention in whiplash-associated disorders: a comparison of two treatment protocols. Spine 25(14):1782–1787.
Schneiders A G, Zusman M, Singer K P 1998 Exercise therapy compliance in acute low back pain patients. Manual Therapy 3(3):147–152.

Schwarzer A C, Wang S C, O'Driscoll D et al 1995 The ability of computed tomography top identify a painful zygapophyseal joint in patients with chronic low back pain. Spine 20(8):907–912.

Scully D, Kremer J, Meade M et al 1998 Physical exercise and psychological well-being: A critical review. British Journal of Sports Medicine 32 (2):111–120.

Selfe J 2004 The Patellofemoral joint: a review of primary research. Critical Reviews in Physical and Rehabilitation Medicine 16(1):1–30.

Selfe J, Callaghan M J, McHenry A et al 2006 An investigation into the effect of number of trials, during proprioceptive testing in patients with patellofemoral pain syndrome. Journal of Orthopedic Research 24: 1218–1224.

Selfe J, Harper L, Pedersen I et al 2001 Four outcome measures for patellofemoral joint problems: Part 1 development and validity Physiotherapy 87(10):507–515.

Sim J, Adams N 1999 Physical and other non-pharmacological interventions for fibromyalgia. Best Practice & Research in Clinical Rheumatology 13(3):507–523.

Sizer P S, Brismee J M, Cook C 2007 Medical Screening for red flags in the diagnosis and management of musculoskeletal spinal pain. Pain Practice 7(1):53–71.

Sjaastad O, Freriksen T A, Pfaffenrath V 1998 Cervicogenic headache: diagnostic criteria. Headache 38:442–445.

Spencer J D, Hayes K C, Alexander I J 1984 Knee joint effusion and quadriceps reflex inhibition in man. Archives of Physical Medicine and Rehabilitation 65:171–177.

Sterling M, Jull G, Vicenzino B et al 2005 Physical and psychological factors predict outcome following whiplash injury. Pain 114 (1–2):141–148.

Stiell I G, McKnight R D, Greenberg G H et al 1994 Implementation of the Ottawa ankle rules. JAMA 271(11):827–832.

Stratford P W, Binkley J M, Stratford D M 2001 Development and initial validation of the upper extremity functional index. Physiotherapy Canada 53:259–267, 281.

Swan K G, Wolcott M 2006 The athletic hernia: a systematic review. Clinical Orthopaedics and Related Research 455:78–87.

Tanaka Y, Kokubun S, Sat T et al 2006 Cervical roots as origin of pain in the neck. Spine 31(17):E568–E573.

Taylor N F, Dodd K J, Shields N et al 2007 Therapeutic exercise in physiotherapy practice is beneficial: a summary of systematic reviews 2002–2005. Australian Journal of Physiotherapy 53(1):7–16.

The Lower Extremity Functional Scale (LEFS): Scale Development, Measurement Properties, and Clinical Application.

Turp J C, Komine F, Hugger A 2004 Efficacy of stabilization splints for the management of patients with masticatory muscle pain: a qualitative systematic review. Clinical Oral Investigations 8(4):179–195.

Verhagen A P, Scholten-Peeters G G, de Bie R A et al 2004 Conservative treatments for whiplash. Cochrane Database Systematic review 1: CD003338.
van der Wees P J, Lenssen A F, Hendriks E J M et al 2006 Effectiveness of exercise therapy and manual mobilization in ankle sprain and functional instability: a systematic review. Australian Journal of Physiotherapy 52 (1):27–37.
van der Windt D A, van der Heijden G J, van den Berg S G et al 1999 Ultrasound therapy for musculoskeletal disorders: a systematic review. Pain 81(3):257–271.
van der Windt D A W M, van der Heijden G J M G, van den Berg S G M et al 2002 Ultrasound therapy for acute ankle sprains.[update of Cochrane Database Syst Rev. 2000;(2):CD001250; PMID: 10796428]. Cochrane Database of Systematic Reviews(1), CD001250.
van Os A G, Bierma-Zeinstra S M A, Verhagen A P et al 2005 Comparison of conventional treatment and supervised rehabilitation for treatment of acute lateral ankle sprains: a systematic review of the literature. Journal of Orthopaedic & Sports Physical Therapy 35(2):95–105.
van Tulder M W, Koes B, Malmivaara A 2006 Otcomes of non-invasive treatment modalities on back pain: an evidence-based review. European Spine Journal 15(Suppl 1):S64–S81.
Waddell G, McIntosh A, Hutchinson A et al 1999 Low Back Pain Evidence Review. Royal College of General Practitioners, London.
Waddell G 2004 The Back Pain Revolution, 2nd edn. Churchill Livingstone, Edinburgh.
Werner R A, Franzblau A, Gell N 2005 Randomized controlled trial of nocturnal splinting for active workers with symptoms of carpal tunnel syndrome. Archives of Physical Medicine and Rehabilitation 86(1):1–7.
Whiplash-Associated Disorder (WAD) Guidelines 2001 Motor Accident Authority NSW.
Zigond A, Snaith R 1983 The hospital anxiety and depression scale. Acta Psychiatrica Scandinavica 67:361–370.

CHAPTER NINE

# Case studies in care of the elderly

*Jennifer Nitz, Susan Hourigan*



## INTRODUCTION

A large proportion of adult physiotherapy practice will focus on older people. Consequently, a clear understanding of how ageing affects all body systems and how these changes might affect your assessment, goal setting and treatment is necessary when working with these patients. Older people often present with a number of medical conditions in addition to the current presenting clinical problem and these need to be identified and considered for their effects on the proposed clinical management. This consideration ensures that a safe and maximally effective treatment programme is developed for the patient. Patients are individuals and it is their innate physical, environmental, social and behavioural characteristics that need to be included in the reasoning processes as their physiotherapy programme of treatment is developed.

With the relocation of sub-acute management of patients from institutions to the community, much of one's practice with older people could be located outside hospitals in day therapy centres, private practice rooms, patients' homes, retirement villages or aged care facilities (nursing homes). The workload will vary and, to some extent, depend on travel time between patient homes if home visiting or if in one location. In a typical community-based day, it would be expected that one would consult with between 6 and 14 patients individually and also may be involved in conducting group sessions. The physiotherapist also has a role in injury prevention which may involve the training and assessment of staff and carers working in this area. It is important that a working day is structured so that all aspects of work can be accommodated. It is essential to consider travel time between clients and try to schedule visits to minimise distances travelled. It is necessary to develop time-management skills in order to leave time for good documentation of clients' notes. This includes assessment findings, goals, treatment, appropriate safety warnings, outcome measures appropriate to the individual and their conditions, expected outcomes and planning for patients' progression to self-management of their condition where possible, and a return to a fulfilling life experience. Other duties may involve communication with older people's family members, liaison with doctors, pharmacists, nurses and other allied health professionals, and the development of policies and practices related to running facilities and centres which care for older people.

Often, the most important part of physiotherapy practice in this area is directly related to assessing functional abilities, e.g. mobility and the treatment may prioritise aspects that will lead to improved independence and safety in activities of daily living. This may often be treatment related to reducing pain, improving balance or rehabilitation of safe independent or assisted walking abilities.



## CASE STUDY 1 COLLES' FRACTURE FROM A FALL

Physiotherapists working in orthopaedic out-patients, fracture clinics or private practice might encounter a patient with the scenario that follows.

### Subjective assessment

| | |
|---|---|
| PC | 64-year-old lady who has just had the cast removed after 6/52 of immobilisation for a Colles' fracture of her right wrist. She has been referred to physiotherapy for exercises |
| HPC | Patient tripped and fell on an uneven section of pavement while hurrying to the bus stop on her way to work<br>After application of the cast on the day of injury, patient did not receive any instruction regarding prevention of joint stiffness or swelling before being sent home<br>She had no problems that she felt were worth reporting during the time of immobilisation |

### Objective assessment

| | |
|---|---|
| Observation | A thin, slightly stooped woman<br>Holding right wrist in left hand in guarded position across her body<br>Her hand and fingers are swollen and quite pink with scaly and flakey skin<br>There is a visible deformity/bulge just above the wrist from the fracture callus |

| | |
|---|---|
| Pain | Present when the fracture site is touched and when moving her hand and finger joints. Also in her shoulder when lifting her arm to dress |
| ROM | Moderately limited from pain and stiffness in the shoulder and from swelling, pain and stiffness in the wrist, hand, thumb and finger joints |
| Grip strength | Right hand is 25% of her left (right dominant)<br>Pinch grip strength 40% compared to her left hand |
| Sensation | Some slight hypersensitivity in the finger and thumb tips |
| Patient's goal | To 'get back to normal' |

## Questions

1. What underlying factors or conditions would you consider in this situation? How might these affect your physiotherapy management?
2. What should you consider about her functional ability?
3. What information is important to find out about the circumstances of the fall the patient had?
4. Is there any other assessment that you might consider important to undertake with this patient?
5. What should you target in your treatment programme?
6. How frequently would you bring the patient back for treatment?
7. What outcome measures would you use to record progress?
8. What would be your criteria for discharge?
9. Do you think there might be any barriers to continuing exercise or changing lifestyle after discharge?
10. Would you consider referral to other health professionals? If so, what professions might be included?

# CASE STUDY 2 BILATERAL OSTEOARTHRITIS IN KNEES

## Subjective assessment

| | |
|---|---|
| PC | 72-year-old man presenting with osteoarthritis (OA) in both knees<br>Causing pain and limiting walking distance to 200 m, then requires rest<br>VAS score: pain constantly at 4 or 5<br>Weight-bearing exercise aggravates the pain, but prolonged rest does too<br>Has consulted you to 'get rid of his pain' |
| PMH | Type 2 diabetes and hypertension both controlled by medication<br>No history of any other medical or surgical conditions |

CHAPTER NINE

| | |
|---|---|
| **DH** | He has been told by his GP not to take non-steroidal anti-inflammatory (NSAID) tablets because they will 'react' with his blood pressure pills<br>Paracetamol only helps the pain 'a bit' |
| **SH** | Retired bank manager<br>Lives in a low set house with his healthy wife<br>Their main leisure activities include watching sport and bus tours<br>He drives a car and receives no community services |

## Objective examination

| | |
|---|---|
| **Observation** | Obese and wears glasses for reading only<br>*Postural alignment* – Shows slight varus deformity of the knees bilaterally but nothing else remarkable. Visible wasting of VMO<br>*Swelling* – On palpation there is a small effusion in the pre-patellar space bilaterally and general thickening of the knee joint area bilaterally<br>*Skin condition* in his legs is good with no evidence of varicose veins or arterial insufficiency |
| **ROM** | Knees – 10° lag on the left and 5° lag on the right<br>Flexion limited to 90° on the left and 100° on the right<br>Passive ROM shows no extension lack and similar flexion range<br>Accessory movements show no ligamentous or meniscal damage<br>Patello-femoral joints are stiff<br>Both hips are limited in abduction and internal rotation range<br>Ankle and foot ROM are normal for age<br>Lumbar spine is stiff but retains a normal curve |
| **Muscle strength** | Hip abductor, adductor, extensor and rotator muscles are all grade 4 or 4+ on manual muscle testing<br>Muscle strength around the knee was not tested due to pain inhibition and visible wasting of VMO |
| **Functionality** | Has to push up with his arms to assist sit to stand<br>Uses the support of the railing/banister when ascending or descending stairs |

## Questions

1. What additional information might you like to find out to assist in your choice of treatment?
2. He mentioned walking is limited to around 200 m before he has to rest and your functional assessment revealed that he uses his upper limbs to assist sit to stand and on stairs. Is there any other aspect related to exercise that you might like to know considering exercise will need to be a large component of his treatment?
3. How will you set your treatment goals to comply with the patients stated goal of 'getting rid of the pain'?
4. What treatment might you choose to help treat the pain?
5. What exercise modalities might you be considering? Does the presence of a knee lag affect the initial choice of exercise?
6. What self-management strategies will you give to manage his knee OA?
7. What outcome measures would you choose to record progress?
8. Would you consider referral to another health professional to complement his physiotherapy management?



## CASE STUDY 3 PALLIATIVE CARE – WORKING IN COMMUNITY AS PART OF A COMMUNITY PALLIATIVE CARE TEAM

### Subjective history

| | |
|---|---|
| PC | 65-year-old lady presents with chest and thoracic pain and fatigue<br>Pain is constant but varies depending on time of day and activity<br>Enjoys daily walks which don't increase fatigue but make her feel 'a bit puffed' when walking up hills and occasionally when getting dressed<br>Worse after washing the dishes when VAS 6/10<br>At most other times VAS is between 2 and 3<br>Resting in a supported slightly reclined sitting position helps relieve the pain when most distressing |
| HPC | History of breast cancer. Had right mastectomy 10 years ago followed by chemotherapy and radiotherapy<br>Two years ago, she presented with chest pain which was found to be due to metastasis in her T7 vertebral transverse process. There were also hialar lymph node enlargement and two metastases in the right upper lung field<br>No other medical conditions |
| DH | Analgesia: oxicodone, naprosin and paracetamol |

| | |
|---|---|
| SH | Moderately active all her life. Played social competition tennis weekly up until 2 years ago<br>Since then has walked 30 minutes/day<br>Lives in a two-bedroom flat with her daughter |

## Objective assessment

| | |
|---|---|
| Observation | Patient alert, but listless. Medium build<br>Right arm – lymphoedema apparent (right arm bigger than left with slight swelling in the hand). Patient reports is not troubling her<br>Thoracic kyphosis that improves when she frequently adjusts her sitting posture<br>Posture is good in standing or sitting up straight but she needs to be reminded to do this |
| Respiratory function testing | FCV 2.4 L (expected 3.2 L)<br>Right upper chest movement is reduced compared to the left<br>Auscultation – reveals an inspiratory and expiratory wheeze and reduced air entry over the right upper lung field. All other lung fields have normal air entry and no added sounds |
| Functional assessment | Bed mobility is independent<br>Rolling to the left causes pain – the lower trunk follows her upper trunk causing considerable torsion to the thoracic spine area<br>Lying to sitting – rolls to the side and pushes up to the sitting position while simultaneously dropping her legs over the side of the bed. Bed height enables the feet to be on the floor when sitting on the side<br>Sit to stand – no trouble but uses her arms to assist<br>Sitting and standing balance are normal<br>Some shortness of breath on exertion |

## Questions

1. How is treating a person with a terminal illness towards the end of their life different from other patients you encounter?
2. What comprises your approach to managing this patient's pain?
3. How will you address the fatigue?
4. What advice will you give the patient about activities she undertakes around the house?
5. Are there any risks associated with her walks that might need to be identified for her so she can increase her awareness and prevent any problems arising?

6. Will you treat the lymphoedema in her right arm? If yes, what management strategies/advice could you give?
7. What advice would you give this patient regarding condition changes she may experience that she should seek assistance to manage?
8. Do you think the patient would benefit from referral to another team member to assist in her care?

## CASE STUDY 4 POST-OPERATIVE HEMICOLECTOMY

### Subjective assessment

| | |
|---|---|
| PC | 86-year-old lady 1st day post-operative laparoscopic assisted right hemicolectomy<br>Surgery done under general and spinal anaesthetic with the epidural cannula at T10<br>Intra-operative blood loss estimated as 1.3 L |
| HPC | Admitted to hospital 2/7 ago with a suspected bowel obstruction |
| PMH | Nil of note |
| DH | Medications are taken for hypertension, left ventricular failure, arthritis and osteoporosis |
| SH | Lives alone in the community<br>Home help assists with house work<br>Visited once weekly by the community nurse (refilled her dosette)<br>Son lives nearby, visits weekly and her daughter phones on most days<br>Patient does own shopping with a neighbour and attends senior meetings once a month<br>Mobilises with wheeled walking frame which helps carry objects and makes her feels 'safer'<br>Able to walk about 1 km on the flat with her walking frame at own pace with rests<br>Vision is good since her cataracts were removed and lenses implanted 10 years ago<br>Hearing is good for her age |
| Pre-operative assessment | Drowsy due to analgesics prescribed to control her abdominal pain<br>Quite lucid and able to answer questions about her home and functional level before admission to hospital |

| | |
|---|---|
| | Chest assessment revealed:<br>Moderate kyphosis<br>Poor basal air entry bilaterally (likely due to abdominal distention) |
| **Handover from nursing staff** | Patient been stable overnight<br>Complained of pain at rest (VAS 6/10) and on movement (VAS 10/10) in the early hours<br>Pain team notified, analgesia adjusted with good effect<br>Current pain VAS 1/10 at rest and 3/10 on movement |

## Objective assessment

| | |
|---|---|
| **Observation** | Naso-gastric tube draining stomach secretions, wound drain and urinary catheter in situ<br>IV line in her left forearm ($KCl^+$ added to normal saline)<br>Epidural in situ delivering fentanyl and bupivicaine to control her pain |
| **Respiratory** | Self ventilating 28% $O_2$ via face mask<br>RR 26<br>$SaO_2$ 90% |
| **Cardiovascular** | HR 72<br>BP 110/70<br>Previous 24-hour fluid balance + 2000 mL |
| **Chest assessment** | Auscultation – decreased air entry bi-basally and in the right mid-zone with fine end inspiratory crackles bilaterally<br>Facilitation of air entry only marginally improves basal chest expansion<br>Supported cough produces 1 plug (5 mL) of thick, yellow sputum |
| **Other information** | DVT check is negative<br>Able to perform circulation exercises well<br>Patients wound dressing needs changing so you decide to mobilise her later in the morning<br>When you return at 1100 hours to mobilise her you find she is agitated and unable to follow instructions |

### Questions

1. What might be contributing to this mild delirium?
2. What do you need to check again even though you did this at 08.30 hours and why?
3. Taking these findings into consideration what is your priority and what treatment could you carry out?
4. Why is it important to liaise with the medical staff in this situation and what further tests or investigations could they carry out to help determine cause of patients behavior?
5. What might you suggest to her son and daughter to do to reduce her confusion?
6. When you get the patient up to mobilise how would you ensure the treatment is safe and effective?
7. In addition to treating her chest and getting her mobile again, what else should you include in the patient's exercise programme and why?

## CASE STUDY 5 NURSING HOME RESIDENT

As the physiotherapist visiting the facility your responsibility is to assess new residents to determine how nursing staff might assist with maintaining functional ability and mobility to enable an acceptable quality of life.

### Subjective assessment

| | |
|---|---|
| PC | 92-year-old lady has been admitted to the nursing home during the last week<br>Has no current complaints<br>She is confused and afraid of standing and being moved by the care staff but responds quite well to one-on-one attention and assisted activity during your visit |
| PMH | Mild CVA 2 years previously<br>Early mild dementia<br>History of multiple falls<br>Sustained a right fracture NOF that was surgically managed 4 years ago<br>Multiple thoracic vertebral fractures from a fall last year<br>Wears a hearing aid in her right ear<br>Glaucoma resulting in 60% visual loss |

### Objective assessment

| | |
|---|---|
| Observation | Fragile skin, poor circulation |
| ROM | Limited in all major joints |
| Strength | Generally grade 3+/5 upper and lower limbs |

| | |
|---|---|
| **Bed mobility** | Can roll using the bed rail or bed stick to assist<br>Moving from lying to sitting on the side of the bed needs assistance from the bed pole and physical assistance to move legs over the edge of the bed |
| **Sit to stand** | Requires maximum assistance from one person |
| **Gait** | Can take two or three steps with maximum assistance from one person to retain balance |

## Questions

1. How might the confusion and fear of movement be overcome when carers assist with mobility?
2. What equipment might you consider using to assist with a sit-to-stand transfer and what will be the key factors driving your decision?
3. In an aged person what can affect skin and circulation condition and make fragility a major problem?
4. What is the importance of maintaining weight bearing?
5. What should the physiotherapist include in patient handling and risk assessment and what might they use in determining competencies of staff in this area?
6. Identify key problems and write an example of an exercise programme bearing in mind that the programme will be applied by the therapy aide or care staff.
7. What might be important to establish about the resident's social support network?
8. What other health care professionals might you consult regarding the resident's care?



# ANSWERS TO CHAPTER 9: CASE STUDIES IN CARE OF THE ELDERLY

## Case Study 1

1. - Osteoporosis (OP) since she is postmenopausal, of slight build, appears slightly stooped and has had a fracture (Kanis 2004, Nguyen et al 2004, Sambrook et al 2002). Education regarding OP and management options including exercise, diet and need for referral to her GP for investigation or pharmaceutical management might be indicated.
   - Cancer (possibility of metastases, contraindications for some electrotherapeutic modalities).
   - Neurological, arthritic or cardiopulmonary conditions (steroids contributing to osteoporosis and fracture risk).
   - What medications is she taking? This will help you decide on referral to her GP if not on OP medications, but there is also a need for consultation if on multiple medications that might have increased her risk of a fall (Andrews et al 2001).

2. There are a number of functional aspects that need to be considered:
   - Has she modified her dress to accommodate for the pain in her shoulder when dressing and moving her fingers? (Counsel her to wear clothing that encourages her to move her upper limb through large ranges of movement and to manipulate small buttons.)
   - Has she any family responsibilities, such as caring for grandchildren or a sick husband?
   - What are her leisure time activities?
   - What type of work does she do?
   - Did she return to work after the fracture?
   - Could she manage to do her work tasks?
   - Work postures need to be considered from the ergonomic and postural perspectives considering her stooped posture and current limitation of her right shoulder movement that might predispose her to developing neck and arm pain.

3. It is important to determine the circumstances of the fall so that the treatment provided has addressed the underlying cause of the fracture and so prevent or limit the possibility of another fall related fracture:
   - What were the weather and light like at the time of her fall? (Contribution of vision, e.g. poor visual acuity and edge perception could have contributed to not noticing the uneven pavement (Lord et al 1991) might suggest that a referral to an optometrist is needed.)
   - Does patient usually wear corrective lenses? Multifocal lenses have been implicated in falls (Lord et al 2002).
   - Was patient multitasking, e.g. carrying groceries or talking to someone (Bloem et al 2001, Shumway-Cook et al 2006)? Even though she is relatively young, multitasking ability is important to elicit.
   - Any previous falls and the circumstances of these falls.

4. Balance assessment:
   - Clinical test for sensory integration of balance (CTSIB)
   - Unilateral stance eyes open and closed
   - Timed up and go (TUAG) with dual tasks. (Compare results to normal values to determine dysfunction.)
   - Berg Balance Scale

5. - Pain – reduce swelling using elevation, active muscle contractions and thermal modalities (remember shoulder, neck and trunk movements).
   - Balance and osteoporosis – integrate upper limb rehab into a functional exercise regime that also targets bone loading and balance training (Chan et al 2004, Hourigan & Nitz 2004, Kelley

et al 2001, Liu-Ambrose et al 2004). (Also included in home exercise programme.)
- Decreased ROM and strength – specific exercises targeting areas affected most.
- Refer her to a community-based exercise group that would target bones and balance.

6. Review patient in the first week to check progress in reduction of swelling and pain, increased ROM and strength, and if she was doing the exercises. If all was progressing well at this first follow-up, the next appointment would be 4 weeks later to reassess the orthopaedic problems and balance.

7. Outcome measures would include:
   - Pain VAS
   - Goniometry for range of movement (optional)
   - Grip and pinch strength
   - Volume of water displacement for swelling
   - Balance measures as above.

8. Discharge criteria:
   - Evidence of steady improvement in outcome measures
   - Achieving goals of pain-free functional activity
   - Back at work
   - Confident in their self-management of their balance and osteoporosis.

9. Barriers to keeping up the exercise or accessing programmes for falls prevention:
   - Denial of a problem and unwillingness to consider falling and injury prevention programmes is possibly the most obstructive barrier
   - Costs involved
   - Reluctance to participate alone (Phillips et al 2004)
   - Person is not at a stage where they are ready to change lifestyle (Dijkstra 2005) and therefore need to be encouraged to progress to this level of readiness with counselling and encouragement.

10. - GP referral is indicated if the patient was taking a number of medications, or was not taking any medication for their bones and had not been investigated for osteoporosis.
    - Optometrist referral is advised if visual acuity or edge perception problems are identified.
    - Referral to an occupational therapist or ergonomist to evaluate the work station may be necessary if it had been identified that these were not optimal for the patient.

    It is tempting to only consider the orthopaedic aspect of the presenting patient, but there are important preventive health concepts associated with the case that need to be addressed in your holistic management.

## Case Study 2

1. Has the patient tried any treatment other than medication to control his knee pain? If so, what has been tried and what was the response to intervention?

2. It is important to know whether exercise or physical activity is only limited by their knee pain and not related to other cardiovascular or respiratory problems. Fitness is obviously a problem needing to be managed.

3. 
   - Factors contributing to pain from OA knees should be discussed.
   - Use a multifocal approach using pain-relieving modalities, exercise and lifestyle modification combined to achieve the patient's primary goal of pain relief.
   - Show how maintenance of a pain-free controlled state will depend on patient's continued adherence to the treatment regime that will be controlled by them, and that only their effort will result in success.

4. Thermal modalities might be used to control pain, but it is crucial to provide any safety warnings. The choice between hot or cold might depend on patient preference and perceived effect. For example:
   - You may consider use of a heat-retaining wrap or splint.

   TENS can also provide pain relief in the community situation as they are cheap to buy or rent.
   - Joint mobilisation may also relieve pain, e.g. Grade III flexion/extension mobilisation and end of range extension mobilisation.

   With either modality chosen, it is necessary to ensure that the patient understands how and when to apply the treatment. Also, any sensory testing should be done and recorded in their notes remembering that diabetes can affect sensory-motor function (Lord et al 1993). Also record any adverse responses, and how these should be managed.

5. 
   - Progressive resisted exercises (PRE) targeting the quadriceps and hamstring muscles have been shown to improve the symptoms of OA (Mikesky et al 2006).
   - Endurance exercise would also be indicated for the patient because of his low fitness state, type 2 diabetes and obesity. Ideally, both these types of exercise should be included in the patient's programme (Pedersen & Saltin 2006). PRE is commonly performed in an open chain when weights are lifted, and this can reduce the strengthening effect at the muscle fibre level and the translation of the effect to functional efficiency. The synergy of muscle recruitment and strength in the lower limb is vitally important for function. Therefore, functional strengthening exercise (incorporating mainly closed-chain activities) is ideally going to be more beneficial to the patient.

- Aquatic physiotherapy is a medium whereby loading during functional activities can be regulated depending on the depth of the water. Resistance can be varied with speed of limb movement and with apparatus such as paddles, and thus great demands are placed on all body muscle groups for stability during function. The buoyancy of the water can also be used to assist strengthening through the range of lag that on land would otherwise reduce the options of position for exercise, until inner range quadriceps strength and outer range hamstring strength was achieved to protect the joint during other PRE or endurance exercises.
- An additional attribute of aquatic physiotherapy is the potential to exercise for longer and with many large muscle groups and this will have a positive effect on diabetes and weight control.

6. Self-management should include the provision of alternate exercise strategies so that once the patient's pain is under control; they are able to vary their exercise regime. In the initial stages, short 5–10 minute bursts of exercise three or four times a day might be tolerated. As endurance and tolerance improves, the duration of sessions should be increased to around 30 minutes and at least twice a day. Frequent exercise sessions with varied focus, e.g. PRE, endurance or aquatic will be more likely to maintain compliance and benefit all the patient's pathologies. It would be beneficial to the patient to encourage their partner to participate too, as exercising with a partner has been shown to maximise continued participation (Yardley et al 2006). Also, demonstrating how the patient's exercise programme can complement their leisure activities would be advantageous.

7. Outcome measures should look at the impairments and cover functional measures that reflect all aspects of patient's presenting problems
   - Pain VAS
   - Functional strength – Oxford muscle scale
   - Lag range – ROM, goniometry
   - Functional – Time to complete five sit-to-stands from a chair without armrests, 6 minute walk test or timed up and go (TUAG).

8. Referral to a dietitian is indicated to control weight and diabetes. An exercise physiologist or personal trainer might be appropriate to encourage a better lifestyle once the patient's knee pain, knee lag and muscle imbalances have been addressed.

   It might also be beneficial to refer the patient to a chronic condition self-management group that is often available through Arthritis Foundations or other community organisations. Considerable autonomy with self-management of chronic conditions has been achieved through this approach and is indicated for the patient (Lorig et al 1993).

## Case Study 3

1. When providing palliative care, the physiotherapist needs to understand that cure is not possible and the aims of treatment are to maximise quality of life and not necessarily quantity of life, by providing treatment that minimises distressing or troublesome symptoms so as to improve comfort (Hourigan & Josephson 2004).

2. Pain management includes:
   - Use of electrotherapeutic modalities such as TENS and thermal applications. (Encourage use of TENS to add to the analgesia from medication. By maintaining the current medication levels, the sedative effect from them will be controlled and the patient will not be restricted due to this complication.)
   - Washing the dishes aggravated the pain. Why? (It might be due to the fact that the lighting over the sink is poor and the patient needs to stoop to see if the dishes are clean, therefore using a sustained flexed upper thoracic position. That is likely to be irritating to their thoracic spine secondary that might be putting additional pressure on the spinal nerve. Investigating the situation and suggesting ways of overcoming the problem would allow the patient to continue their daily tasks, thus helping to maintain normality in both physical and emotional function.)

3. Keeping active is very important for this patient:
   - Since she does not experience increased fatigue after her walk each day, the patient should be encouraged to do exercise in the other half of the day as well.
   - Encourage gentle exercises that aim to reduce the lymphoedema in the right arm (Didem et al 2005, Moseley et al 2005).
   - Discuss energy-saving strategies including work simplification and the importance of adequate rest periods.

4. Good posture during activities is paramount:
   - Avoid sustaining flexed postures involving the upper trunk. Activities such as washing up, peeling vegetables or preparing meals might be better undertaken sitting at the kitchen table or bench rather than at a work surface that is too low and forces the patient to bend.
   - Rolling to the left in bed causes pain. (Suggest log rolling to reduce the torsion on the vertebral structures that is likely the origin of pain during this movement.)

5. Age-related changes in low-contrast visual acuity and edge perception increase the risks of slips, trips or falls when light is poor (Lord & Webster 1990, Low Choy et al 2003), so raising the patient's awareness of this situation is important so that they can be more

careful or ensure that when the light is poor, they are walking where it is well lit. Care with slippery or uneven surface is also important, as any jerk from a slip or trip can cause a fracture in the region of bony metastases and increase the pain. Safety might be enhanced and the option for walking in all terrains retained by using 'ski poles' for support.

6. The patient is not concerned by her right arm swelling at present, however:
   - strategies should be provided to reduce or prevent an increase in the lymphoedema
   - the problems associated with lymphoedema need to be raised. These include reduced function, the difficulty in lifting the weight of the arm, and how this might causes extra stress on the patient's thoracic spine. Pain is also experienced by the swelling in the arm if it becomes excessive
   - discuss the reasons why the problem needs to be addressed now when it is not causing any real problems enabling her to reflect and decide to participate in management. This can reduce the stress associated with coping with this additional problem. Intervention may at this stage include advice regarding elevation during rest times and self massage of axillae and groins to enhance drainage while in elevation and is simple for the patient to do. Adding gentle exercises to facilitate drainage will also help (Moseley et al 2005). A sleeve or glove might be useful to reduce the additional swelling that occurs during walking when the arm is dependent. Using 'ski poles' and the gripping and upper limb activity might also reduce this dependency oedema.

7.
   - Any increase in pain should be reported immediately so that the patient remains comfortable.
   - Change in bladder or bowel control or weakness and changed sensation in their lower limbs might indicate spinal stenosis and needs to be reported so that safe mobility is retained and continence control assistance provided as needed.

8. Working in a palliative care team, the patient should have access to:
   - occupational therapist and social worker. (Liaising to ensure appropriate aids are installed in the home and ensuring that the patient's daughter has appropriate support to help care for her mother.)
   - the pain team should be actively involved to ensure control of pain
   - pastoral assistance might be accessed too.

## Case Study 4

1. • Delirium in the post-operative time is common in older people who have undergone major surgery (Olin et al 2005). Other factors that might lead to delirium include:
   - Inter-operative blood loss (Demeure & Fain 2006, Olin et al 2005)
   - Method and efficacy of pain relief (Beaussier et al 2006, Fong et al 2006, Vaurio et al 2006). Therefore, all these aspects need to be looked at.
   - In this patient's case:
     - positive fluid balance
     - decreased air entry to their right mid-zone and bi-basally might be more likely to cause hypoxia and therefore contribute to her delirium.
2. Therefore you will need to check:
   - $SaO_2$ (which is 80% and she is pulling her oxygen mask off in agitation)
   - respiratory rate (32 per minute)
   - auscultation and observation of the patient's chest:
     - Poor air entry to the mid-zone and reduced bi-basal breath sounds
     - End inspiratory crackles in lower lung fields
     - Slight supra-clavicular recession on inspiration increased use of accessory respiratory muscles of inspiration.

   You decide that these findings are indicative of a combination of fluid retention and possible aspiration in the post-operative period causing the right middle lobe collapse and consolidation and reduced basal expansion exacerbated by some abdominal distention and discomfort.

   The least likely cause of the respiratory symptoms is pulmonary emboli from a DVT.

3. Treatment priority is to improve aeration and remove any sputum plugs that might be causing the right middle lobe signs.

   Treatment should involve:
   - positioning in a more upright position
   - improving air entry using tactile facilitation and staged breaths with inspiratory holds if the patient could cooperate to achieve this
   - vibration during expiration, which has been suggested to assist with improving air entry and expiratory forces that might help secretion removal (McCarren et al 2006). (Remember that the patient is osteoporotic and vigorous application of sputum clearing methods should be applied with care.)
   - trying to ensure that they keep their Venturi mask in place during these manoeuvres

CHAPTER NINE

- supported huff and cough, which will be encouraged after these actions
- assisted arm elevation, if patient is unable to participate in the breathing exercises, timed to coincide with inspiration, which might be effective in improving air entry and facilitating a spontaneous cough
- mobilisation, which should be commenced as soon as possible depending on patient co-operation.

4. Liaison with the medical staff is important to:
   - see if they were aware of her deteriorated condition
   - ensure the chest assessment findings and interpretations are known
   - see if the positive fluid balance has been considered (e.g. stat dose of diuretics)
   - carry out a chest X-ray (to rule out PE)
   - repeat blood tests (to check electrolytes and for the presence of blood loss anaemia)
   - see if urine microscopy had been ordered as a method of eliminating infection as a factor contributing to the delirium (Demeure & Fain 2006).



5. The son and daughter might be encouraged to stagger their visits during the day so that they could sit with their mother for longer periods and encourage orientation to her surroundings, time and place. Having familiar people and orientating conversation, making eye contact and frequently touching helps reduce confusion and enable better treatment compliance with keeping their oxygen mask on for example (Demeure & Fain 2006). The family might also encourage deep breathing and leg exercises to enhance the physiotherapy treatment effect.

6. Efficient and safe mobilisation will be attained by ensuring:
   - use of a walking frame that is similar, if not the same, as the one the patient previously used. Familiarity with an object and its use is very important if the person you are working with is unable to follow instruction or is having problems with thought processing (Demeure & Fain 2006)
   - a family member or assistant is present during mobilisation to help with carrying drainage bags and perhaps push the drip stand to ensure safe ambulation
   - that talking during the walk is limited as this would interfere with the patient's concentration on the task in hand and increase the likelihood of her losing balance (Lundin-Olssen et al 1997).

7. Before discharge and when the patient was able to participate in the task, the following would be introduced:
   - Gentle abdominal muscle exercises including transversus abdominus recruitment. Also encourages pelvic floor muscle function that will enhance their continence (Sapsford et al 2001). Incontinence can be worsened after a period of catheterisation. Incontinence (Dingwall & Mclafferty 2006) and delirium are risk factors that commonly precipitate admission to long-term nursing care (Demeure & Fain 2006).
   - Ensure that the patient and their family was given ergonomic advice appropriate to abdominal surgery, for example regarding when lifting can be resumed. This is generally around 6 weeks post operatively.
   - The patient should continue all their current exercises and add more walks.

## Case Study 5

1. - Ensure clear and simple instructions to the patient.
   - Ensure good eye contact with the patient and explain exactly what it is that they are going to assist them to do, what they need to do to help, and where they will be moving to before assisting with the transfer.
   - Use confident and steady handling to reassure the patient that they will not fall while they are there and encourage the patient positively to do as much as they can to help.

2. Equipment:
   - A walking belt might be used around the patient's waist/hips to increase safety for both resident and staff member. This will enable the carer to control balance and to guide the movement.
   - If performing a standing transfer to a chair, a pivot disc might be used to aid the turn if stepping is unsafe. Pivot discs have their own inherent dangers, however, and must be used correctly to avoid injuries.
   - If these aids prove to be insufficient to allow all carers to safely transfer the patient a standing hoist might be introduced.

   Key factors affecting decisions:
   - The resident's ability to cooperate and assist the transfer.
   - The safety of both resident and staff (to avoid injuries from falls, skin trauma, possible fractures and back care during movements).
   - The staff members' abilities to communicate and assist the resident.
   - The resident's physical status, including reduced range of movement in limb joints, decreased strength, increased bone fragility and the need to retain bone loading and standing considering her osteoporosis status.
   - Continuation to stand in some manner for transfers will also help maintain some self-esteem for the resident.

3. - There is loss of collagen and elasticity, reduction in the number of blood vessels, sub-cutaneous fat, hair follicles, sebaceous glands and free nerve endings in the dermis of older people that contribute to skin fragility and poor sensation which puts the resident at greater risk of accidental injury.
   - Circulation is compromised by cardiac and peripheral arterial and venous changes due to ageing. Increased thickness of the ventricular walls, dilation and stretching or calcification of valves affects cardiac output and in effect failure of the cardiac pump. Atherosclerotic changes in the arteries can contribute to postural hypotension that is most problematic during sit to stand and reduction in distal perfusion of tissue including the skin. This might contribute to poor healing of injuries (Nitz & Hourigan 2004).

4. Retaining the ability of the resident to stand helps:
   - maintain bone mineral density, joint range and strength
   - manage continence by assisting renal drainage, encouraging bowel motility, allowing transfers to the toilet or commode and enables easier access to allow for clothing changes
   - dispel feelings of complete dependency and helplessness, it may greatly influence quality of life.

5. Physiotherapists generally undertake the manual handling and risk assessment education for workers in nursing homes. The important components of such an education programme are:
   - ensuring that the language used is at a level that is understood by the staff. Asking questions of the staff such as: 'What do you think I mean by that?' can help to get optimal understanding
   - identification of what entails an injury risk, e.g. wet floors, assisting a resident to stand by pulling on the arm
   - identification of when, how and why the resident is needing close supervision or help with a task, which will clarify the need for specific instructions regarding an instruction
   - emphasising the importance of re-assessing the awareness level and physical status of the resident every time they are undertaking a transfer, especially where participation in the transfer is expected of the resident
   - emphasising the responsibility of management to protect staff from injury and of the staff to adhere to safety procedures
   - emphasising the responsibility of staff to report malfunctioning or broken equipment and ensure repair before use
   - ensuring that staff are familiar with what equipment is available for assisting residents, know how to use the equipment and are aware of safety precautions during use, e.g. care with applying hoist slings to residents with frail skin

- identification of how much to assist a resident to ensure they are not being helped too much and understanding that each resident is an individual and will require individual care plans and instructions that relate to their medical status
- emphasising the importance of reporting and recording accidents and injuries to residents and themselves.

6. A simple exercise programme might include:
   - Assisted range of movement exercise for arms and legs, e.g. arm raises × 10, once a day
   - Sit-to-stand exercise at a rail or with assistance, e.g. standing at rail with assistance where necessary × 6 at once, once a day
   - Posture correction exercise and trunk extension in sitting by encouraging sitting upright and not slumping.
7. - Does the patient have any family? What is their involvement in care?
   - How willing are they to assist with the provision and organisation of additional devices to enhance quality of life such as a supportive recliner chair with pressure-relieving features or an individualised wheelchair?
   - What is their impression of the goals and wishes of the patient?
   - What might be their own goals for their mother?
   - If there is no family does the patient have friends who visit and are caring for her needs?
   - How much might the friends be willing to participate in the patient's management?
8. Case conferencing and communication between health care workers is a key aspect in achieving best practice care. It is necessary to communicate with the nursing staff, GP, pharmacist, geriatrician, dentist, podiatrist, dietitian, speech pathologist, occupational therapist and audiologist as required.



### References

Andrews H P, Gilbar P J, Wiedmann R J et al 2001 Fall-related hospital admissions in elderly patients: contribution of medication use. Australian Journal of Hospital Pharmacy 31:183–187.

Beaussier M, Weickmans H, Parc Y et al 2006 Postoperative analgesia and recovery course after major colorectal surgery in elderly patients: a randomized comparison between intrathecal morphine and intravenous PCA morphine. Regional Anesthesia and Pain Medicine 31(6):531–538.

Bloem B R, Valkenburg V V, Slabbekoorn M et al 2001 The multiple tasks test. Development and normal strategies. Gait & Posture 14:191–202.

Chan K, Qin L, Lau M et al 2004 A randomised prospective study of the effects of Tai Chi Chun exercise on bone mineral density in postmenopausal women. Archives of Physical Medicine and Rehabilitation 85:717–722.
Demeure M J, Fain M J 2006 The elderly surgical patient and postoperative delirium. Journal of American College of Surgeons 203(5):752–757.
Didem K, Ufuk Y S, Serdar S et al 2005 The comparison of two different physiotherapy methods in treatment of lymphedema after breast surgery. Breast Cancer Research and Treatment 93(1):49–54.
Dijkstra A 2005 The validity of the stages of change model in the adoption of the self-management approach to chronic pain. Clinical Journal of Pain 21(1):27–37.
Dingwall L, Mclafferty E 2006 Do nurses promote urinary continence in hospitalized older people?: An exploratory study. Journal of Clinical Nursing 15:1276–1286.
Fong H K, Sands L P, Leung J M 2006 The role of poetoperative analgesia in delirium and cognitive decline in elderly patients: a systematic review. Anaesthesia and Analgesia 102(4):1255–1266.
Hourigan S R, Josephson D L 2004 Physiotherapy in palliative care. In: Nitz JC, Hourigan SR, eds. Physiotherapy Practice in Residential Aged Care. Butterworth Heinemann, Edinburgh, p. 332–347.
Hourigan S R, Nitz J C 2004 Osteoporosis. In: Nitz JC, Hourigan SR, eds. Physiotherapy Practice in Residential Aged Care. Butterworth Heinemann, Edinburgh, p. 239–250.
Kanis J A 2004 Assessment of fracture risk and its application to screening for postmenopausal osteoporosis: synopsis of a WHO report. WHO Study Group. Osteoporosis International 4:368–381.
Kelley G A, Kelley K S, Tran Z V 2001 Resistance training and bone mineral density in women: a meta-analysis of controlled trials. American Journal of Physical Medicine and Rehabilitation 80(1):65–77.
Liu-Ambrose T, Khan K M, Eng J J et al 2004 Resistance and agility training reduce fall risk in women aged 75 to 85 with low bone mass: a 6-month randomised, controlled trial. Journal of the American Geriatric Society 52:657–665.
Lord S R, Webster I W 1990 Visual field dependence in elderly fallers and non-fallers. International Journal of Aging and Human Development 31:269–279.
Lord S R, Caplan G, Colagiuri R et al 1993 Sensori-motor function in older persons with diabetes. Diabetic Medicine 10:614–618.
Lord S R, Clark R D, Webster I W 1991 Visual acuity and contrast sensitivity in relation to falls in an elderly population. Age and Ageing 20:175–181.
Lord S R, Dayhew J, Howland A 2002 Multifocal glasses impair edge-contrast sensitivity and depth perception and increase the risk of falls in older people. Journal of the American Geriatrics Society 50:1760–1766.
Lorig K, Lubeck D, Kraines R et al 1993 Outcomes of self help education for patients with arthritis. Journal of Arthritis Rheumatology 28:680–685.

Low Choy N L, Brauer S G, Nitz J C 2003 Changes in postural stability in women aged 20 to 80 years. Journals of Gerontology Medical Science 85: M825–M830.
Lundin-Olssen L, Nyberg L, Gustafson Y 1997 'Stops walking when talking' as a predictor of falls in the elderly. Lancet 349:617.
McCarren B, Alison J A, Herbert R D 2006 Vibration and its effect on the respiratory system. Australian Journal of Physiotherapy 52(1):39–43.
Mikesky A E, Mazzuca S A, Brandt K D et al 2006 Effects of strength training on the incidence and progression of knee osteoarthritis. Arthritis & Rheumatism 55(5):690–699.
Moseley A L, Pillar N B, Carati C J 2005 The effect of gentle arm exercise and deep breathing on secondary arm lymphedema. Lymphology 38(3):136–145.
Nguyen T V, Center J R, Eisman J A 2004 Osteoporosis: underrated, underdiagnosed and undertreated. Medical Journal of Australia 180 (Suppl 5):S18–S22.
Nitz J C, Hourigan S R 2004 Physiological changes with ageing. In: Nitz JC, Hourigan SR, eds. Physiotherapy Practice in Residential Aged Care. Butterworth Heinemann, Edinburgh, p. 7–31.
Olin K, Eriksdotter-Jönhagen M, Jansson A et al 2005 Postoperative delirium in elderly patients after major abdominal surgery. British Journal of Surgery 92:1559–1564.
Pedersen B K, Saltin B 2006 Evidence for prescribing exercise as therapy in chronic disease. Scandinavian Journal of Medicine & Science in Sports 16(Suppl 1):3–63.
Phillips E M, Schneider J C, Mercer G R 2004 Motivating elders to initiate and maintain exercise. Archives of Physical Medicine and Rehabilitation 85(Suppl 3):S52–S57.
Sambrook P N, Seeman E, Phillips S R et al 2002 Preventing osteoporosis: outcomes of the Australian Fracture Prevention Summit. Medical Journal of Australia 176 (Suppl 8):1–16.
Sapsford R R, Hodges P W, Richardson CA et al 2001 Co-activation of the abdominal and pelvic floor muscles during voluntary exercises. Neurology and Urodynamics 20:31–42.
Shumway-Cook A, Guralnik J M, Phillips CL et al 2006 Age-associated declines in complex walking task performance: the walking InCHIANTI Toolkit. Journal of the American Geriatrics Society 55(1):58–63.
Vaurio L E, Sands L P, Wang Y et al 2006 Postoperative delirium: The importance of pain and pain management. Anaesthesia and Analgesia 102(4):1267–1273.
Yardley L, Bishop F L, Beyer N et al 2006 Older people's views of falls-prevention interventions in six European countries. Gerontologist 46(5):650–660.

# Case studies in mental health

*Lead author Caroline Griffiths, with contributions from Clare Leonard, Sharon Greenshill, Jean Picton-Bentley, Victoria Welsh Hamelin, Josephine Bell*



## INTRODUCTION

Physiotherapy should 'promote, maintain and restore physical, psychological and social well-being' (Chartered Society of Physiotherapy 2002a).

'Mental health problems affect one in four of us at some time in our lives. They can also be the result of drug or alcohol dependency, illness or long-term physical disability' (Chartered Society of Physiotherapy 2005).

From these descriptors given by our professional body, The Chartered Society of Physiotherapy (CSP), it is clear that the influence over wellbeing of both psychological and physical health is recognised. However, the history of physiotherapy within mental health is a recent one compared to the work done in physical specialties. Still many people both outside and within the profession wonder what physiotherapists' role in mental health might involve.

Physiotherapists working in mental health may be working as part of a Community Mental Health Team (CMHT) or as a member of a larger physiotherapy team. Some will be employed directly by a mental healthcare trust and some by a Primary Care Trust (PCT) or may work in the private or charity setting.

Provision of, and access to, a specialist, physiotherapy, mental health service varies dramatically dependent upon geographical location. Some services focus on older adults while others have input into all age groups.

'Care-group'-specific services may occur for eating disorders, personality disorder, primary care anxiety disorders or addictive behaviours. There are specific facilities for forensic mental health, which deal with people who are detained in a special hospital or secure unit following a court judgement that their offence was wholly or partially due to their mental ill health.

Patients/clients may be in hospital voluntarily or may have been admitted under a section of the Mental Health Act in order to safeguard themselves or others. The majority of people with a mental health diagnosis, e.g. bipolar disease, depression, anxiety are treated by their GPs. If more specialised treatment is required then the CMHT may be involved. Initiatives to enable people to stay in the community include: Intensive Home Support Teams; Crisis Intervention Teams and Assertive Outreach Teams whose remit is to engage those clients whom have long-term enduring mental illness and may have difficulty maintaining concordance with treatment.

Clinical specialist physiotherapists in mental health have developed roles in orthopaedic and rheumatology clinics and may act as liaison specialists for physical health services in both primary and secondary care settings.



Wherever the physiotherapist works effective input occurs when the wider team together with the client and carers are involved, as stated in 'New Ways of Working for Psychiatrists, Enhancing Person Centred Care by...True Multidisciplinary Working' (DoH 2005).

Skills transfer between other specialties and mental health can range from musculoskeletal to continence, from neurological to respiratory but specific skills of anxiety management, massage, communication in challenging situations may best be learnt in the mental health environment. Our work correlates with the government drivers of the wellbeing agenda which include the National Service Framework (NSF) for Mental Health (DoH 1999) and the NSF for Older Adults (DoH 2001) along with Our Health, Our Care, Our Say (DoH 2006).

Evidence for physical interventions and effects are most prolific in terms of the positive outcomes of exercise in depression and anxiety. Other studies which have, by nature of their size, given evidence but have acknowledged flaws include studies of massage, acupuncture and falls prevention with general mobility for older adults.

Examples include:

- Exercise for people with dementia improves cognitive functioning (Fox 2000, Laurin et al 2001)
- Exercise reduces falls risk (Skelton 1999) and in depression (Liu et al 1998)
- Regular activity reduces incidence of depression (Mutrie 2000)
- Exercise may alleviate secondary symptoms of schizophrenia (Faulkner & Biddle 2002)
- Exercise has a positive effect on self esteem (Fox 2000)

- Exercise is an effective treatment for depression (Lawler & Hopker 2001)
- Exercise has a low-to-moderate anxiety reducing effect (Taylor 2000)
- Exercise brings benefits to problem drinkers (Donaghy & Mutrie 1999).

The outcomes of a student placement or junior post should be to develop a clear knowledge of three key facts: (i) the interaction of physical and mental health, (ii) the effects of our core skills on mental disorder and (iii) the need to provide equitable access and quality of physical care to clients who also have a mental health diagnosis. Alongside those gems of knowledge an inspired physiotherapist who wants to use skills learnt to help bridge the gap, which still exists, between physical and psychological health provision would be deemed a great and successful outcome.

The following case studies give a glimpse of the variety of client group, clinical settings, and skills required and the professional opportunity offered in physiotherapy in mental health. They include cases from primary, secondary and tertiary care and range from somatisation to anorexia.

## CASE STUDY 1 BACK PAIN AND LIFESTYLE, A HOLISTIC APPROACH

### Subjective assessment

| | |
|---|---|
| **Psychiatric history** | 37-year-old man experiencing a psychotic depression<br>He has been under the care of mental health services for the past 5 years following an unsuccessful suicide attempt. As a result of which the patient was admitted to an acute psychiatric ward under a section 3 of the Mental Health Act 1983. This allowed a period in which to assess and treat him<br>He was discharged from the ward after 3/12 and has since been under the care of a CMHT<br>He is seen regularly by a community psychiatric nurse (CPN) who helps him to take his medication<br>The patient has regular reviews with a consultant psychiatrist who reviews the medication and monitors his mental health state<br>He has had ongoing input from a social worker who helped him to get accommodation with a local housing association. The social worker, who is his care co-ordinator, continues to offer support and is responsible for setting up, monitoring and reviewing the overall care package through the Care Programme Approach (CPA)<br>He is currently reviewed at 6/12 intervals. The CPA meeting is an opportunity for all people involved |

| | |
|---|---|
| | in the patients care to come together and discuss his progress and ongoing needs (Mental Health Act 1983 Code of Practice (1999))<br>He has been referred to a mental health physiotherapist by the CPN for back pain |
| **HPC** | 2-year history of back pain<br>Has gained approximately 4 stone over the past 3 years since starting an antipsychotic medication<br>Pain is present in the morning on rising. It reduces as the day progresses but playing snooker once a week seems to increase pain |
| **Investigations** | X-ray – taken 2 years ago at the initial onset of back pain. This showed no abnormality |
| **DH** | Anti-depressant medication<br>Anti-psychotic medication |
| **PMH** | Mild asthma diagnosed aged 16<br>Fractured tibia 10 years ago |
| **SH** | Lives alone in a one-bedroom flat and has few friends<br>Once a week he plays snooker at a voluntary sector mental health drop-in centre<br>Has a very sedentary life and does not engage in any other physical activity<br>His social worker has also referred him to a befriending scheme and a volunteer visits him once a week<br>Sleeping pattern is erratic and he reports staying up most nights watching television. He generally sleeps from 4am to midday on his sofa<br>Diet consists entirely of takeaways<br>Unable do his own shopping as he gets very anxious in busy environments<br>Ex-smoker and no longer drinks alcohol |

## Objective assessment

| | |
|---|---|
| **Posture/ observation** | Overweight gentleman, standing with a forward head position slumped shoulders and flattened lumbar lordosis |
| **Lumbar ROM** | Flexion was half normal range as was side flexion bilaterally |

| | |
|---|---|
| | Extension was approximately three-quarters normal range<br>Pain was reported at end of available range flexion and extension |
| **Muscle power** | Normal |
| **Neurological examination** | NAD |
| **Palpation** | Moderate muscle spasm in lumbar area<br>Antero-posterior mobilisation L3–5 = stiff |
| **Patient's attitude** | Frustrated with being overweight as prior to being unwell he was an average weight<br>Wants to be more fit and active and to pursue a healthier lifestyle<br>Doesn't know where to begin and feels like there are too many problems in his way. For example he could not imagine coming to a gym at the moment as he feels too self-conscious<br>Appears really motivated to change and willing to take advice and work with therapist to solve problems. He also revealed he had an exercise bike in a cupboard at home |



## Questions

1. What may have contributed to his recent weight gain?
2. The patient has a 2-year history of low back pain. From the information provided what lifestyle factors may contribute to this?
3. Suggest what could be done to tackle some of these? What could be done initially and what may be a long-term goal?
4. What treatment is indicated specifically for the treatment of the back pain?
5. What other professionals could be involved to help him with the broader issues?
6. What outcome measures could be used?
7. How can social inclusion be incorporated into the overall management approach of this client?

## CASE STUDY 2 CHRONIC BACK AND LEG PAIN

This patient was referred to the CMHT by his GP with depression and chronic pain. Referral was allocated to the clinical specialist physiotherapist working within the team.

He was also referred on by the physiotherapist to the psychiatrist for further assessment of his mental health.

## Subjective assessment

| | |
|---|---|
| PC | 44-year-old man with a 12-month history of low mood, which has not responded well to medication prescribed by the GP<br>4-year history of leg and back pain following an accident at work<br>Constant low back pain and leg pain radiating from buttock to posterior upper thigh with no variation in intensity of pain<br>Patient reports he is unable to stand or sit for prolonged periods; however, he was able to sit for the whole of the interview without moving or adjusting position |
| **Patient's perception** | Feels unable to cope with the pain and the disability as he is in pain when doing 'everything'<br>Avoids doing a great deal because of the pain and rarely goes out due to fear of falling or being unable to get home<br>Believes the reason for his condition worsening is general deterioration |
| **Daily routine** | Avoids mornings as this seemed to increase his pain<br>Gets up late then spends the day in his chair which is placed in a selected position with everything he needs within easy reach<br>His wife is able to visit her parents in the morning when the patient is in bed but she is unable to leave him the rest of the time due to fear of him falling, despite the patient not falling once within the last 4 years |
| **Mental health** | No previous history of mental health problems<br>The recent condition has been treated by his GP with numerous antidepressants but found no improvement in symptoms, patient is currently not on any medication |
| SH | Lives with his wife, no children<br>His wife has given up her job to look after him. She is extremely supportive and admits to having a major role in supporting and assisting 24 hours per day, including all aspects of daily living including driving him to appointments with his |

| | |
|---|---|
| | solicitor or to hospitals, making all meals and drinks, managing his medication, dealing with solicitor and appointments<br>He has no social life, no hobbies and spends little time out of the home<br>He has no contact with his family but does see his mother and father-in-law weekly<br>The patient worked as a car mechanic for 15 years but has been off sick for the last 4 years<br>He has a claim against employers for an accident which is being dealt with by his solicitor<br>Patient is receiving Disability Living Allowance, Incapacity benefit and his wife receives carer's allowance |
| **PMH** | High cholesterol, irritable bowel syndrome<br>Past psychiatric history – none<br>Both his wife and mother have a history of back problems |
| **Investigations** | X-rays, bloods and MRI all normal<br>Has been given a diagnosis of mechanical back pain and muscle spasm. He sought a private second opinion but was given the same diagnosis |
| **DH** | Tramadol<br>Paracetamol<br>Simivastatin |
| **Mental health assessment** | Patient casually dressed<br>Good eye contact and speech normal in flow and content<br>Gives a comprehensive picture of his symptoms<br>Concentration was good throughout the assessment<br>Orientated to time, place and person<br>There were no thoughts or plans of suicide or self-harm<br>He describes feeling hopeless about his situation<br>His sleep is broken and he wakes frequently, managing between 3 and 7 hours per night, which was attributed to pain<br>Has no enjoyment of meals but no weight loss<br>States that his mood is low, and he has little motivation |

## Objective assessment

On questioning no evidence of any red flags.

Thoracic spine: unable to achieve full extension. Pain at half range.

Lumbar spine: unable to achieve full extension. Pain at half range.

SLR right = 40° left = 30°.

Distracted straight leg raise – knee was extended when seated on the edge of the chair. He did not report any pain or discomfort.

Axial loading was positive – eliciting pain when pressing down on the top of the patient's head.

He complained of superficial tenderness – skin discomfort on light palpation.

Pain on simulated rotation – rotating the shoulders and pelvis together should not be painful as it does not stretch the structures of the back.

No altered sensation.

Reflexes normal.

**Screening tools** The distress and risk assessment method (DRAM; Main 1992) combines screening tools of the modified somatic perception questionnaire (MSPQ; Main 1983) and the Zung self-rating depression scale (Zung 1965).

Scores:

- Zung Score 40, suggesting an element of clinical depression which required treatment with anti-depressant medication.
- MSPQ Score 25, suggesting a high level of anxiety and a combined assessment of distress and somatization.
- Oswestry Disability Questionnaire (Fairbank et al 1980) Score 80%, which indicates the patient felt 80% disabled by his back pain.
- Fear avoidance beliefs questionnaire (FABQ) score 87, which suggests a significantly high level of fear avoidance beliefs and behaviour.

## Questions

1. What can be deduced from the symptoms described in the objective assessment?
2. What behaviours does the patient present with?
3. What factors in the patient's life reinforce his behaviour?
4. Why is the development of a therapeutic relationship so important?
5. Why was it necessary to ask the patient about suicidal thoughts or plans?
6. What treatment interventions could you use in this situation?

## CASE STUDY 3 SOMATIZATION

### Subjective assessment

| | |
|---|---|
| PC | 20-year-old woman admitted to a specialist mental health unit for a period of assessment and rehabilitation<br>Using an electric wheelchair with straps to maintain her back and neck position and a strap to prevent her right arm from becoming too extended<br>Functional movement in right arm sufficient to drink through a straw and to eat<br>Presented no movement in her left arm and legs<br>Extensive investigations failed to identify an organic cause for this level of disability |
| HPC | Previously had a very healthy lifestyle then developed a rash and fatigue-like symptoms when she was 15 and was admitted to hospital where she had a cardiac arrest<br>Immediately afterwards she described shakes and tremors that she referred to as making her think of herself as a thunderbird puppet<br>This progressed to loss of function in first her legs and then her left arm. As her disability increased she was catheterised<br>Has become totally wheelchair dependent, although her father had secretly obtained video footage of walking 3/12 and 2 years before her present admission |
| PMH | Fractured right arm falling out of a tree age 11 |
| SH | 2 years ago moved into a boarding school for disabled children<br>Presently awaiting her A level results prior to taking up a university place<br>Parents divorced when she was 3 years old<br>Initially she would regularly see her father but they moved away when the patient was 12 following an allegation of rape by her brother's friend<br>Prior to her illness there were some difficulties in her relationship with her mother as the patient had become increasingly rebellious<br>Her premorbid personality was one of a bright teenager, although somewhat rebellious at times, with a keen interest in sport and competing at badminton for her school |

| | |
|---|---|
| **DH** | Had become involved in illicit drugs in social settings from the age of 13<br>Since illness began she was on a high dose of painkillers and antidepressants plus a variety of herbal remedies |
| **Patient's behaviour** | Would display long periods of inactivity, then would then take herself out in the wheelchair for hours at any one time<br>She believed that a miracle cure may occur |
| **Attitude** | An angry young lady who resented instruction<br>Acquisition and use of illicit drugs resulted in episodes of disruptive behaviour<br>Perceived motivation on admission:<br>Reports that she was very eager to get better<br>Tearful and looking for quick fixes<br>Did not undertake her exercise routinely<br>Poor insight |



### Objective assessment

Dependent on nursing staff using the hoist to transfer her from bed to chair

No apparent movement in her legs and poorly defined muscle bulk throughout lower limbs

Weight 6 stone

Specific muscle testing was not carried out as the patient was unable to produce a contraction on request

Barthel Index score (indicates how independently patient is managing ADLs) – 15/20

Poor trunk control in sitting

Writhing movements of her right arm frequently taking her out of her base of support

Her head moved continuously in a nodding motion

Right shoulder and arm also moved constantly

Predominant posture – flexed elbow with flexion and medially deviation at the wrist

Full ROM when supporting right arm with movement's uncontrolled and poor stabilisation at the shoulder girdle

| | |
|---|---|
| **Motivation after input** | Admits that it is much harder to do things after her initial illness. After admitting her difficulty she became much more involved with her physiotherapy programme<br>Progression was stepwise and though directed by the multidisciplinary team was led by patient progression |

| | |
|---|---|
| **Outcome** | This renewed period of cooperation resulted in the lady leaving the unit able to run and dance, although there was still occasionally a fine tremor when she was tired |

## Questions

1. What physical consequences may have resulted from the client's period of immobility?
2. What might be the primary gain and secondary gain factors for this patient in developing this very dependent lifestyle?
3. What immediate needs and support might the multidisciplinary team require from the physiotherapist?
4. How might you start to plan a rehabilitation programme with this lady?
5. Why is multidisciplinary team working vital?
6. Which professions may be involved with this patients care? What would be their role?
7. What could a physical rehabilitation programme include?



## CASE STUDY 4 ANOREXIA NERVOSA, BACK PAIN

### Subjective assessment

| | |
|---|---|
| PC | 23-year-old woman with anorexia nervosa, presents with back pain<br>She is a patient on a specialist eating disorders unit |
| HPC | Has suffered from chronic, insidious onset low back pain for about 5 years<br>Has had a constant dull ache in the upper thoracic spine since sustaining spontaneous wedge fractures while studying for her 'A' levels<br>Both pains have worsened since being admitted to the ward and ceasing all her usual activities<br>Unable to identify specific aggravating and easing factors, but reports difficulty sitting still for the duration of therapeutic groups (usually an hour) and difficulty standing for more than 15–20 minutes |
| **Past medical and psychiatric history** | Patient first diagnosed with anorexia nervosa by her GP when studying for her GCSEs, but this is her first episode of specialist treatment<br>She has just completed 16/52 of in-patient treatment where she achieved her target BMI of 17<br>On admission she weighed 38 kg with a BMI of 14.3 |

| | |
|---|---|
| | In the year prior to admission she had become increasingly preoccupied with minimisation of her weight and shape, restriction of her diet and excessive exercising<br>She also developed depressive beliefs about herself and the future<br>Osteoporosis diagnosed aged 18<br>Spontaneous wedge fracture of T4–5<br>Spondylolisthesis of L5–S1 (asymptomatic second degree slip)<br>Anaemia<br>Asthma since early teens (currently well controlled) |
| **Investigations** | DEXA scan indicates low bone mineral density with intermediate risk of fractures |
| **Social and family history** | Very sporty as a teenager. Enjoyed long-distance running and competed in gymnastics competitions at national level<br>High achiever at school, attaining five A grade 'A' levels and gaining a place at university to study law<br>The symptoms of her eating disorder escalated when studying for her final year law exams, which she failed to complete, resulting in her deferring third year at law school<br>Has a supportive family<br>Smokes 20–30 cpd and is a social drinker (approximately 6–8 units per week) |
| **Maladaptive lifestyle developed** | For 6/12 prior to admission patient increasingly avoided social activities due to social anxiety and body image disturbance: she stopped attending lectures, going to the gym and meeting all but the closest of friends. She also began exercising more covertly: getting up early to go for long runs, stair climbing at home and practising 1000 abdominal crunches a day (100 at hourly intervals throughout the day) when her flat mates were out |
| **Drug history** | Antidepressant medication<br>Inhalers for asthma (bronchodilators and corticosteroids)<br>Bisphosphonate (to slow bone metabolism)<br>Calcium supplements |

## Objective assessment

Patient was reluctant to undress for objective assessment but agreed if the mirror was removed from the room.

| | |
|---|---|
| **Observation** | Sway-back posture (Kendal et al 1993):<br>■ Forward head position with upper cervical extension and lower cervical flexion<br>■ Upper thoracic kyphosis with posterior placement of upper trunk<br>■ Shoulder protraction<br>■ Flattened lumbar spine and forward sway of posteriorly tilted pelvis<br>■ Hyperextended knees<br>Poor muscle bulk throughout due to low weight |
| **Active ROM** | Cervical spine: full ROM<br>Thoracic spine: unable to achieve full extension actively or passively<br>Lumbar spine:<br>■ Hands to floor on forward flexion. Complains of pain in lumbar spine approximately half way through returning to upright position: uses hands on thighs for support<br>■ Normal range of lumbar extension but with pain at end of range<br>Chest expansion: 2 cm<br>Upper and lower limbs: Full functional ROM with hyperextension noted at knees, elbows and at metacarpophalangeal joints |
| **Muscle strength** | Generalized weakness: Grade 4 muscle power throughout |



## Questions

1. What are the indicators in the patient's history that she is at increased risk of future fractures?
2. What is the significance of her having hyperextended knees and elbows and being able to touch the floor, and what does this indicate?
3. What should be the aims of the treatment programme? What should also be considered in her treatment programme? (Consider one or two short-term and long-term goals within this answer.)
4. How could you help manage the pain of osteoporosis?
5. What type of exercises would be beneficial as part of the treatment programme?
6. Are there any types of exercise that you should advise the patient to avoid?

7. What outcome measures would be appropriate?
8. Why is close liaison with the eating disorders team necessary throughout physiotherapy intervention?

## CASE STUDY 5 DEPRESSION

The patient was referred from the crisis team after presenting at A & E following an overdose.

Reasons for overdose were low mood, weight gain, poor self-esteem, neck and shoulder pain, and social isolation.

### Subjective assessment

| | |
|---|---|
| PC | 45-year-old lady with a history of depression following divorce from her husband and the death of her mother for whom she was the main carer. She was treated for depression by the GP but states that she has gained 3 stone in weight due to her medication |
| SH | Lives alone in a terraced house since her divorce 4 years ago<br>She is currently unable to work due to her depression |
| PMH | Nil |
| DH | Mirtazapine 30 mg<br>Paracetamol |
| Mental health assessment | Casually dressed with brushed hair and wearing a little make up<br>Eye contact was good and speech was normal in its content but she spoke quietly<br>During the assessment she became weepy at times in particular when speaking of her losses<br>Is able to give a good history and to articulate her difficulties<br>Reports poor sleep with early morning wakening and comfort eating<br>She described feelings of worthlessness and loneliness<br>Denies any thoughts or plans of suicide or self-harm stating that her overdose had been an impulsive act and that she would not consider this again |
| Key issues identified | ■ Weight gain – since being on medication the patient reported that she has gained 3 stone in weight. Is unable to fit into most of her clothing, and due to her financial situation cannot buy many new clothes |

- Has difficulty going up stairs and hills as she gets breathless
- Participation in exercise in the past had been sporadic. Has attended the gym in the past but this stopped due to her caring for her mum. As a child she had enjoyed sports and exercises. She reported that she had become very inactive over the past 5 years
- Low mood – has suffered from low mood particularly since the death of her mother
- Smoking – has increased due to her mood and to boredom
- Poor self-esteem – since gaining weight and also since her husband left her
- Social isolation – since the death of her mother she has lost her sense of purpose and her role. Following her split from her husband she found that she lost contact with many 'friends' and now rarely sees anyone and only goes out of the home when attending appointments or going shopping
- Neck and shoulder pain – pain over the whole of the posterior aspect of her neck and her upper shoulders with no referred pain or neurological symptoms



## Questions

1. Why would the physiotherapist receive this referral?
2. What would you need to ensure had happened before commencing any intervention?
3. What interventions would you offer and what benefit would they be for the patient?
4. Outline the important aspects of an exercise programme for this client?
5. What other professions might also be involved?
6. What would be your long-term goals?

## CASE STUDY 6 OLDER ADULT WITH LEWY BODY DEMENTIA

### Subjective assessment

| | |
|---|---|
| PC | 83-year-old woman who is immobile following a DHS to her left NOF 5/7 ago as a result of a fall<br>Nursing staff are finding her difficult to manage on an acute ward and the orthopaedic physiotherapists are struggling to get this lady mobile and have asked for specialist mental health physiotherapy assessment |

| | |
|---|---|
| **HPC** | Patient fell at home while independently mobilising around her house<br>She is always on the move at home, constantly up and down the stairs<br>Not orientated in time but in familiar surroundings can orientate herself<br>Has visual hallucinations and has been noted to be unsteady and has had previous falls<br>Following her latest fall the ambulance was called by daughter and she was admitted to hospital for surgery |
| **PMH** | Lewy body dementia<br>Osteoporosis<br>Fractured bilateral wrists on separate occasions<br>Fractured right NOF 3 years ago |
| **SH** | Lives with husband in a two-storey house, which they own<br>Husband is not fit and struggles to manage his wife but wants her home again<br>Has daughter is 1 hour away but tries to support at least once a week doing shopping, cleaning, etc.<br>Patient has had respite recently to give her husband a break but it was not successful as patient became very agitated and did not sleep or eat while there and became more challenging on her return home |
| **Handover** | Ward staff report that patient can be aggressive at times and agitated which makes it difficult for them to carry out any interventions<br>As patient was trying to get out of bed independently the nursing staff have put cot sides up<br>Patient's mood has been noted as changing rapidly from happy to agitated and challenging and appears to be constantly anxious on the whereabouts of her husband<br>Nursing staff unable to mobilise patient and she has therefore been nursed in bed |

## Objective assessment

| | |
|---|---|
| **Observation** | Sitting in bed with cot sides up with catheter in situ and attempting to get out of bed over the cot sides<br>Mini mental state examination (MMSE)<br>This test is the most commonly used test for complaints of memory loss or when considering a diagnosis of dementia |

| | |
|---|---|
| | Unable to carry out due to level of cognitive impairment and agitation |
| **Behaviour and communication** | Verbal response appears unreliable, despite being vocal it is difficult to comprehend her speech<br>Able to respond to commands but becomes agitated very quickly, appears to express fear as aggression<br>Responds to tone of voice, if loud then will become more agitated and challenging in her behaviour but then calms down when she hears a calm voice<br>Does not appear to remember her operation, but could point to area of surgery with some insight into discomfort but not apparently to the reason<br>Follows clear short commands and appeared to dislike a lot of touch<br>Responds to gesture and allowing time for response |
| **ROM** | Ankle movement good<br>Knee flexion: right knee able to achieve 90°, left knee able to achieve 45° but then became agitated |
| **Bed mobility** | Good if allowed to do independently: possibly pain denoted by grimace when she moves noticed |
| **Sit to stand** | Requires support of one<br>Appears to be in pain on weight bearing, expressing as agitation and occasionally aggressively pushing staff away |
| **Mobility** | Mobile between two people a short distance of 6 m but unable to manage frame as carrying it and not putting all feet down safely<br>Became agitated and aggressive when wanted to sit but calmed quickly using calm manner and voice |

## Questions

1. What should you consider before assessing this lady?
2. How do you think her pain level could be assessed appropriately?
3. Considering her surgical intervention how do you think you may support this lady when mobilising?
4. What would your recommendations be to the staff on the ward with regards to mobility and management?
5. Who else would you involve in giving advice to the staff?
6. When planning for discharge who could be involved in her follow-up and how would you assess the future risks?
7. Which physiotherapy service should be involved in this patient's care?

# ANSWERS TO CHAPTER 10: CASE STUDIES IN MENTAL HEALTH

## Case Study 1

1. The patient takes antipsychotic medication. Some antipsychotics cause weight gain as a result of increasing appetite. Therefore most clients who take this medication put on some weight. It is a well-documented side effect (BNF 2007). It is important that clients are made aware of this as they start the medication so that they can make positive choices about food and are aware of healthy living principles.

2. a. Poor diet and weight gain
   b. Sedentary lifestyle
   c. Sleeping on sofa
   d. Poor posture

3. a. Dietary advice:
      i. Educate as to the main food groups and nutritional needs.
      ii. Encourage to shop and cook his own food. As he has anxiety in busy places perhaps he could go initially with someone from the befriending scheme.
      iii. Encourage to reduce frequency of takeaways.
      iv. Reduce portion sizes. It is important changes are made gradually so as not to overwhelm the patient. For example, only once he has established healthier eating principles should portion sizes be mentioned.
   b. Strategies to improve sleep patterns:
      i. Advise to try and sleep in a more regular pattern. One way of making these changes is to set an alarm progressively earlier. The patient must commit to getting up at the alarm time. This is done in small steps over a period of weeks until the target time is reached. Patients often find that this approach leads to both falling asleep more easily at night and earlier.
      ii. Reduce caffeine intake.
      iii. Increase physical activity.
      iv. Increase exposure to daylight.
      v. Sleep in a bed rather than the sofa.
   c. Encourage increased activity levels. Following a health screen to assess suitability for an exercise programme the following plan could be implemented:
      i. Initially exercise at home using his exercise bike.
      ii. Other ways to exercise at home could be instigated for example, he could be given a pedometer to increase his walking in the local area.

iii. He could set a goal to attend the hospital gym. Initially there are barriers to overcome such as his anxiety of busy places, disordered sleep making morning sessions difficult and lack of confidence about exercising in public. However, it is important that the client has goals such as this to work towards.
iv. A long-term goal may be to use the gym at the local leisure centre.

4. Specific treatment for back pain may include:
   a. Lumbar mobilisations
   b. Posture advice
   c. Specific mobilising exercises
   d. Postural stability exercises
   e. Heat to reduce muscle spasm.

   The other interventions such as exercise, weight loss and sleeping in a bed will also have a significant impact on his back pain.
5. It may be necessary to refer to a dietician for expert advice on weight loss and dietary needs.
6. Examples of suitable outcome measures used in this instance include:
   a. VAS to record pain levels
   b. Oswestry low back pain disability index (Fairbank et al 1980)
   c. Active range of movement
   d. Pedometer readings.
7. Social inclusion is an area receiving increasing attention in mental health services. When a client is very unwell they need the expert help of mental health professionals; however, as they recover clients can be helped to access support from other sources not under secondary care services. For example in the case of this client, he initially planned to exercise at home and with one-to-one input from a mental health physiotherapist. The next step would be to exercise in the hospital gym supported by exercise professionals. As his confidence grows he may progress to using the local leisure centre gym. It is important that there are clear pathways through services so that patients increase the chances of sustaining their lifestyle changes independently. This approach also helps to normalise mental health problems, reduce stigma and keep the person integrated in society.

## Case Study 2

1. The symptoms of distracted straight leg raise, axial loading, skin tenderness and pain on rotation all fall under Waddell's signs, first described by Waddell et al in 1980, that may indicate non-organic or psychological component to chronic low back pain.

The significant level of pain reported does not correspond to the diagnosis made and the results of the investigations. As a result he uses maladaptive ways to manage his condition.

2. 
   - Negative irrational beliefs about his condition, which has led to fear avoidance behaviour and beliefs surrounding the thought that activity increases damage. The patient believes that by restricting his activity he is protecting himself.
   - Lack of activity resulting in an increase in stiffness resulting reinforces fear.
   - Over-generalising (Ciccone & Grzesiak 1984), e.g. 'everything causes pain'. Rest reduced the pain and reinforced belief that movement was harmful (Vlaeyen & Linton in 2000).

3. The main reinforcers:
   - His wife's role as the full-time carer
   - Attention from the medical profession and his solicitor
   - Prospect of financial gain from the claim against his employers
   - Home modification for role as 'disabled'.

4. The development of a therapeutic relationship is important to establish initially, to emphasise that the clinician does not think that the problem is 'all in his head' but that he/she understands the patient's situation and believes it is real. Once trust has been built between the patient and therapist the patient is more likely to take on board advice and education regarding his condition, which will result in better outcomes of treatment.

5. This is a normal part of the mental health assessment; however, suicide risk is increased in chronic physical illness. In addition, there is generally an increased rate of psychiatric disorder, especially depression, in people with physical illness.

6. 
   - Cognitive behavioural therapy (CBT)
   - Cognitive restructuring discussion with the patient to link physical and psychological health
   - Education about links between the physical and psychological aspects of pain and maladaptive fear avoidance beliefs
   - Activity scheduling to assess level of activity and compare to beliefs (Hawton et al 1989)
   - Discussion around activity/pain cycle to address negative beliefs and fears. Butler and Moseley (2003) book explains pain in an easy to understand way and may help you to teach the patient about pain mechanics
   - Pacing and increasing activity
   - Graded task assignment and the aim to replace inactivity with activity

- Activity planning to allow him to test out the therapist's hypothesis that activity would not lead to damage. Increase in tasks done would increase self-efficacy beliefs that he could do more (Bandura 1977)
- Setting of small achievable goals
- Identification of the key things that aggravated/decreased pain
- Challenging his negative beliefs
- Hydrotherapy.

## Case Study 3

1. General muscle deconditioning, exercise tolerance muscle shortening, poor neck and trunk control, bladder control would be negligible after years of disuse.

2. Primary gain for this individual appeared to be attention. Secondary gain covers the aspects of life that have now developed around the initial disability, e.g. sympathy of others and financial in terms of benefits received.

3. The physiotherapist can support the manual handling coordinator and nursing team in devising risk assessments and forming care plans for safe physical management, i.e. transferring patient.

4. - Set clear goals/tasks, for example walking in the parallel bars twice a day and following a specific exercise regime
   - Establish a rapport and empathise with the client
   - Try not to ignore bad behaviour, instead reward good and reinforce and focus on what client is doing well.

5. Clients presenting with complicated non-organic physical illness can have very complex needs. This requires extremely close team working, particularly with the therapy team in order to support and reinforce the total treatment programme. Treatment may be long term.

   Clients can display quite manipulative behaviours such as splitting of the teams. There are various forums to assist, such as weekly ward rounds and smaller therapy meetings as and when required.

   There are discharge-planning meetings and in addition some clients will have their care programme approach (CPA) review. The CPA is used in the mental health setting for clients who can be with services for many years. It is held 6-monthly and the client is the central figure saying whom he/she wants to invite with their key worker organising it. People involved with care will come together to review progress and identify any further needs for the coming 6 months.

6. - Psychiatrist and medical team – lead on treatment and approach and formulate or confirm a diagnosis on discharge. Alter drug

regimes. Undertake diagnostic tests and liaise and refer to other agencies.
- Mental health nurse – to support in the ward environment helping her to engage in the new environment, set care plans which reinforce the aims of the multidisciplinary approach.
- Psychologist – diagnostic psychometric tests to assess cognitive functioning and processing skills.
- Occupational therapist – assess ADLs. Provide meaningful activity within structured timetable. Introduce functional daily activity, e.g. cooking, photography and travelling independently.
- Cognitive therapist – identifying learned behaviours that have contributed to the development of this disabled state. Devise management strategies to deal with issues and encourage a more active lifestyle. Encourage use of symptom diaries to discuss progress.

7. A physical rehabilitation programme could include:
   - Teaching control of trunk and neck muscles in a lying position
   - Working through progressive stages including supported kneeling exercise to regain further trunk and head control
   - As limb function returns, helping to build muscles, mat work in kneeling, standing exercise, walking and running
   - Providing a graded programme of exercise
   - Functional activity, e.g. swimming, gym, short walks.



## Case Study 4

1. The indicators for increased risk of future fractures are:
   - DEXA scan result (confirming poor bone mineral density)
   - long history of amenorrhoea: one of the diagnostic criteria for anorexia nervosa (American Psychiatric Association 1994, WHO 1992)
   - previous spontaneous fractures
   - long-term steroid use (for asthma)
   - reduced dietary intake
   - smoking 20–30 cigarettes daily
   - lack of exposure to sun
   - increasing age (naturally reducing bone mineral bank).

2. Significance:
   - For many people being hypermobile is not problematic (ARC 2005), but inherent laxity of tissues increases vulnerability to the effects of injury and can contribute to abnormal biomechanics (Ferrell et al 2004).
   - It is likely that the patient's spondylolisthesis resulted from a combination of excessive joint range, soft tissue extensibility and decreased

bone mineral density (as well as possible repetitive strain caused by participating in competitive gymnastics).

- Individuals with hypermobility have also been shown to have decreased proprioceptive acuity, which may affect motor control and result in movement abnormalities, in turn contributing to abnormal biomechanics (Ferrell et al 2004).

What this indicates: That the patient is generally hypermobile and there is a need to incorporate joint stabilising exercises as well as proprioceptive exercises in her programme.

3. Aims of treatment should be to:
   - reduce/control pain
   - improve posture
   - improve muscle strength and joint stability
   - improve proprioception and kinaesthetic sense
   - provide education and advice on both osteoporosis and joint hypermobility, including information on national associations and/or local support networks. Education about osteoporosis could be delivered as part of a health education programme on the eating disorders unit, as it is a common complication of anorexia nervosa.

   The following may also be considered:
   - Lifestyle advice such as pacing, ways to avoid lifting, appropriate exercise and ergonomic advice
   - Promoting a healthy attitude to exercising
   - Promoting relaxation techniques.

   Cardiovascular fitness should also normally be considered in an individual with osteoporosis (Chartered Society of Physiotherapy 2002b); however, this may be problematic in this case, as it involves more calorific output and may jeopardise her weight control and/or contribute to her problem of excessive exercising. This may be more appropriate to include later in the recovery process.

   Short-term goal example:
   - To reduce pain to a manageable level, e.g. to be able sit through a therapeutic group on the unit comfortably.

   Long-term goal example:
   - To gain sufficient confidence to attend a Pilates class at the local gym.

4. The following interventions may assist with pain management:
   - Liaising with the team regarding initial adequate oral analgesia to enable participation in the physiotherapy process
   - Transcutaneous electrical nerve stimulation (TENS)
   - Interferential therapy
   - Heat
   - Hydrotherapy

- Postural correction/advice in standing, sitting and lying
- Advice on pacing
- Ergonomic advice.

5. The following exercises should be incorporated into the programme:
   - Spinal stabilisation exercises and postural re-education
   - Strength training exercises, starting with short levers and body resistance only (such as half squats and lunges) and progressing to long levers and light weights. All major upper and lower limb muscle groups should be included. To help maintain improved posture, rhomboids and trunk extensors should be strengthened. This should be carefully conducted to prevent shearing forces in the thoracic spine or excessive compensatory movement in the lumbar spine
   - Endurance work on the deep neck flexors to improve head and neck posture
   - Exercises to improve joint position sense and proprioception
   - Specific stretches: the patient's posture indicates that the muscle groups most likely to be tight are the paraspinal muscles in the upper cervical spine, pectoral muscles, hamstrings, gastrocnemius and soleus. However, this should be confirmed with the appropriate muscle length tests prior to incorporating specific stretches into the programme
   - Low-impact activities should be performed at least three times a week for 20–30 minutes to help increase bone mineral density. These activities should build to medium impact in the longer term (Chartered Society of Physiotherapy 2002b). However, due to the patient's eating disorder this may not be appropriate so early on in the recovery process. Such a programme would require careful monitoring and liaison with the team and the patient would need to increase calorie intake on those days to allow for increased energy output.

6. The following exercises should be avoided:
   - High-impact activities, such as jogging, skipping, aerobics and any contact sports
   - Exercises that involve loaded trunk flexion or trunk rotation
   - Exercises that involve excessive repetition (especially trunk rotation and forward flexion of the lumbar spine)
   - Ballistic stretches
   - Heavy lifting or heavy weight training.

7. Examples of appropriate outcome measures:
   - VAS for pain (Scott & Huskisson 1976)
   - Oswestry low back pain disability index (Fairbank et al 1980)
   - Tragus to wall (Laurent at al 1991)

- Trunk extension endurance (Chartered Society of Physiotherapy 2002b): pillow under abdomen and not to exceed 20 seconds.

8. Close liaison with the team is necessary throughout physiotherapy intervention:
   - so that the team is informed about any physical problems and made aware that there is a valid reason why she may be finding some of the therapeutic groups a challenge
   - to familiarise the team with the patient's exercise programme and to reassure them that this level of exercise is appropriate and not part of her eating disorder behaviour or maladaptive lifestyle
   - so that the physiotherapist is fully aware of the psychopathology associated with anorexia nervosa and can be alert to any manifestations of this
   - so that the patient is aware that the team is working collaboratively to ensure the best outcome.

   To allow time for physiotherapy to be incorporated into the patients current weekly programme.



## Case Study 5

1. As the physical health experts in the team physiotherapists are best placed to assess and offer a programmed of graded exercise (Biddle 2000, NICE 2003, 2007).

2. Complete a health-screening questionnaire to ensure she is medically fit.

3. a. Exercise programme including:
   - Gym group within the leisure centre run by a technical instructor (TI) working alongside the centre staff. Many service users are unable to access gym or leisure facilities as they do not have the confidence to go on their own or the motivation to exercise alone
   - Ladies hydrotherapy/aqua aerobics session.

   *Benefits*
   - Physical activity and weight management
   - Hydrotherapy to manage pain and promote relaxation and reduction of tension
   - Social contact.

   b. Massage:

   *Benefits*
   - Reduction of muscle tension and pain
   - Promotes relaxation.

c. Tai chi and relaxation sessions:

*Benefits*

- Reduced base-line stress
- Promotion of motivation and enjoyment
- Improved sleep patterns, combats fatigue and helps reduce pain (Heptinstall 1995).

4. Exercise programme needs to:
   - be flexible, thus enabling individuals to progress at their own rate, with graded exercise which is introduced slowly and based on individual tolerance
   - have achievable goals to avoid feelings of failure, worthlessness and hopelessness
   - be appropriate to level of motivation and concentration
   - be easily accessible for the patient and involve a group number the patient feels comfortable with.
5. - Dietician – for advice on weight management and healthy eating
   - Smoking cessation advisor – to support her to stop smoking
   - Bereavement counsellor.
6. Long-term goals should be driven by client, who has ownership of recovery/rehabilitation plan:
   - For the patient to become a member at the leisure centre and attend independently
   - For the patient to integrate into sessions and classes within community services
   - Establish a return-to-work plan.



## Case Study 6

1. Considerations:
   - How to communicate appropriately. Establish what she likes to be called. Spend some time just talking to assess her communication level and to build a therapeutic relationship. Explain what you are going to do slowly and clearly only one person talking at a time.
   - How to approach the patient. It is best to approach from the front using a friendly face and non-threatening posture (Oddy 2003).
   - Issues over consent and capacity (Mental Capacity Act 2005) need to be considered as the patient will not have been deemed to have capacity over some decisions, whether to have tea or coffee and what she may like for lunch are different to going home or being placed in supported care. The patient's care plan will state the decision-making process.

2. Pain management is poor in this population, as they cannot verbalise their pain and therefore it is forgotten (Warden et al 2003).

   Using pain assessments that are non-verbal may give an indication of the probability of pain. As pain is a very individual experience sometimes people with advanced dementia may tolerate high levels of pain.

   Non-verbal pain scales use all aspects of pain assessment (Abbey et al 2004) from biological, physiological and psychological factors and will enable you to make a decision on the probability of pain and to request regular analgesia for this patient group. Prorenata medication is not recommended as people with cognitive impairment have a poor ability to request analgesia appropriately and there is difficulty in perceiving their pain both from staff and the patient perspective.

3. It may not be possible for the patient to understand why she may benefit from using the frame – she may be prompted to use it while staff are present but then forget. You may find that she will mobilise independently and with a greater degree of risk and this must be documented. Risks should be minimised by the provision of hip protectors, greater supervision from staff and ensuring good footwear. It may also be considered possible that a walking aid may be used as a weapon in some circumstances so this may need to be considered and the aid only given when supervision is present.

4. Establish why this lady is catheterised. Is it for ease of care? Or a medical reason? If appropriate, recommend that the catheter be removed as soon as possible because people often do not have an understanding of what it is or why it is there. They can pull them out and also become a hazard to people who are attempting to mobilise unaided. There is also the risk of infection and in turn this can increase cognitive impairment. Staff should be advised to mobilise the patient as often as possible and instructed to encourage the patient to sit up in the chair in the safest way.

5. Carers often know the person the best so ask them how best to manage them. They may be able to share prompts, likes and dislikes, terms of phrase that they use and understand. Carers will also be able to share nutrition preferences and life history of the person which may enable better communication and understanding of that individual as a person. Carers are also important in helping to make decisions if the patient is deemed not to have capacity (Mental Capacity Act 2005).

6. If the person is known to the mental health team then the care co-ordinators should be involved in discharge planning. Many acute hospitals have a liaison team that can advise on care of those with mental health issues, it may be more appropriate that the mental health physiotherapists follow-up at home or that discharge

is planned sooner rather than later to prevent increased disorientation. Future risks can be assessed and reduced as possible on a home visit by the appropriate staff in discussion with the relevant carers.

7. Mental health physiotherapists have more time to spend with their patients due to the nature of the illness but this does not mean that all people diagnosed with a mental health issue should be seen by the mental health team. People should be referred to the generic services but if the mental health issues appear to be a block for their rehabilitation then it may be appropriate for the mental health physiotherapist.

### References

Abbey J A, DeBellis A, Piller N et al 2004 One minute indicator for people with late stage dementia. International Journal of Palliative Nursing 10(1):6–13.

American Psychiatric Association 1994 Diagnostic and Statistical Manual of Mental Disorders, 4th edn. American Psychiatric Association, Washington DC.

Arthritis Research Campaign (ARC) 2005 Joint Hypermobility. An Information Booklet.

Bandura A 1977 Self efficacy: toward a unifying theory of behavioural change. Psychological Review 84:191–215.

Biddle S J H 2000 Emotion mood and physical activity. In: Biddle S J H, Foc K R, Boutcher S H (Eds) Physical Activity and Psychological Well-being. Routledge, London, p. 63–87.

British National Formulary London (BNF) 2007 BMJ Publishing Group Ltd/RPS Publishing: London.

Butler D, Moseley L 2003 Explain Pain. Noigroup Publications, Australia.

Chartered Society of Physiotherapy (CSP) 2002a Curriculum Framework. CSP, London.

Chartered Society of Physiotherapy (CSP) 2002b Physiotherapy Guidelines for the Management of Osteoporosis. CSP, London.

Chartered Society of Physiotherapy (CSP) 2005 Mental Health Review. CSP, London.

Ciccone D S, Grzesiak R C 1984 Cognitive dimensions of pain. Social Science and Medicine 19:1339–1345.

Department of Health (DoH) with Royal College of Psychiatrists 2005 New Ways of Working.

Department of Health 1999 National Service Framework for Mental Health.

Department of Health 2001 National Service Framework for Older Adults.

Department of Health 2006 Our health, our care, our say. White Paper, TSO, Norwich.
Donaghy M E, Mutrie N 1999 Is exercise beneficial in the treatment and rehabilitation of the problem drinker? A critical review. Physical Therapy Reviews 4:153–166.
Fairbank J, Couper J, Davies J B et al 1980 The Oswestry Low Back Pain Disability Questionnaire. Physiotherapy 66(8):271–273.
Faulkner G, Biddle S 2002 Mental health nursing and the promotion of physical activity. Journal of Psychiatric and Mental Health Nursing 9(6):659.
Ferrell W, Tennant N, Sturrock R 2004 Amelioration of symptoms by enhancement of proprioception in patients with joint hypermobility syndrome. Arthritis & Rheumatism 50(10):3323–3328.
Fox K R 2000 The effect of exercise on self-perceptions and self-esteem In: Biddle S J H, Fox K R, Boutcher S H (eds) Physical activity and psychological well being. Routledge, London, p. 88–117.
Hawton K, Salkovskis P M, Kirk J et al 1989 Cognitive Behavioural Therapy for Psychiatric Problems – A Practical Guide. Oxford Medical Publications, Oxford.
Heptinstall S T 1995 Relaxation Training in Physiotherapy in Mental Health a Practical Approach.
Kendall F, McCreary E, Provance P 1993 Muscles Testing and Function. Lippincott Williams & Wilkins, Pennsylvania.
Laurent M, Buchanon W, Bellamy N 1991 Methods of assessment in ankylosing spondylitis clinical trials: A review. British Journal of Rheumatology 30:326–329.
Laurin D, Verreault R, Lindsay J et al 2001 Physical activity and risk of cognitive impairment and dementia in elderly persons. Archives of Neurology 58(3):498–504.
Lawler D, Hopker S 2001 The effectiveness of exercise as an intervention in the management of depression. British Medical Journal 322:1–8.
Liu B, Anderson G, Mittmann N et al 1998 Use of selective serotonin reuptake inhibitors or tricyclic antidepressants and risk of hip fractures in elderly people. Lancet 351(9112):1303–1307.
Main C J 1983 The modified somatic perception questionnaire. Journal of Psychosomatic Research 27:503–514.
Main C J, Wood P L, Hollis S et al 1992 The distress and risk assessment method. Spine 17:42–52.
Mental Health Act 1983 HMSO, London.
Mental Health Act 1983 Code of Practice 1999 HMSO, London.
Mental Capacity Act 2005 HMSO, London.
Mutrie N 2000 The relationship between physical activity and clinically defined depression. In: Biddle S J H, Fox K R, Boutcher S H (eds) Physical Activity and Psychological Well being. Routledge, London, p. 88–117.
National Institute for Clinical Excellence 2003 Depression, NICE guidelines. NHS, London, p. 19, 21.

National Institute for Health and Clinical Excellence 2007 NICE clinical guideline 23 (amended). National Collaborating Centre for Mental Health, London.
Oddy R 2003 Promoting Mobility for People with Dementia; A Problem Solving Approach, 2nd edn. Age Concern, London.
Scott J, Huskisson E 1976 Graphic representation of pain. Pain 2:175–184.
Skelton D A, Dinan S M 1999 Exercise for falls management: rationale for an exercise programme aimed at reducing postural instability. Physiotherapy Theory and Practice 15:105–120.
Taylor A H 2000 Physical activity, anxiety, and stress. In: Biddle S J H, Fox K R, Boutcher S H (eds) Physical Activity and Psychological Well being. Routledge, London, p. 88–117.
The Mini Mental State Examination – Factsheet for Patients and Carers 2002 The Alzheimer's society. London.
Vlayeyen J W S, Linton S J 2000 Fear avoidance and its consequences in chronic musculoskeletal pain: a state of the art. Pain 85(3):317–332.
Waddell G, McCulloch J A, Kummel E et al 1980 No organic physical signs in low-back pain. Spine 5:117–125.
Warden V, Hurley A C, Volicer L 2003 Development and psychometric evaluation of the Pain Assessment in Advanced Dementia PAINAD scale. Journal of the American Medical Directors Association 4(1):9–15.
World Health Organization 1992 The ICD-10 Classification of Mental and Behavioural Disorders: Clinical Descriptions and Diagnostic Guidelines. World Health Organization, Geneva.
Zung W W K 1965 A self-rated depression scale. Archives of General Psychiatry 32:63–70.



### *Further reading*

Everett T, Donaghy M, Feaver S 2003 Interventions for Mental Health. Butterworth Heinemann, Edinburgh.
Keer R, Grahame R 2003 Hypermobility Syndrome: Recognition and Management for Physiotherapists. Butterworth-Heinemann, Oxford.
Petty N, Moore A 1998 Neuromusculoskeletal Examination and Assessment. A Handbook for Therapists. Churchill Livingstone, Edinburgh.
Richardson C, Jull G, Hodges P et al 1999 Therapeutic Exercise for Spinal Segmental Stabilization in Low Back Pain. Churchill Livingstone, Edinburgh.
Schmidt U, Treasure J 1997 A Clinician's Guide to Getting Better Bit(e) by Bit(e): Survival Kit for Sufferers of Bulimia Nervosa and Binge Eating Disorders. Psychology Press, East Sussex.
Sran M, Khan K 2005 Physiotherapy and osteoporosis: practice, behaviors and clinicians' perceptions – a survey. Manual Therapy 10:21–27.

### Bibliography

Maynard C 2003 Assess and Manage somatisation. The Nurse Practice 28(4):20–29.
Reid S, Wessely S, Crayford T 2001 Medically unexplained symptoms in frequent attendees of secondary health care: retrospective cohort study. British Medical Journal 322(7289):745–746.
Ron M 2001 Explaining the unexplained: understanding hysteria. Oxford University Press. Brain 124(6):1065–1066.
Stone J, Sharpe M, Hothwell J 2003 Twelve-year prognosis of unilateral functional weakness and unilateral weakness. Journal of Neurology, Neurosurgery and Psychiatry 74(5):591–596.

### Useful websites

www.edauk.com (Eating Disorders Association).
www.nos.org.uk (National Osteoporosis Society).
www.hmsa.org (Hypermobility Syndrome Association).

# Case studies in women's health

*Maureen Gardiner, Lauren Guthrie*



## INTRODUCTION

Women's health (WH) is a very specialised and diverse area of physiotherapy which covers problems pertaining to obstetrics (may also be referred to as maternity) and gynaecology. A WH physiotherapist may also treat women with breast cancer and men with continence issues. A placement or rotation in WH may involve one or all of these sub groups depending on the service provision within the NHS Trust.

Obstetrics is the term that refers to the care of women during their pregnancy (antenatal period) and just after the delivery of their baby (post-natal period). Antenatal care from the physiotherapist 'aims to prevent or alleviate the physical and emotional stresses of pregnancy and labour' (ACPWH 2007). Care may involve teaching relaxation, breathing awareness and comfort positions for labour individually or in a group setting as part of antenatal or preparation for parenthood classes with other professionals such as midwives, dieticians, speech and language therapists and agencies such as the child benefit agency. It should be noted that the provision of antenatal education and the involvement of physiotherapists varies greatly throughout the NHS. Physiotherapists also have an important role to play in treating women who have musculoskeletal problems relating to their pregnancy. Women may be seen in an out-patient department or as an in-patient in a maternity hospital. Common problems encountered during pregnancy include low back pain, pelvic girdle pain (including lumbosacral, sacroiliac and symphysis pubis pain) disc problems, hip pain, coccygeal pain, thoracic pain, carpal tunnel syndrome (CTS), lower limb oedema, varicose veins and diastasis recti. Women may also be treated for bladder and bowel dysfunction, including constipation.

The physiotherapists' role in the post-natal period is to assist in the recovery of the mother by treating a painful perineum, incontinence problems or any presenting musculoskeletal issues associated with childbearing mentioned above. Teaching exercises and general back care and advising the mother on returning to exercise is also important. The care of the post-natal woman begins after the delivery of her baby when she is still in the obstetric unit/maternity hospital and can extend to a number of months after the birth when the patient will be seen as an outpatient. The involvement of physiotherapy services with post-natal women vary within the NHS. Treatment of musculoskeletal problems by an obstetric physiotherapy service may stop as early as 6 weeks after delivery. However, involvement by the physiotherapist may continue through post-natal exercises classes for example, where on-going advice regarding exercise can be provided as well as progressions of exercises covered in the immediate post-natal period.

Gynaecology refers to 'the science of dealing with the diseases of the female reproductive system' (Brooker 2003). Depending on local services, the physiotherapist working in this area of women's health may be involved with the pre-operative assessment and post-operative intervention of women undergoing gynaecological surgery, where care would take place within an in-patient hospital setting. The role of the physiotherapist in treating patients immediately post gynaecological surgery is similar to that of a respiratory physiotherapist treating a patient post anterior resection, for example, in that 'the immediate objectives are to achieve good respiratory and vascular function and early mobilization' (Cook 2004). The reader should refer to Chapter 5 cases 5–8 for more information in dealing with respiratory problems post surgery. Depending on the type of gynaecological surgery the woman has had, the physiotherapist may progress post-operative intervention to teaching pelvic floor muscle exercises, abdominal muscle exercises and advising on posture and back care. The physiotherapist may also have to help the patient deal with the psychological reactions they may have to their surgery. Treatment of women (and men) suffering from bladder and bowel dysfunction at any stage of life may also be included in the area of gynaecology and will usually take place in an out-patient setting within a specialised department or within a general out-patients department. Treating continence problems requires specialised post-graduate training and, therefore, students and junior members of staff are not usually as involved with this aspect of women's health other than in an observatory capacity.

Due to the similarities between the role of the physiotherapist treating patients post-gynaecological surgery and other forms of abdominal surgery and the specialised role of the physiotherapist treating continence problems, only obstetric cases have been included in this chapter. The reader is referred to Mantle et al (2004; Chapter 10, Gynaecological surgery) for more information on specific types of gynaecological surgery and associated physiotherapy input.

## CASE STUDY 1 ANTENATAL OUT-PATIENT

### Subjective assessment

| | |
|---|---|
| SH | Currently 32 weeks' pregnant in her second pregnancy<br>Age 27 in full-time employment as a Training and Development Officer. Planning to work to 37 weeks of pregnancy<br>Postural stresses at work – sitting for long periods at computer and group teaching which involves being on her feet and moving around departments within the office<br>Postural stresses at home – driving child of 20 months to and from her nursery. Transferring her in/out car seat and all other duties involved in childcare. Partner and family are very supportive |
| HPC | 2/12 history of intermittent central low back and posterior pelvic pain with occasional shooting pains down back of the thighs but more frequent in the right thigh. Symptoms worsening since the onset of pain. No referral of pain below the right knee but the patient states that she 'feels as if leg could give way'. She has therefore ceased carrying her 20-month-old child downstairs due to fear of falling |
| Sleep pattern | Sleep disturbed as she is unable to get comfortable in bed |
| Aggravating factors | Prolonged sitting especially at work – 'feels as if back stiffens up', rising from sitting, initiating walking (as the right leg feels stiff after prolonged resting), in/out of bed, turning in bed (aware of clicking/crunching sensation in back), prolonged walking (tending to use the pram for support) |
| Easing factors | Nothing in particular |
| Special questions | Bladder/bowel changes – has noticed she is emptying her bladder more often and when she does it is usually a small volume of urine but no other altered function<br>No altered sensation or saddle anaesthesia<br>No accidents, slips or falls recently |
| PMH | Mid-cavity forceps delivery with a large blood loss 20 months ago. Has experienced intermittent problems with low back pain where she felt as if it locked or seized. This was relieved by moving around, but |

CHAPTER ELEVEN

| | |
|---|---|
| | after-effects were short lived. Returned to work when baby was 6 months and has no sickness record noted |
| | No other medical conditions and is not currently on any medications |

## Objective assessment

| | |
|---|---|
| **Observation** | Posture in sitting/standing: reasonable |
| | Lordosis: reduced |
| | No shift detected |
| | Gait abnormal at times. Feels unable to fully weight bear on her right leg due to pain and fear of it giving way. Also feels she waddles at times |
| | Neurological tests – no abnormality detected |

**TABLE 11.1 MOVEMENT LOSS AND PELVIC ASSESSMENT**

| | |
|---|---|
| Standing | Flexion and extension within normal limits for the third trimester. Right iliac crest, PSIS and ASIS higher than left<br>Stork/step test abnormal showing right sacroiliac (SI) joint blocked<br>Palpation of pelvic and lumbar area shows tenderness and muscle spasm in right quadratus lumborum muscle and non-specific tenderness over right SI joint area |
| Sitting | Right PSIS higher than left and moves upwards when flexing showing right SI joint is blocked |
| Supine lying | Apparent leg length by comparing medial malleoli levels shows right leg shorter<br>Posterior ilial glide test (Squish test) blocked or hypomobile on right<br>Right and left active SLR reduced due to discomfort in lower back<br>No irritability detected<br>Levels of pubic symphysis normal and no tenderness apparent |

## Questions

1. What do you think may be wrong with this patient?
2. What considerations would you give to the altered bladder function symptom the patient is reporting?
3. What physiological changes that happen during pregnancy may have lead to this patient's problem?
4. Do you think her previous history of episodic posterior pelvic pain may be relevant?
5. What are this patients functional problems and what advice would you give her to help overcome them?

6. What other treatment could you offer her as well as advice regarding her functional problems?
7. What advice could you give to this patient with regard to her labour and immediate post-natal period?

## CASE STUDY 2 ANTENATAL OUT-PATIENT

### Subjective assessment

| | |
|---|---|
| SH | Age 23. Currently 29 weeks' pregnant in her second pregnancy. Owns her own dance school and teaches ballet and modern dancing to children and adults. Currently planning to work till 36 weeks. She also has a 30-month-old toddler<br>Postural stresses at work – On feet for extended periods of time and demonstrating dance routines to children all ages<br>Postural stresses at home – All activities required to look after active 30 month old toddler, and all other activities at home. Husband, family and friends are very supportive |
| HPC | Was aware very early into this pregnancy of pelvis feeling very lax and unstable at the front and also noticed a clicking sensation. Four weeks ago the symptoms started to increase and she now describes a feeling of pressure deep inside over her symphysis pubis which also feels tender to touch. This pain sometimes travels down the inside of her thighs to just above the knee. No reports of low back or posterior pelvic pain<br>24-hour pain pattern – feels stiff and finds it difficult to get going in the morning, gets worse as day goes on especially if she has been doing lots of standing and walking |
| Aggravating factors | In/out of the car, in/out of the bath, going up and down stairs, getting dressed and rising from sitting and lying |
| Easing factors | Resting in sitting or lying position |
| Special questions | No bladder/bowel changes<br>No altered sensation or saddle anaesthesia<br>No history of any accidents recently or outwith any of her pregnancies |

| | |
|---|---|
| PMH | During first pregnancy 30 months ago had mild anterior pelvic pain from around 30 weeks. She noticed occasional discomfort associated with higher activity levels. This type of discomfort was also noticed pre-menstrually. She had a mid cavity forceps delivery of a baby weighing 9 lb 3 oz and sustained a 2nd degree tear to her perineum. On returning to work after 6 months she became aware of left sided anterior pelvic pain. This was assessed and treated at a sports injury clinic and states had her pelvis 'fixed' on five occasions along with advice and an exercise programme but she never returned to her pre-pregnancy level of fitness<br>No other medical conditions |
| DH | Taking paracetamol only when really necessary. |

## Objective assessment

| | |
|---|---|
| Observation | Posture in standing sitting good<br>Lordosis increased but normal for gestation<br>No shift noted<br>Gait pattern: patient equally weight bearing on left and right but has a wide stance, short stride length and patient reports she feels she is waddling<br>Recti diastasis noted when patient was getting on and off the bed. Appears as a bulging or doming centrally around umbilicus |

**TABLE 11.2 MOVEMENT LOSS AND PELVIC ASSESSMENT**

| | |
|---|---|
| Standing | Flexion and extension within normal limits for this gestation in pregnancy. Iliac crest, PSIS and ASIS levels equal. Step test normal but very unsteady. Finds standing on one leg very painful |
| Sitting | Iliac crest and PSIS levels equal. Seated flexion test normal |
| Supine lying | Medial malleoli levels equal. ASIS levels equal. Posterior ilial glide test (Squish test) normal. Pubic rami and pubic tubercle levels equal but symphysis pubis very tender and feels puffy/swollen<br>Active SLR – painful left and right. Easier with compression of the pelvis at the ASISs |

## Questions

1. What diagnosis would you give to this patient?
2. How would you explain this condition to the patient?
3. What is the prognosis for this type of condition?
4. From the assessment it was noted the patient has a recti diastasis. How would you explain what this is and what problems can it cause to the pregnant woman?
5. What concerns do you think the patient may have and how would you help the patient to overcome these problems?
6. What advice could you offer the patient to help make her symptoms improve?
7. What exercises could you prescribe in this situation and how would you progress them? Are there any positions you should avoid when pregnant and why?
8. The patient asks you if she can continue swimming. What should you recommend?
9. What advice would you give to this patient with regards to labour and delivery?



## CASE STUDY 3 PAINFUL PERINEUM AND RECTI DIASTASIS FOLLOWING MID-CAVITY FORCEPS DELIVERY

### Subjective assessment

| | |
|---|---|
| SH | Age 38. This is her first pregnancy and it was unplanned. She commenced her maternity leave at 36 weeks of pregnancy. Her occupation is a manager in a large company. She did not attend any antenatal preparation classes and has been supported by two female friends who were her named birthing partners; her partner left her when he was informed of the pregnancy. Her mother and father live far away and do not keep in close contact with her |
| HPC | Patient admitted to a six-bedded bay in a postnatal ward following a mid cavity forceps delivery subsequent to a labour that lasted approximately 17 hours the previous day. She had an episiotomy, and sustained a 2° tear to her perineum. She has a catheter *in situ* for 48 hours as per hospital protocol as she was unable to void urine for 10 hours after the delivery. This is causing her extreme distress as she is worried she will become incontinent. The patient reports that she is unable to get comfortable due to the discomfort she is in |

| | |
|---|---|
| **Handover from the midwives** | Patient is not mobilising very well and does not seem motivated to care for her baby independently. She has not been taking her painkillers; the staff keep finding them at her bedside |
| **PMH** | History of depression 4 years ago. Received counselling and was on medication for 6/12. Problems resolved after this |
| **DH** | Previously not on any medication. She had an epidural for the delivery of her baby. Currently prescribed brufen 400 mg 6 hourly, paracetamol every 4 hours if required and enoxaparin to reduce the risk of a DVT |

## Objective assessment

| | |
|---|---|
| **Observation** | The patient was sitting slumped in bed, tilted awkwardly to the side. She appeared to be very uncomfortable, distressed and tearful with oedematous feet and ankles. On movement causing any strain there is a bulging of her abdomen centrally around the navel area. When she stands her abdomen looks distended and pendulous<br>On examination of her perineum it is found that it is extremely oedematous, bruised and she also has prolapsed bruised haemorrhoids |

## Questions

1. What are the main problems for this patient?
2. What advice could you give this patient to improve her mobility and comfort?
3. Are their any electrotherapy modalities you could use with this patient?
4. What advice should this patient be given with regard to exercising her pelvic floor and the long-term benefits of this?
5. How would you explain what the bulging of the patient's abdomen is to her?
6. What advice and exercises would you give this patient to help reduce her diastasis?
7. What risk factors for postnatal depression does this patient have?
8. Is the patient displaying any of the signs and symptoms of having baby blues and is there anything you could do to help or support her?

## CASE STUDY 4 EMERGENCY CAESAREAN SECTION

### Subjective assessment

| | |
|---|---|
| **SH** | 24-year-old primary school teacher. Been on maternity leave from 37 weeks' gestation. This is her first baby. She has attended a 5-week course of antenatal classes with input from the midwife and physiotherapist. Prior to pregnancy she attended the gym regularly and enjoyed running |
| **HPC** | Patient admitted to a post-natal ward following an emergency lower segment caesarean section (LSCS) after a trial of forceps the previous afternoon at 39 weeks' gestation<br>The patient had been in active labour (actively pushing) for 1 hour and 10 minutes prior to a trial of forceps with a subsequent LSCS. She also sustained an episiotomy, 2° tear to her perineum, which was sutured. The midwives documented in her medical notes that her perineum looks bruised and slightly swollen but that the suture line looked satisfactory. She lost 450 mL of blood and her baby weighed 9 lb (4.1 kg)<br>She currently has a catheter and a wound drain *in situ*. She is also connected to an intravenous drip which has almost finished. TED stockings are in place and she has not been out of bed yet since her section<br>The patient reports that she is currently very painful, uncomfortable and distressed at not being able to get out of bed and look after her baby. She appears overwhelmed by the whole experience she has been through |
| **DH** | Spinal anaesthesia given, therefore the patient was awake for the LSCS, the effects of this have now worn off. Prior to this the patient received a dose of morphine and was using entonox for pain relief during her labour contractions<br>The patient is on her regular doses of insulin and has also receiving enoxaparin, an antithrombotic to prevent deep venous thrombosis |
| **PMH** | Type 1 diabetic. Pregnancy uneventful, mild nausea during first few months. Did not suffer any back or pelvic problems during pregnancy |

### Objective assessment

Patient appears pale and tired. She is lying slumped on the bed in an awkward position.

| | |
|---|---|
| **Observations** | Blood pressure – 115/75 mmHg<br>Heart rate – 85 bpm<br>$SaO_2$ – 99% on room air<br>Blood sugar level – within normal limits |

## Questions

1. You notice that the patient's feet are very oedematous and her TED stockings are creasing and cutting into her ankles. What would you recommend in this situation?
2. What considerations would there be for mobilising this patient for the first time?
3. What advice could you give to the patient to help her get up? Is there anything you could ask her to do before getting up?
4. When you visit the patient the next day she is sitting slumped on the edge of the bed breast-feeding her baby. She is complaining of cramping pains in her stomach and a sore low back. How would you explain why she is having these symptoms and what advice would you give her?
5. What factors related to her delivery may have contributed to her perineal pain?
6. What advice and treatment options could you consider to help this complaint?
7. What long-term advice would you give this patient for when she is discharged home with regard to carrying out normal activities?
8. The patient asks you about returning to exercise as she in concerned about how much weight she has gained. What recommendations would you give her?



# ANSWERS TO CHAPTER 11: CASE STUDIES IN WOMEN'S HEALTH

## Case Study 1

1. The history shows that the patient has pelvic dysfunction in the form of a right upslip. This means that her right sacroiliac joint has become hypomobile due to the right ilium slipping upwards on her sacrum. As active straight leg raise was reduced this may also indicate pelvic instability.

2. Altered bladder and bowel function in patients with low back pain should be carefully questioned as it can indicate cauda equina syndrome, a serious pathology and a red flag. However, urinary frequency is common in pregnancy due to pressure on the bladder by the pregnant uterus. An increase in nocturia frequency (waking to void) is also common due to an increase in sodium excretion and mobilisation of dependent oedema when in lying (Chaliha 2006). The patient should be thoroughly questioned about other red flag issues on the initial assessment and each subsequent assessment to ensure that no further symptoms arise that are indicative of serious spinal pathology.

3. There are hormonal changes in pregnancy with action and interaction between oestrogens, progesterone and relaxin. Increased joint laxity has been shown, but these changes do not correlate well with hormonal levels (Marnach et al 2003). This is the body's natural way of preparing for the growing fetus and subsequent delivery as the pelvis must have more 'give' in it to allow the baby to pass through (Rote 1995). The hormonal changes (especially relaxin) cause gradual replacement of collagen in the pelvic joints with a remodelled modified form that has a greater pliability and extensibility (Haslam 2004). As a result of this, the locking mechanism of the joints of the pelvic girdle become less effective with a resultant increased strain on the ligaments of those joints (Lee 1999) thus resulting in a pelvic dysfunction and pelvic girdle pain.

   As the pregnancy progresses the increase in body mass as a result of the growing fetus alters the body's centre of gravity. The abdominal muscles also become progressively more stretched. This extra stress placed on the body results in compensatory postural changes of an increase in thoracic kyphosis and lumbar lordosis which results in pelvic anterior rotation (Bullock-Saxton 1991). It has been suggested that these alterations in posture can be linked to backache and pelvic pain (Danforth 1997 as cited in Bullock-Saxton 1991).

4. Yes. This may have been during her normal menstrual cycle as women with posterior pelvic pain have higher detectable serum relaxin levels than healthy women do (Wreje et al 1995). If relaxin hormone levels rise it may cause pelvic girdle laxity but less than in pregnancy.

5. See Table 11.3.

6. Additional treatment options are:
   - self-stretch technique which aims to lengthen the muscles between the ribcage and ilium and help reduce spasm which may result in correction of the upslip. See Figure 11.2
   - muscle energy technique (MET) to realign the ilium on the sacrum thus attempting to normalise the function of her right sacroiliac joint. This is a hold–relax technique requiring specialised training that many physiotherapists are now using
   - stabilising exercises, including transversus abdominis exercises in side lying or four-point kneeling and pelvic floor exercises
   - pelvic rocking/tilting exercise in sitting and side lying would help to ease off stiffness in her back
   - heat over the painful area may help to relieve pain and reduce muscle spasm.

| TABLE 11.3 ADVISE ON FUNCTIONAL PROBLEMS | |
|---|---|
| **Functional problem** | **Advice** |
| Prolonged sitting at work | Ensure correct posture at work with firm supportive seating with adequate support at back. Use a foot stool to bring level of knees higher than hips to stabilise the pelvis in sitting. Advise the woman to obtain a risk assessment from her employer |
| Rising from sitting | Contract the gluteals on rising and use arms to help push off the chair. Getting out of a more supportive chair will be easier than a soft sofa |
| Prolonged walking/ standing | Reduce time spent on feet as much as possible. Avoid stairs by using lifts and escalators. Sit to dress, put shoes on, do ironing, etc. |
| Comfort in bed/ turning in bed | Always sleep on side to take pressure of abdomen off internal organs. Place a pillow between knees and use a pillow to support the 'bump' in side lying which has been shown to reduce back pain (Young & Jewell 2002) (see Figure 11.1)<br>When turning in bed, keep knees together, contract gluteals and role on to back then to other side. Alternatively, move round on to all fours and then onto other side. Further information can be found in ACPWH (2006) |
| Getting in and out of bed | Roll onto side, bend knees up and push up into sitting using arms as legs slip out of the bed Reverse to get into bed |



7. Labour advice – stay mobile during labour and change position frequently. Standing in a forward lean position, on all fours or kneeling over a birthing ball are all examples of safer positions for the pelvis.

   Avoiding the use of stirrups if possible and do not push against anyone's hips as these positions increase the strain on the pelvis (ACPWH 2007b). If the patient decides to have an epidural a side lying position is best with the uppermost leg resting in a leg support.

   Immediate post-natal advice – correct posture when feeding and changing should be reinforced. Feed in a firm supportive chair with pillows on the lap to support the baby to ensure good posture during this repetitive activity. Changing and bathing the baby should be done at a waist level height in a cot or changing unit.

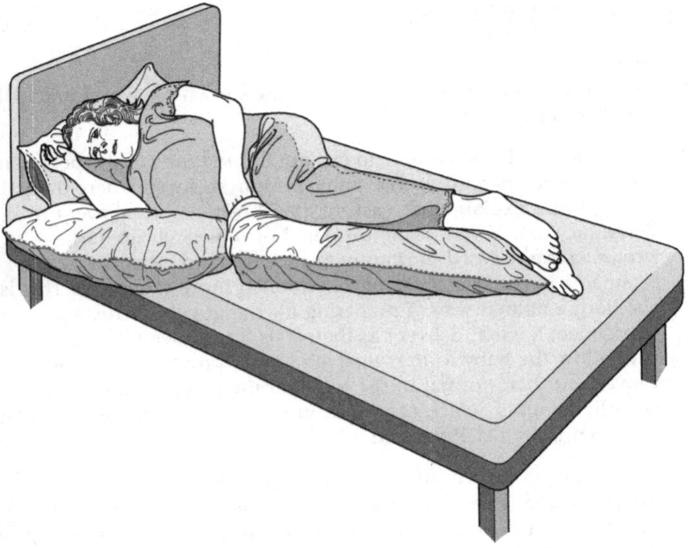

**FIGURE 11.1** Comfort position in bed.

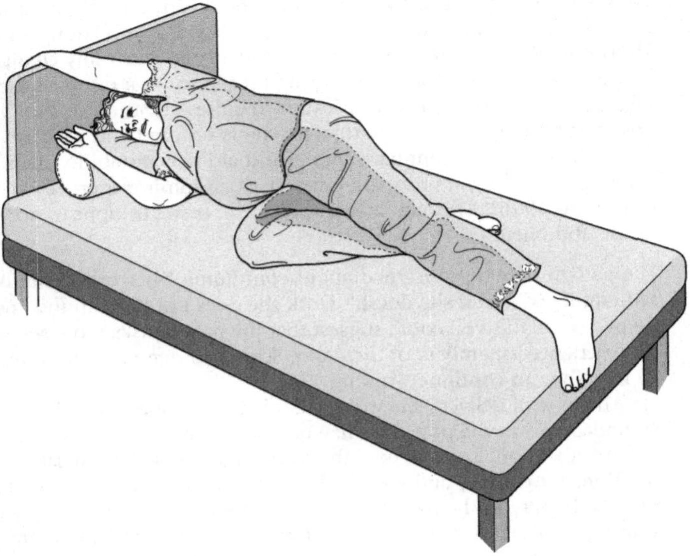

**FIGURE 11.2** Upslip self stretch technique.

## Case Study 2

1. Symphysis pubis dysfunction (SPD) now known as pelvic girdle pain (PGP) (Vleeming et al 2007).

2. Use a model of a pelvis to help explain the anatomy of the pelvis and with specific reference to the pubic symphysis joint, where the pain comes from. Explain and reassure that this is a normal event in pregnancy and is very common. The hormones relaxin and progesterone released during pregnancy have an effect on all the ligaments in the body making them much more extensible. This is the body's natural way of preparing for the growing fetus and subsequent vaginal delivery as the pelvis must have more 'give' in it to allow the baby to pass through. The hormones allow more movement than normal in the joints of the pelvis including the symphysis pubis, which can result in the pelvic girdle joints moving asymmetrically (ACPWH 2007b).

3. PGP can be classified into various sub groups dependent on the joints affected (Alberts et al 2001). There is an excellent chance of post-partum recovery in the majority of women. Those with pain in all three pelvic joints have the worst prognosis (Alberts et al 2001).

4. From the assessment it was noted that the patient has a diastasis (divarication) recti abdominis. It is thought that the lack of support during pregnancy and labour caused by the divarication may cause problems with active pushing during 2nd stage labour (Thornton & Thornton 1993). There is no research evidence to show any change in digestion or other condition during pregnancy as a result of the divarication. However, the divarication requires attention in the post-partum period to ensure that activity is restored and the gap decreased to gain abdominal support and aid pelvic stability. This is best achieved by appropriate transversus abdominis exercise (Sheppard 1996). This will also improve the cosmetic appearance of the abdomen.

5. The patient may be concerned about continuing her work as she is self-employed and if she doesn't work she does not have an income. To overcome this you could suggest that the patient asks more senior or experienced members of the dance school to demonstrate moves so that she can continue working.

   The type of delivery she will have this time as she has had complications in the past. She may be considering an elective caesarean section. To overcome this you could advise her on safe positions for delivery and reassure her that just because she has had a forceps delivery in the past doesn't mean she will have another one. Liaising with the obstetric consultant and midwifery staff about any concerns regarding delivery and other possible options for delivery would be appropriate.

6. Advice you could offer the patient may include:
   - Rest as much as possible and avoid any activity that increases the PGP. This may include altering working patterns, asking family and friends to help out more, sit to do things you would normally do standing for example ironing or preparing a meal, getting dressed, putting shoes on. Avoid stairs and take lifts and escalators where available. Going up stairs one at a time leading with the leg on the least painful side can help minimise the strain put on the SP
   - Avoid heavy lifting especially lifting 30-month-old child. As a compromise getting the child to climb onto a chair and then lifting them up from a higher level as opposed to bending down to the floor. Suggest partner or whomever available helps with transferring child in and out of car
   - Keep knees together when getting in and out of the car, in and out of bed and turning in bed, again to reduce the strain on the SP. To get out of bed, roll onto side, bend knees up and push up into sitting with arms. When turning in bed squeeze knees together and contract the gluteal muscles to help stabilise the pelvis
   - Sitting in a firm supportive chair is important and in bed placing a pillow between the knees and under the 'bump' will help keep the back and pelvis in a good position (refer to Figure 11.1)
   - Shower instead of bath as it can be too much strain on the SP getting in and out of the bath
   - Consider alternative positions if wanting sexual intercourse. Try side lying or kneeling on all fours (ACPWH 2007b)
   - Activate transversus abdominis by drawing tummy in when moving to reduce doming of the abdomen.

7. Exercises to stabilise the pelvis should be recommended including pelvic floor muscles and transversus abdominis exercises. Pelvic floor muscle exercises can be progressed by starting off with a small number of repetitions and gradually increasing the number of seconds that you can hold a contraction and the number you can do with a 4 second rest between each one.

   Transversus abdominis exercises can be started in crook side lying and again can be progressed by increasing the number of seconds you can hold the muscle tight for and the number of repetitions you can do in a row. This exercise can also be done in four point kneeling as a progression.

   Positions to avoid – prone lying is uncomfortable during pregnancy. Supine lying is not advised after 16 weeks' gestation as there is an increased likelihood of obstruction to venous return resulting in a decreased cardiac output due to the increased weight and size of the pregnant uterus. A feeling of claustrophobia or breathlessness and heartburn can also occur. With patients who have a large recti diastasis four point kneeling should be avoided due to the extra stretch placed on the abdominal muscles in this position.

8. Swimming is safe but the patient should avoid the breast stroke as the action of kicking the legs apart will put the SP under strain. Front crawl or using a float and kicking with the legs straight diminishes this problem. Supervised aquanatal exercise classes are also to be recommended.

9. Reassure her that it is still possible to have a normal delivery but she should inform her midwife on arrival at hospital that she has suffered from SPD (PGP). It is important for the patient to know her pain-free range of hip abduction as this should not be exceeded during labour and delivery. The patient should be advised to stay mobile during labour and change position frequently. Standing in a forward lean position, on all fours on kneeling over a birthing ball or the back of the bed are all examples of safer positions for the pelvis.

   If the use of stirrups is essential, both legs should be lifted into them at the same time. At no time should the woman push against someone's hips as it would increase the strain on the pelvis. If the woman decides to have an epidural a side lying position is best with the uppermost leg resting in a leg support. It is advisable for any woman with SPD (PGP) to have her condition and her pain-free range of hip abduction noted in her birth plan for labour and delivery.



## Case Study 3

1. • Poor mobility/unable to get comfortable and therefore finding it hard to care for her baby
   • Oedematus ankles and feet
   • Painful swollen perineum and haemorrhoids
   • She may have a large divarication of abdominal muscles
   • Psychosocial problems as she has no partner or close family to support her. She is also distressed at having a catheter *in situ* and the damage that has happened to her pelvic floor.

2. The advice you could give this patient to improve her mobility and comfort could include:
   • Circulatory exercises for oedematus ankles and feet. Often abbreviated to TAQs, meaning exercising the toes, ankles and quads.

These should be done when the patient is resting with her feet up
- Reinforce the importance of taking regular medication for her pain
- Comfort positions: side lying with a pillow between her knees and ankles, sitting in a supportive chair on a pillow and using a pillow on her lap to help support the baby when feeding (refer to ACPWH 2006) (refer to Figure 11.3)
- Ice pack application for her swollen perineum (Moore & James 1989) and haemorrhoids.

3. Ultrasound is known to increase blood flow and assist the repair process (McMeehan 1994). There should be an infection control protocol in place to cover the use of ultrasound on a perineum. If one is in place, treatment usually takes place in crook or side lying, a cleansed perineum and the ultrasound head covered appropriately with couplant gel (Barton 2004).

   Pulsed short-wave diathermy has also been used in this condition; however, parameters used and the evidence for its use is not conclusive.

4. Once the catheter is removed and normal voiding restored it is advisable for the physiotherapist to observe the perineum to see that the woman is able to contract her PFM. If she is unable to contract the PFM, or is bearing down she should be told to cease trying and be given an out-patient WH physiotherapy appointment for 6 weeks post natal. Meanwhile she can be given healthy bladder information and instructions regarding safe moving and handling. If there is any concern regarding the woman not being able to fully empty her bladder, it is advisable for a bladder scan to be performed by the appropriately trained person.

   It has been shown that PFM training is the most effective conservative therapy for pelvic floor dysfunction and has been recommended by NICE (2006). She would be best advised to attempt to achieve at least eight contractions three times a day when possible. She should start at whatever level she is able and gradually increase the length and number of contractions that she is able to do while pain free until she is able to do 10 contractions each lasting 10 seconds. She should also be advised to try up to 10 short co-ordinated contractions at each exercise session.

5. The bulging and distended abdomen is termed diastasis or divarication of recti. This is a common occurrence in pregnant and postnatal women and is caused by the stretching and subsequent separation of the left and right sides of the rectus abdominus muscle. It is caused by the increasing girth of the pregnant uterus, although the change in hormone levels during pregnancy making the musculature and connective tissue more pliable and stretchy, the

linea alba (the central connective tissue between the recti) will often disrupt causing separation of the recti. When these muscles are separated it is more difficult to increase abdominal pressure during coughing, sneezing or trying to sit up or move, during these activities the abdominal contents bulge due to the lack of support.

The amount of separation can vary and may extend the whole length of the recti muscle and is determined by palpation and examination.

6. Advice and exercises to help reduce the recti diastasis:
   - To get out of bed roll onto your side, bend your knees and push yourself up into sitting using your arms to prevent straining or pulling on the muscles. Reverse for getting in to bed
   - Pull in your tummy muscles (by imagining drawing your navel towards your back to hollow out your tummy) before: moving, sitting up, getting in/out of bed or lifting anything
   - Exercising the transverse abdominis in side lying, supine or in sitting by pulling the pelvic floor muscles and focusing on tightening and pulling in your abdominal muscles below your navel. There are many ways to teach this exercise and your individual technique will come with practice and watching others teach the exercise.



7. The risk factors that this patient has for post-natal depression are:
   - her partner recently left her and she lacks support from her close family
   - she has a history of depression
   - she experienced birth complications (forceps delivery) (Johnstone et al 2001).

8. Generally the 'baby blues' presents itself on day 3–5 and usually resolves and is short lasting. The WH physiotherapist must be aware that a woman with a sore perineum, catheterised, having swollen breasts, etc., is more likely to be unhappy with her situation. She may not feel that she is bonding with her child and be tearful and uncooperative. Supportive, empathetic care is needed, with out-patient appointments given when and where necessary. In some women the 'baby blues' will develop into full post-natal depression which will require skilled trained professional help.

## Case Study 4

1. The TED stockings may need pulling up to correctly position them or may be the wrong size for her. If this is the case they should be removed then the patient should be re-measured. The patient should be encouraged to rest on the bed with her feet up and do circulatory exercises to help the circulation and therefore reduce swelling.

It may also be possible to tip the bed to raise her legs slightly higher than her body. She should be advised to have her legs dependent for minimal periods and not sit or lie with her knees or ankles crossed.

2. Considerations for mobilising this patient for the first time are:
   - ensuring the catheter and wound drain are not going to be pulled on when she moves
   - her intravenous drip. As this has almost finished it may be possible to ask a midwife to remove it
   - the patient's blood pressure. As her last reading was slightly low, care should be taken when standing the patient as she may become lightheaded or nauseous
   - making sure the patient has adequate pain relief
   - ensuring that the patient's blood sugar level is normal and checking that she doesn't feel faint or light headed.

3. Emphasise the need to get up slowly and reassure that despite it possibly feeling sore, she won't be doing any damage to her wound.

   To get out of bed the patient should be instructed to role onto her side, bend her knees up and push her self into sitting as her legs come over the edge of the bed.

4. The cramping pains in her stomach, also described as being like 'period pains', are caused by the involution of the uterus contracting back to its original size after childbirth. These 'after' pains are commonly associated with breast feeding due to the hormones that are released when the baby suckles having a direct effect on the uterus. Pelvic rocking exercises are advisable as they may help with the cramps. Ensuring adequate pain relief is also important.

   Her back pain is probably due to her poor posture as she feeds. Advising the patient to sit in a firm chair with her back supported and pillows on her lap to support lay the baby on should be more comfortable for her (ACPWH 2006) (Figure 11.3). The 'rugby ball' hold for breast feeding may also be recommended as this means the baby is not as close to the wound. Advising her to ensure good posture while changing and bathing the baby by doing these at a waist level height should also be explained. Again, doing pelvic rocking can also help to ease low back pain in this situation.

5. The factors that may have contributed to her perineal pain are: episiotomy, second degree tear, forceps delivery, large baby (>4 kg), and the fact that this is her first pregnancy (Albers 1999, Thompson 2002).

6. Advising the patient to side lie with a pillow between her knees and ankles may help to reduce any discomfort arising from direct pressure onto the perineal area for example in sitting.

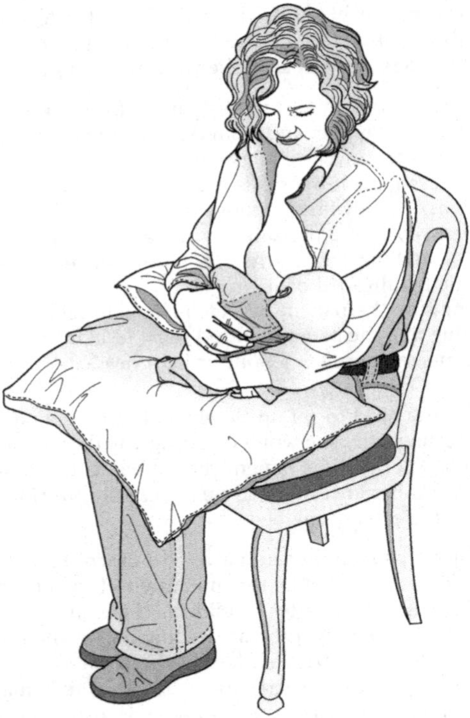

**FIGURE 11.3** Safe feeding position in chair.

- When sitting in a firmer chair the patient may find sitting on a normal pillow more comfortable. When moving into sitting contracting the gluteals and pelvic floor can help to reduce discomfort.
- Once her catheter is out the patient can be advised to start doing pelvic floor muscle exercises (Haslam & Pomfret 2002). She should be reassured that it is safe to do pelvic floor muscle exercises when she has stitches in her perineum and that it can help reduce swelling and promote healing in the area due to the increased blood flow (Barton 2004).
- There is limited evidence that the application of pulsed electromagnetic energy helps to reduce the severity of perineal pain when applied at 6, 12, 24 and 30 hours post-delivery (Gaille et al 2003). However, the use of this modality may depend on local protocols.

- Ice packs are widely recommended in clinical practice to help reduce pain and swelling in the perineal area. The effectiveness of this intervention is in the process of being evaluated through the Cochrane Library.

7. Advice you could give to this patient with regard to carrying out normal activities once she gets home is:
   - check with insurance company with regard to going back to driving. Six weeks is usually given as a rough guide but the patient should be confident that they can concentrate, turn to look over their shoulder and most importantly do an emergency stop. When wearing a seat belt it can help to put a towel or jumper between the LSCS wound and the seat belt for comfort
   - changing and bathing the baby should be done at a waist level height. On a changing unit for example, or else using a changing mat on a table or chest of drawers
   - avoid heavy lifting and housework for the first few weeks. When starting to lift things again, advise the patient to bend the knees, keep the object close to the body, lead up with the head and tighten the pelvic floor muscles.

8. The recommendations for exercising post LSCS are:
   - building up core stability and pelvic floor muscle strength, which is important before starting more high-impact exercise
   - begin with working the deep abdominal muscles, i.e. transversus abdominis. This can be done in side lying, supine or sitting
   - pelvic floor muscle exercises should be started, as there is some limited evidence to show that they are linked to core stability
   - the patient should also be advised to carry out pelvic tilting
   - the above three exercises can be progressed for the first 6 weeks by gradually increasing the number of repetitions and sets and length of a pelvic floor and transversus abdominis contraction in seconds
   - the patient can progress onto small crunches, i.e. supine with knees bent up, pulling in the pelvic floor and abdominal muscles and lifting head off the floor, then progressing on to shoulders as well
   - for the above exercise the patient should ensure that there is no bulging of the abdomen, as this would indicate a divarication of the recti. In this situation the patient should continue with more basic core stability exercises
   - attending a post-natal exercise class run by an obstetric physiotherapist or a fitness instructor with specialised training, which could

be recommended after a post-natal check by a Doctor (usually about 6 weeks if this is still the practice in the local area)
- high-impact activities, such as running/jogging or aerobics classes, should not be started until after 2–3 months depending on core stability and pelvic floor muscle strength.

***References***

ACPWH (Association of Chartered Physiotherapists in Women's Health) (2006) Fit for Motherhood. Available http://www.acpwh.org.uk 21 May 2007.

ACPWH (Association of Chartered Physiotherapists in Women's Health) (2007a) What do members of the ACPWH do? Available http://www.acpwh.org.uk 21 May 2007.

ACPWH (Association of Chartered Physiotherapists in Women's Health) (2007b) Pregnancy related pelvic girdle pain; guidance for health professionals. Available http://www.acpwh.org.uk 21 May 2007.

Albers L, Garcia J, Renfrew M et al 1999 Distribution of genital tract trauma in childbirth and related postnatal pain. Birth 26(1):11–15.

Alberts H, Godskesen M, Westergaard J 2001 Prognosis in four syndromes of pregnancy-related pelvic pain. Acta Obstetricia et Gynaecologica Scandinavica. 80(6):505–510.

Barton S 2004 The postnatal period. In: Mantle J, Haslam J, Barton S (eds) Physiotherapy in Obstetrics and Gynaecology, 2nd edn. Butterworth Heinemann, Edinburgh, p. 222–224.

Brooker C 2003 Pocket Medical Dictionary, 15th edn. Churchill Livingstone, Edinburgh, p.133.

Bullock-Saxton J 1991 Changes in posture associated with pregnancy and the early postnatal period measured in standing. Physiotherapy Theory and Practice 7:103–109.

Chaliha C 2006 Pregnancy and Childbirth and the effect on the pelvic floor. In: Cardozo L, Staskin D (eds) Textbook of Female Urology and Urogynaecology, 2nd edn. Informa Healthcare, UK, p. 683–684.

Cook T 2004 Chapter 10 Common gynaecological conditions. In: Mantle et al (eds) Physiotherapy in Obstetrics and Gynaecology, 2nd edn. Butterworth Heinemann, Edinburgh.

East C E, Marchant P, Begg L et al 2006 Local cooling for relieving pain from perineal trauma sustained during childbirth. (Protocol) Cochrane Database of Systematic Reviews, Issue 4.

Gallie M, Pourghazi S, Grant J M 2003 A randomised trial of pulsed electromagnetic energy compared with ice-packs for the relief of postnatal perineal pain. Journal of the Association of Chartered Physiotherapists in Women's Health 93:10–14.

Hansen et al 2000 Pregnancy associated pelvic pain. II: symptoms and clinical findings Ugeskr Laeger 162(36):4813–4817.

Haslam J 2004 Physiology of pregnancy. In: Mantle J, Haslam J, Barton S (eds) Physiotherapy in Obstetrics and Gynaecology, 2nd edn Butterworth Heinemann, Edinburgh, p. 32–33.
Haslam J, Pomfret I 2002 Should pelvic floor muscle exercises be encouraged in people with an indwelling urethral catheter in-situ? Journal of the Association of Chartered Physiotherapists in Women's Health 91:18–22.
Johnstone S J, Boyce P M, Hickey A R et al 2001 Obstetric risk factors for postnatal depression in urban and rural community samples. Australian and New Zealand Journal of Psychiatry 35(1):69–74.
Lee D 1999 Biomechanics of the lumbo-pelvic-hip complex. In: Lee D The Pelvic Girdle. Churchill Livingstone, London, p. 65–66.
Mantle et al (eds) 2004 Physiotherapy in Obstetrics and Gynaecology, 2nd edn. Butterworth Heinemann, Edinburgh.
Marnach M L, Ramin K D, Ramsey P S et al 2003 An KN. Characterization of the relationship between joint laxity and maternal hormones in pregnancy. Obstetric Gynaecology 101(2):331–335.
McMeehan J 2004 Tissue temperature and blood flow – a research based overview of electrophysical modalities. Australian Journal of Physiotherapy 40th Jubilee Issue, p. 49–55.
Moore W, James D K 1989 A random trial of three topical analgesic agents in the treatment of episiotomy pain following instrumental vaginal delivery. Journal of Obstetrics and Gynaecology 10:35–39.
National Institute for Health and Clinical Excellence (2006) Urinary incontinence; the management of urinary incontinence in women. NICE, London, p. 59.
Rote B 1995 The Pregnant Exerciser. The risks and rewards of a prenatal exercise program. American Fitness. Jan-Feb www.findarticles.com accessed 5th Feb 2007.
Sheppard S 1996 A case study. Management of postpartum gross divarication recti. Journal of Association of Chartered Physiotherapists in Women's Health 79:22–26.
Thompson J F, Roberts C L, Currie M et al 2002 Prevalence and persistence of health problems after childbirth: associations with parity and method of birth. Birth 29(2):83–94.
Thornton S I, Thornton S J 1993 Managemnt of gross divarication of the recti abdominis in pregnancy and labour. Physiotherapy 79:457–458.
Vleeming A, Albert H B, Ostgaard H C 2007 European guidelines on the diagnosis and treatment of pelvic girdle pain. Working group 4, concept version. Available: http://www.backpaineurope.org 21 May 2007.
Wreje U, Kristiansson P, Aberg H et al 1995 Serum levels of relaxin during the menstrual cycle and oral contraceptive use. Gynaecology Obstetric Investigation 39(3):197–200.
Young G, Jewell D 2002 Interventions for preventing and treating pelvic and back pain in pregnancy. Cochrane Database of Systematic Reviews, Issue 1. Art. No.: CD001139. DOI: 10.1002/14651858.CD001139.

# INDEX

## B

## C

## D

## G

## I



## J

# O

## T

Printed in the United States
By Bookmasters